Food and the Risk Society

T0362070

This book offers a comprehensive understanding of the current scientific knowledge concerning risks associated with food preparation, processing and consumption, with particular attention to the gap between scientific research and public perception. Examining the effects of food on the body from both micro and macro levels, it covers a range of broad themes and current concerns, including obesity and the 'obesity epidemic', the benefits or otherwise of dietary supplements, caffeine consumption, GM food, alcohol, organic food, the consumption of fruit and vegetables, and pathogens and contaminants.

Thematically arranged according to the application of broad theoretical approaches in sociological theory – the socio-cultural perspective, the risk society perspective and the governmentality perspective – each chapter focuses on a particular area of interest or concern in relation to food, covering the existing literature in detail and offering illustrative empirical examples, whilst identifying gaps in knowledge and areas for further research. An accessible and rigorous examination of food and health, and the discrepancy between scientific opinion and consumer perception of safe food – the real risks versus the perceived risks – this book will appeal to scholars and students of sociology, geography, food, nutrition and environmental ecosystems, as well as health professionals.

Charlotte Fabiansson has a PhD in Sociology and is a Senior Lecturer in Sociology and Criminal Justice at Victoria University Melbourne, Australia. She is the author of *Pathways to Excessive Gambling: A Societal Perspective on Youth and Adult Gambling Pursuits*.

Stefan Fabiansson has held positions as Professor in Food Safety at the Swedish University of Agricultural Sciences, and leading food safety positions in Swedish, Australian and EU organisations.

Food and the Risk Society

The power of risk perception

**Charlotte Fabiansson and
Stefan Fabiansson**

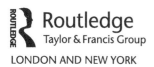

Routledge
Taylor & Francis Group

LONDON AND NEW YORK

First published 2016 by Routledge

2 Park Square, Milton Park, Abingdon, Oxfordshire OX14 4RN
52 Vanderbilt Avenue, New York, NY 10017

*Routledge is an imprint of the Taylor & Francis Group, an informa
business*

First issued in paperback 2020

British Library Cataloguing in Publication Data
A catalogue record for this book is available from the British Library

Library of Congress Cataloguing in Publication Data
A catalog record for this book has been requested.

ISBN: 978-1-4724-7896-2 (hbk)
ISBN: 978-0-367-59652-1 (pbk)

Typeset in Times New Roman MT Std
by Out of House Publishing

Contents

Figures and Tables

Preface

This book is a collaborative work combining two distinctly different disciplines: sociology and public health. It analyses one of the most common and essential everyday activities humans engage in – eating. Food is a complicated and multifaceted essential part of life with three main stages: production, processing and consumption. The three stages are interlinked, and all involve phases that can potentially cause harm. The book focuses on risks across the food chain; especially the gap between scientific experts' definition of risk and the public's perception of risk.

The different stages of food production, processing and consumption are analysed from three different sociological risk discourse perspectives: the socio-cultural, the risk society and the governmentality risk discourses, as food relates to all societal levels.

This work builds on findings from numerous research projects and publications by scientists from diverse disciplines to give a holistic perspective about food; from production and processing to consumption. Why there is such a wide gap between the views of scientists, public health experts and the public is explored. Risks can be found everywhere or nowhere, and the interpretation of risk depends on who is defining the food product as a risk and who is considering it safe. Social, cultural and religious environments, levels of knowledge and the societal context will all influence the definition of risk. Without the research, documentation and scientific journals there would not have been such comprehensive knowledge to utilise. The authors are grateful and indebted to all scientists and experts behind the research and publications.

The overall aim of the book is to enhance the debate and develop knowledge about food risks; food is an area that concerns everyone. The text is extensively referenced, hence is a source for further research and knowledge development for experts in various fields and laypeople having an interest in issues of food.

We thank the reviewers for their pertinent and thoughtful comments; their help has enhanced the quality of the discussion. Furthermore, we express our gratitude to the Ashgate Publishing Group and especially to Neil Jordan and his wonderful team who prepared the text in its final form. Additionally, we would like to acknowledge the financial contribution in the final stage of the book by the College of Arts, Victoria University, Melbourne.

The book should not be seen as giving medical or health advice. Where such issues are discussed, they are in a generalised form and should not be considered as individual recommendations. Readers should always seek independent medical advice concerning individual health issues.

Food and risk cover an enormous field; we have only focused on a small part, as it would have been impossible to include in one book the vast range of issues that relate to this area. We, as authors, come from different disciplines. We do not agree about all of the issues that are discussed, and we have tried to present different viewpoints to enhance knowledge about food and risk.

Charlotte Fabiansson
Stefan Fabiansson

Acronyms

AA	Alcoholics Anonymous
ACS	American Cancer Society
AD	After common dating
AICR	American Institute for Cancer Research
BC	Before common dating
BMI	Body Mass Index
Bt	Bacillus thuringiensis
CAC	Codex Alimentarius Commission
CAERS	CFSAN Adverse Event Reporting System
CDC	United States Centers for Disease Control and Prevention
CFSAN	United States Center for Food Safety and Applied Nutrition
Crispr	A method of precisely modifying the DNA code by using RNA to introduce new heritable traits
DASH	Dietary Approaches to Stop Hypertension Diet
DNA	Deoxyribonucleic Acid that carry the genetic instructions for life
EC	European Commission
EFSA	European Food Safety Authority
EPA	United States Environment Protection Agency
EU	European Union
FAO	Food and Agricultural Organization of the United Nations
FAOSTAT	The Statistics Division of FAO
FDA	United States Food and Drug Administration
UK FSA	United Kingdom Food Standards Agency
FSANZ	Food Standards Australia New Zealand
GFC	Global financial crisis
GI	Glycaemic Index used to measure how quickly carbohydrates raise glucose blood levels
GM	Genetically modified
GMO	Genetically modified organism
HACCP	Hazard Analyses Critical Control Point system used by industry to assure that food is safe
HDL	High-density lipoprotein cholesterol
IAASTD	International Assessment of Agricultural Knowledge, Science and Technology for Development
IARC	International Agency for Research on Cancer
IFOAM	International Federation of Organic Agriculture Movements
ILO	International Labour Organization
IOGT	International Organisation of Good Templars

IOMC	Inter-Organisation Programme for the Sound Management of Chemicals
IPCS	International Programme on Chemical Safety
LDL	Low-density lipoprotein cholesterol
Lite	Food products lower in fat than their conventional counterparts
MoE	Margin of Exposure
NADH	Nicotinamide Adenine Dinucleotide
NIH	United States National Institutes of Health
OECD	Organisation for Economic Co-operation and Development
OGTR	Australian Office of the Gene Technology Regulator
PCB	Polychlorinated biphenyls
RNA	Ribonucleic Acid carries information from DNA to other cell components
SCF	European Commission Scientific Committee on Food
SCFS	European Union Standing Committee on Foodstuffs
Talens	A method of precisely cleaving DNA to introduce new heritable traits
TDI	Tolerable Daily Intake used to set a maximum daily lifetime intake of a contaminant that will not cause appreciable health effects
TLC	Therapeutic Lifestyle Changes Diet
TV-dinner	A frozen ready-made meal on a tray intended to be re-heated and consumed in front of the television
UNCTAD	United Nations Conference on Trade and Development
UNEP	United Nations Environment Programme
USDA	United States Department of Agriculture
vCJD	Variant Creutzfeldt-Jakob disease
WHO	World Health Organization
WTO	World Trade Organization
€1=US$1.24	The exchange rate used in comparisons of euro vs. US dollars

Part I

Food and risk in sociological discourse

In the twenty-first century society, risk has become a common concept used in diverse situations – risks are everywhere but nowhere to be seen. What actually is a risk is debatable in many settings as it depends on the context, the social and cultural environment and who is defining the situation or action as a risk: the expert or the layperson.

The risk concept is well grounded within food production, processing and consumption, defined by experts, scientific research, but also by consumers. Some common ground between these areas exists about what food is safe and what food is risky to eat, but there is also a wide gap between what the experts assess as a food risk or hazard and what a layperson considers a risk, especially in regard to food that is not classified as 'natural'. The gap between real or perceived risk within the food area is the focus of this book.

Food is one of the fundamental components of human existence, thus the perception of risk in relation to food is a significant everyday issue. Good health and wellbeing in their most broad definitions are core human values, and food consumption is also one of the most socially, culturally and religiously influenced activities we engage in daily.

The final food product for consumption has a complex history because of the many different stages involved from production, processing and retailing, to food preparation and consumption where hazards can enter the food chain at any point. It is difficult for laypeople and even experts to understand and to gain a holistic view of the whole food handling chain.

Consumers make decisions based on knowledge gained in their social and cultural environment. They interpret and assess which food is safe to eat and which to avoid based on their social networks and previous experiences, but also about what is presented in the mass media. Scientific advice and information can be difficult to interpret; hence, consumers often disregard the knowledge.

Additionally, consumers often judge their exposure to a risk situation with a focus on the severity of *possible* consequences, rather than the *probability* of its occurrence. This anomaly is at the root of the disparity between technical and social definitions of risk, and the reason why technical assessments of risk have proved an inadequate basis for the management of societal risks, including food safety issues.

The risk concept has progressed from covering not only situations that can be calculated through a mathematical model, but extended to all other societal risk areas interlinking different disciplines; hence the risk concept has become of particular significance within sociological research of food production, processing and consumption, and ultimately people's wellbeing.

This book explores a range of real and perceived risks posed by hazards found in the food chain and their potential impact on the consumer of the food. Some of the risks are inherent to the food product and are often called 'natural risks', while others are introduced by interventions during food production, food processing or even through the final food preparation stage and are commonly referred to as 'introduced' or 'manufactured risks'.

Frequently, manufactured risks are seen as posing a greater risk to health than natural risks. The use of a preservative to prevent mould growth can be seen by some as being more dangerous than mould growth in itself. This is a questionable assumption, as some moulds produce potent toxins that can cause cancer, while preservatives should be safe if used as directed before they enter the consumer market.

Although science can be fallible, it provides the most current information available at the time. This book utilises the best scientific food safety information available in presenting current knowledge for a number of threats to food safety.

The book is divided into four sections, with the initial section providing the sociological theoretical framework to explore risk within the field of food. This is followed by three sections that focus on individual examples of risks throughout the whole food chain, from food choice and dieting, to pesticide use in agriculture and chemicals formed during heating of food in the kitchen; each from a different sociological risk perspective.

People's social and cultural environment, ethnicity and traditions strongly influence their food consumption habits and any adjustment to change food customs is a slow process, but furthering knowledge provides a big step forward to improving food safety.

Each chapter can be read in isolation or the book can be read as a whole to gain an augmented understanding of how, rightly or wrongly, risks are perceived by experts and by the lay populace.

The first two chapters discuss risk from the sociological perspective to provide a theoretical framework for risk discourses in contemporary society and the changing public perception of risk.

1 Food and health from a risk perspective

Introduction

Food habits are among the most deeply ingrained forms of human behaviour. Food and beverages, although central to life and very pleasurable, can also carry some inherent or introduced risks of causing harm. Risk is an all-encompassing but nebulous concept applicable to many facets of life. In the twenty-first century, risk has become an everyday concern, referring to real and perceived situations that can be seen as dangerous. However, from a historical perspective, the risks humans face today are different from ancient times and the ability to survive injuries and illnesses have dramatically increased.

It is easy to perceive contemporary life as more dangerous than in ancient times given the prevalence of negative mass media stories, as well as a political and policy emphasis on risk and security. The societal risk debate has reignited a focus on risk discourses. Risk is not a new concept (Rose 1996), but it gained renewed interest after the publication in 1986 of Ulrich Beck's book, first in German *Risikogesellschaft – Auf dem Weg in eine andere Moderne,* but especially when the book was translated into English in 1992 as *Risk Society, Towards a New Modernity*. The publication generated an intensive debate and encouraged new research in the area of risk within the modern, increasingly industrialised society (Beck 1992).

Within the sociology discipline, risks have been analysed from three theoretical perspectives: the socio-cultural risk discourse, the risk society discourse and the governmentality risk discourse. In this book, we take a sociological perspective to explore the interconnectivity between scientific knowledge and public perception about risks in relation to food production, processing and consumption, where scientific knowledge and public perception often contradict each other in what constitutes a risk of harm.

This introductory chapter is followed by a more detailed discussion of the three sociological risk discourse perspectives in the next chapter.

Food production and consumption within societal risk discourses

There has been a shift from an initial focus on quantification of risks associated with property insurance and banking, to applying the risk discourse to other fields of research and using it in analysing new emerging issues. Everyday activities are analysed through the interpretation of social and cultural constructs of activities, which have emerged within the modern industrialised twenty-first century society. Certain foods and related food production methods, as well as food preparation and consumption habits, are all phases in the food production process that include the potential of a detrimental impact on health and wellbeing of individuals and the society as a whole. As a result, regulation of the whole food chain is now largely based on official risk assessments where human and animal health, as well as environmental and commercial interests are balanced, but also compete against each other. Analysing food production and consumption from the societal risk discourse perspective will enhance understanding of food's place within society, from raw material to consumption.

The categorisation of food as safe or unsafe as seen by the consumer is not necessarily based on scientific discoveries and research. Risk perception measures people's emotional response to an anticipated risk, and their subjective experience of being or living in a risk prone environment (Beck 1997a, 1992; Ewald 1991; Douglas 1985; Douglas and Wildavsky 1982; Slovic 1987). Thus, there is often a disconnection between consumer perception of risk and scientifically documented risk pertaining to food product safety.

Risks in relation to food are defined as anything that can potentially be harmful to a person's life or health. Research focusing on the perception of risk around food production, processing and consumption has shown that the perception of risk is influenced by socio-demographic variables, such as gender, age, ethnicity, level of education, occupation and prior experiences of risks (Ekberg 2007; Slovic 1986, 1987). Although it is nominally mentioned in the food safety risk discourse, food safety scientists commonly prefer to focus on scientific discoveries, hence mostly disregard the consumers' perception of risk.

The ways in which government food safety officials or the industry communicates risk scenarios to consumers are often misconstrued, as the risks perceived by consumers are not necessarily understood or embraced by authorities and experts (Beck and Holzer 2007). Expert assessments of available scientific information that demonstrates insignificant risks generally do not make people less concerned. Rather, if consumers perceive that their concerns are being dismissed too lightly, they may trust those in authority less and worry more (Beck 1992). The presumption of a risk may require more precautions and planning by people than the harm the risk will eventually cause, as 'riskiness means more to people than expected number of fatalities' (Slovic 1987:285; Ewald 1991:199).

The risk discourse perspective can be applied to diverse activities in society and has lately seen an increased focus on individual responsibility. Risk management has become a subject that people need to consider in their private and public life. Everyday life is hardly without risky situations, but there are also different perceptions of what constitutes a risk for the individual or to the wider society. Preparing and eating food is an everyday activity necessary to maintain life and serve as an important social function that creates cohesion and bonds people together. Even if consuming food is an essential but unremarkable activity, food preparation and consumption also involve some risks to human health and wellbeing, which includes eating too much or too little, eating the 'right' or the 'wrong' food, or eating food that has been prepared incorrectly or has an unknown history. The commercial history of food products can sometimes be obscure and difficult to penetrate before it enters the private sphere and becomes an individual risk discourse.

Not surprisingly, given the centrality of food to human health, there is a divisive ongoing debate in mass media and in the research community that embraces numerous aspects of appropriate food consumption behaviour. Concerning food and health, a topic discussed extensively in mass media, the influence of increasing portion sizes and energy-dense food consumption on obesity prevalence is contrasted against the favouring of a slim body ideal achieved through extensive dieting. Coincidently, an influential and powerful food and advertising industry has been established around different diet strategies, with the emergence of 'light' or low calorie food being one example of addressing consumer anxieties.

In a broader sense of risk, questions are raised about the ethics surrounding the production of food, including organic versus non-organic food production, and the humane treatment of animals with debate around cage-laid versus free range egg production.

It is worth asking why food and health need to be explored from a risk society perspective when it is possible to claim that we live in a safer society than previous generations (Giddens 1991). This is a society where, for the majority of people in the industrialised world, contact with food is restricted to conveniently displayed packages in the supermarket without linkage to its history and no requirements for individuals to hunt or individually grow food for survival.

With food production systems becoming considerably more complex and difficult to understand by individual consumers, many citizens have become so far removed from the origin of the food they consume that they have started to question what they eat. Modern food production has become a confusing conundrum causing societal discontent that should be better explored.

Contemporary society and risk

In contemporary society, introduction of novel food products, issues around healthy living, and risks associated with eating unhealthy food, are common mass media topics. However, at the individual level, many of the risks associated with food and health are difficult to thwart as the knowledge about the origin and prior handling of the food and possible threats to health are limited. The link between dangerous food ingredients, the misuse of toxic pesticides, or accumulation of heavy metals and their influence on short or long term healthy living can take years or decades to be scientifically proven, officially acknowledged and regulated (Beck 1992).

As this book analyses contemporary food and health issues from societal risk perspectives, it is worthwhile to reflect on how the notion of a risk society encompassing food hazards arose out of Beck's (1992) thoughts about the repercussions of the catastrophic meltdown of the Chernobyl nuclear power plant in April 1986. The explosion and the fire at Chernobyl released large quantities of radioactive particles into the atmosphere which spread over much of the then western USSR and northern Europe and contaminated plants and animals. It has and will continue to have long term consequences for food production in several affected countries and in particular for people living close to the nuclear plant. The risk of similar events happening is not insignificant, as was proven with the catastrophic failure of the Fukushima nuclear power plant in March 2011. It contaminated fish and the surrounding agricultural land. Although such extreme events are rare, Beck found that the risk concept was equally applicable to more mundane food safety hazards, which could involve growth of harmful microorganisms or common chemical contamination across societies.

At the individual level, healthy living is very much about food choice, food preparation methods employed and the amount of food consumed on a regular basis. Occasional overindulgence or risky food habits will not pose a threat to health as long as acute toxicity limits are not exceeded and basic food knowledge is adhered to. Nonetheless, experimentation with food production methods might create inherent risks that challenge accepted societal norms and a broader concept of human wellbeing.

How to define risk in contemporary society

To understand the whole food chain is difficult. We all know that everyday life is full of risks that pose some kind of dangers to our equilibrium. What is considered a significant risk is related to the circumstances in which it occurs and whom it affects (Ewald 1991). A 'risk' is defined differently depending on societal level, whether judged by governments, independent organisations or by individuals. Governments and independent organisations look at the overall probability of harm to the society based on Margin of Exposure (MoE) calculations and, if appropriate, issue Tolerable Daily Intake (TDI) recommendations to protect a majority of the public. Individuals are more circumspect and assess their personal risk based on the seriousness of the harm and attempt to reduce risk ambience by adopting risk mitigation strategies derived from their own or trusted networks' assessments.

Risk can be expressed in general terms as the probability that the threat will cause damage, injury, loss or any other negative occurrence caused by external or internal vulnerabilities, and that the risk situation may be avoided through pre-emptive action or management of the situation (Beck-Gernsheim 1996; Beck and Beck-Gernsheim 2009). Even in our most trivial activities we can incur a level of risk, such as the risk of harm from slicing the breakfast bread with a sharp knife (Hamstra *et al.* 2011). Some risks are clearly individual risks, like the potential of falling down a set of stairs after a night of heavy celebration. Other risks can be considered collective risks, which need to be addressed at the societal level, for example, setting speed limits to reduce careless driving threatening the lives of other drivers. Nonetheless, a detailed definition of the risk concept will vary from circumstance to circumstance and the individual's ability to assess the risk situation, but also in relation to scientific discipline and theoretical perspective.

Appropriate and suitable food choices are an integral part of a healthy life. It is a truism that we have to eat and drink to sustain life, but in choosing what to consume we sometimes ignore potential risks that could pose a danger to our health and wellbeing. This could be due to a misconstrued perception of the actual level of benefit versus risk, but could equally be a deliberate choice. An example of the former is high consumption of predatory fatty fish (shark, swordfish, tuna, king mackerel and orange roughy) by pregnant females in the belief that high levels of omega-3 fatty acids will support foetal brain development, while they might be unaware of the high levels of accumulated methyl mercury that could have the opposite effect on the brain growth of the foetus. An example of the deliberate choice is choosing to consume the poisonous pufferfish, or *fugu* in Japanese, that can cause death unless prepared by highly skilled chefs trained over several years in removing the liver and ovaries without contaminating the edible meat with the deadly tetrodotoxin. This is an example where the risks are known within the Japanese culture and where the trust in the chef is absolute.

The effects of eating habits, food choices, food safety and lifestyles on our health and wellbeing have been principal research areas within food science, public health and medicine for many years. It is also a growing research field in sociology, where sociologists have focused on food diversity in cultural and social environments, festive season celebrations, healthy living, body image and food as a social class issues (Bourdieu 1984; Lindsay 2010; Cova 1997; Bekin *et al.* 2007; Adams and Raisborough 2010). The choice of food and what is considered good health are social constructs. We do not necessarily think about what we eat, who we eat it with, and where and how we eat the food.

A focus on food by both researchers and the public has been developed by an increased awareness of the global character of agricultural markets and politics, heightened concerns with health and safety, and the ways those areas have become topics for media coverage. The risk society discourse exposes the complexity when trying to understand the wider commercialisation and the influence of global corporations over societies. Issues include the difficulty identifying people responsible along the food chain, gaps in the regulation of the international food trade and the shift from government to individual responsibility, but also the growing environmental concerns about food security, safe products and production methods. Giddens (1991) and Beck (1992) argue that whilst humans have always been subjected to a level of risk – such as natural disasters – these have been perceived as produced by non-human forces. Modern societies, however, are exposed to risks such as largely untested production methods and products, newly discovered illnesses and superbugs, illegal procedures that are the result of shortcuts applied in the modernisation process itself, as well as air and soil pollution. Volcanic eruptions are examples of natural disasters that can influence the food supply by releasing arsenic into the atmosphere. High levels of arsenic in food can cause skin, bladder and lung cancer. An example of a new disease due to industrial changes in cattle feeding practices is the bovine spongiform encephalopathy that came from 'nowhere' in the mid-1980s. It was initially thought to be limited to cattle, but it soon proved to be transmissible to humans, causing the variant Creuzfeldt-Jakobs disease. Beck (1992) and Giddens (1991) define these two types of risks as external risks and manufactured risks. A high level of human agency is involved in manufactured risks, and the agency influence is in both producing and mitigating such risks. As manufactured risks are the product of human activity, it is possible for societies to assess the level of risk that is being produced, or what is about to be produced. Beck's (1992, 2007; Beck and Holzer 2007) research highlights the politics of risk as a key feature of the critical analysis of life in the global village.

While agreeing that 'the idea of risk has recently risen to prominence in political debate, and has become the regular coinage of exchange on public policy', Mary Douglas (1992:x) held a less optimistic view of the widening gap between the government attempts to manage risk and the public's emotionalised responses to threats and dangers. From the point of view of science, risks are estimated from calculations of probabilities of events in defined circumstances of time and place. As such, empirical risks transcend the ideologies of those that wield them and assert their status as facts, which must be contested scientifically. Yet, once they enter the public realm they are 'cultural facts' whose meanings, as Douglas points out, become publically contested. The problem that Douglas sees in current approaches is that it puts too much faith in the abstracted and instrumental science of risk experts, but has forgotten that 'in all places at all times the universe is moralized and politicized. Disasters that befoul the air and soil and poison the water are generally turned to political account: someone already unpopular is going to be blamed for it' (Douglas 1992:5).

Risk controversies, therefore, do not exist in a cultural vacuum, but find themselves re-articulated within the legal disputes about whom to blame and political mobilisations around how to reduce them.

Governmental risk strategies

Government efforts to manage risk depend highly on the regulation of the industry and the research of risk scientists, but also on how mass media presents the information. Governments but also risk scientists, manage official publication of risk information. However, what information and how it is presented in the public arena comes down to the coverage by the mass media. Creating a moral and political blame game can work against the presentation mode and the nature of politically sensitive information, hence a blameworthiness scenario that favours mass media in reporting risks, crime and health issues (Furedi 2005; Sorenson *et al.* 1998; Harrabin *et al.* 2003) to increase media news circulation.

Even if the assessment of the probability and severity of risk is a strictly scientific discipline, communicating risks through mass media is often the only manner in which citizens are informed. Public opinion has traditionally an important role in the politics of managing risks (Sandman *et al.* 1992; Kasperson 1992). While acknowledging multidimensional and often conflicting interpretations between scientific facts, political ideology and public perception, several attempts have been made in the food area to address the complexity of societal risk discourses. The risk concepts and analysis of risks are grounded in structured decision-making processes.

Risk analysis within the food sector is used to identify potential hazards in the food supply, to assess the risks to human health and the danger posed by the threats, to design and implement appropriate measures to control the risks, and to communicate with stakeholders about the risks and measures applied. The risk paradigm applied within the food and health area has become an almost universally accepted stratagem, which was initially developed by the Codex Alimentarius Commission (CAC) in the early 1990s to incorporate three distinct but closely connected components: risk assessment, risk management and risk communication (Codex Alimentarius Commission 2007). The three components are complementary measures of the overall risk assessment discipline within the food safety discourse. During the past two to three decades, the three components have been formalised, refined and integrated into a unified discipline, and applied at both national and international levels. The three main components of risk analysis within food science have been defined by CAC as follows:

- *Risk assessment*: A scientific process consisting of the following steps: i) hazard identification ii) hazard characterisation iii) exposure assessment and iv) risk characterisation. The outcome is a quantification of the public health risks posed by a potential hazard.
- *Risk management*: The process, distinct from risk assessment, of weighing policy alternatives in consultation with all interested parties, considering risk assessment and other factors relevant for the health protection of consumers and for the promotion of fair trade practices and, if needed, selecting appropriate prevention and control options.
- *Risk communication*: The exchange of information and opinions throughout the risk analysis process concerning risk, risk-related factors and risk perceptions, among risk assessors, risk managers, consumers, industry, the academic community and other interested parties, including the explanation of risk assessment findings and the basis of risk management decisions.

Risk analysis can be used to support and improve the development of food standards, as well as to address food safety issues that result from emerging hazards or breakdowns in food control systems. It provides food safety regulators with the information and evidence they need for effective decision-making, contributing to better food safety outcomes and improvements to public health. Regardless of the institutional context, the discipline of risk analysis offers a tool that food safety authorities at different levels and stages of the process can use to make significant gains in securing food that are safe to consume. However, in contemporary society where food production and food processing involve global industries and are increasingly dominated by international corporations that can afford targeted advertising, and where business and political interests might have higher priority than consumer safety, the information presented to the public might not be easily construed and not necessarily presented in plain language. In the current information overflow of the technological society, it is difficult for most people, to know what represents safe and healthy food.

Communicating risk strategies

There is a growing acceptance among risk communication experts that dietary risk has a different meaning and is something inherently different seen from the public's perception of risk compared to the scientific view. This includes how scientists and regulators define risk (Beck 1997a, 1992; Ewald 1991; Douglas 1985; Douglas and Wildavsky 1982; Slovic 1987). For example, to be able to target consumer perception of diet deficiencies and food threats, scientists and regulators must address the real concerns and attitudes of the public. Even food safety risk communication in its present form is lacking in proper consideration of consumer perceptions and attitudes.

According to Ropeik (2007), the term 'risk communication' arose largely because of environmental controversies in the 1970s, when public concern was high about some relatively low threats to human health and the environment. Scientists, regulators and industry described people as irrational, and they became frustrated in not being able to convey their message. Similar discrepancies between the message and the understanding of the message prompted governments to establish educational campaigns to educate the public about the food facts and thus to defuse controversies surrounding food production and consumption. This proved to be a too simplistic strategy, as individual and societal perceptions of health risks are multidimensional and often convoluted. Social, political, psychological and economic factors interact with technological factors and affect people's perceptions in complex ways. Education alone is most often not sufficient to change public perception and to convey knowledge of underlying factors. Attributes, like trust, dread, control, uncertainty and cultural traditions are also factors that individuals take into account when judging what to be afraid of and how afraid to be (Ropeik 2007).

Attempts in the past to identify and review the factors influencing consumer perception of food safety risks have found that the extent to which a risk is perceived to be unnatural, dreaded or to which an individual perceives exposure to be involuntary, are important dimensions. Consumers' societal and individual perceptions of risk are diverse and how people respond to potential risks associated with safety across different risk and danger domains, including that of food hazards, depends on their risk perceptions. Research shows that the two most important determinants of perceived risks associated with food were the extent to which the potential danger was seen to have technological or naturally occurring origins, together with the temporal dimension in which the potential risk was presented: immediate or long term (Kaptan *et al*. 2014).

On the one hand, novel technologies applied to food production and processing tend to be associated with higher levels of perceived risk and seen as unnatural. For some risks involving novel biological manipulation, like genetically modified food or cloning of animals, moral, ethical or environmental concerns may become more important determinants of consumer responses than direct risk or benefit perceptions.

On the other hand, because of consumers' often low level of risk perception associated with naturally occurring food dangers, like microbial contaminants, risk communication has had limited success in improving public health associated with the adoption of self-protective measures for foodborne microorganisms causing illness (Nauta *et al*. 2008).

Further complexity is provided by the temporal context in which the potential risk occurs. More is known about reactions to acute effects of a food safety incident compared to long term impacts, in particular when examining changes in risk perceptions and subsequent consumption behaviours. Presenting even a naturally occurring risk in an acute or crisis context may generate an immediate surge in perceived risk (Pidgeon *et al*. 2003).

Other important factors influencing risk perception include consumer demographics, country of residence, as well as reliance on, and trust in, alternative food safety information sources. Tonsor *et al*. (2009) showed how consumers in Canada, Japan and the United States had risk perceptions shaped by their level of reliance on observable and credible information. Personal and indirect food safety experiences substantially affected risk perceptions. Factors such as household income, number of children, gender, age and voting preferences were strong predictors of an individual's risk perceptions.

Differences in familiarity with food products may influence how information about the risks and benefits of some food is conveyed, how food is used in creating risk scenarios and influence perceptions. It is argued that risks and perceptions of risks associated with food may be dependent on social and cultural traditions and different psychological processes, as risk perception is more likely to be derived from deliberative information processing, while the perception of the food's benefit is derived from heuristic information processing and personal experience (Fischer and Frewer 2009).

The research findings point to the importance of better exploring and integrating consumer risk perception, whether irrational or not, into the food safety risk analysis paradigm. Potential solutions for rebuilding consumer confidence in food safety and bridging the gap between consumer and expert opinions regarding food risks, might include traceability and labelling, segmented communication approaches, and public involvement in risk management decision-making (Verbeke *et al.* 2007).

Although considerable uncertainty is often associated with the outcome of any risk assessment, the findings are most often seen as incomprehensible science for a layperson. Sociological analyses of the food context are almost completely forgotten. The use of pesticides, although deemed safe to humans, might lead to monocultures, lack of diversity, and environmental destruction threatening the society. The safe use of preservatives might produce sliced bread that can be kept for months, but lacks artisan craft to create eating satisfaction. Genetically modified food might be a short lived advantage for the agriculture industry, but there is a forgotten ethical aspect and consideration for long term public and animal health and wellbeing. The public might not be ready for salmon modified to grow twice as fast as natural salmon, while increasing environmental pressure and threatening animal welfare.

As we combine two different disciplines in this book: a sociological and a public health perspective, definitions of certain concepts might create some confusion. It is particularly important to point out that health, which can be seen as having a strictly medical definition from a public health point of view, has a much wider meaning when seen from a sociological perspective. It involves social, mental as well as physical wellbeing, how the individuals feel about themselves and how happy and satisfied they are in their private and public space. It thus encompasses much more than a sole focus on a medical illness. As the book is written from a sociological perspective, health and wellbeing concepts are defined in this broader social sense. Another concept that can cause confusion is the difference between risk and hazard. In sociological terms, a risk is 'a distinct, outlined and calculated uncertainty which is a side effect of actions of particular individuals' (Sørensen and Christiansen 2013:24). A hazard is incalculable, erratic and difficult to delimit. It does not affect a special group and the causes are external, for example, nature and gods. Luhmann (1990:143) describes the differences between risks and hazards by referring to the different position between a smoker and a non-smoker: 'It is only for the smoker themselves that cancer is a risk; for anybody else it will always be a hazard'. Beck did not initially differentiate between risk and hazard, but did so in later writings where he stresses that:

> 'Risks' are understood...to be determinable, calculable uncertainties; modernity itself produced them in the form of foreseen or unforeseen secondary consequences, for which social responsibility is (or is not) taken through regulatory measures....There is, accordingly, a consensus in

international social-scientific literature that one should distinguish here between pre-industrial hazards, not based on technological-economic decisions, and thus externalizable (onto nature, the gods), and industrial risks, products of social choice, which must be weighed against opportunities and acknowledge, dealt with or simply foisted on individuals. (Beck 1995:77)

Food safety scientists use a more limited definition. The International Programme on Chemical Safety (IPCS) defines a hazard as an inherent property of an agent or situation having the potential to cause adverse effects when an organism, system, or (sub)population is exposed to that agent. Risk is the probability of an adverse effect in an organism, system, or (sub)population caused under specified circumstances by exposure to an agent (International Programme on Chemical Safety 2004). However, in this book the broader sociological perspective on health and wellbeing is adopted. The risk concept will be discussed in more detail in Chapter 2.

Conclusion

It is postulated that the current food system interpretation of the societal risk paradigm would benefit from better inclusion of significant sociological perspectives in analysing food production, distribution and consumption, as well as how food and eating are integrated into social institutions, systems and networks. Sociological perspectives of food production and processing will contribute to exploring social and cultural inequalities, social class differences, food market differences, politics and power exerted by governments, global corporations, work and health implications and local and global environmental issues. It should include the whole process from how we produce food to what we eat, who benefits, with whom we eat, what we think about food, and how food fits with contemporary social life. It would widen the debate about body weight to include the social consequences of diet-related diseases and the so called 'obesity epidemic' and build an understanding of food and health from a more holistic perspective rather than the current sole focus on food intake and exercise (Dixon and Broom 2007; Gard and Wright 2005).

Research points to the importance of better exploring and integrating consumer risk perception, whether irrational or not, into the food safety risk analysis paradigm. Sociological perspectives on food can assist in confronting the various crises that surround the food supply. These include the relationship between food and environmental problems, escalating food costs, and national, community and domestic food security (Lawrence *et al.* 2009). Questions around quality of life, healthy living, but also about the right to correct information and being able to make educated decisions, are essential parts in each of these areas.

Chapter 2 provides further explanations of the theories developed around the risk society framework and the overall risk concept; the socio-cultural, the risk society and the governmentality risk discourses. It discusses the socio-cultural perspective of the risk discourse, how it is grounded within the anthropological discipline, and how theorists representing the socio-cultural risk discourse are concerned with the basic principles that determine how people see themselves and how their understanding of themselves influences their behaviour and actions. Furthermore, the chapter discusses the risk society discourse, which examines modern industrialisation from a socio-logical perspective, and the governmentality risk discourse, which explores the ideology of how individuals' everyday life is governed.

2 Sociological risk discourse frameworks

Introduction

The concept of risk can be traced back to the middle of the seventeenth century. It stems from the French word 'risque' and from the Italian word 'rischio' meaning risk or danger. In general terms, the risk concept describes the possibility or anticipation that something unpleasant or unwelcome will happen. The situation has not occurred yet, but it might happen if the indications are trustworthy and if the actions continue in the anticipated direction. The outcome from these actions is considered dangerous or at least have adverse effects for the people exposed to the anticipated risk event (Oxford Dictionaries Online 2013).

Risk can also be described from a strictly mathematical point of view as a combination of the probability of an event occurring and the magnitude of the consequences should it happen, or in simpler terms, the likelihood of an incident happening and the severity of its effects. The calculations include the uncertainty aspects of the probability and the magnitude risk components, as they are important elements in the decision-making process. Uncertainty is based on deductions from gained knowledge and experience, but also on the limitations of the proposed risk model, the analysed system and an understanding of its behaviour (Montewka *et al.* 2014). The outcome of the analysis should be an objective and technical description of the anticipated risk.

Food and beverages are not devoid of risks and the ramifications of dangerous hazards that under unfavourable conditions could be harmful to public health and wellbeing. Scientific tools from the toxicology, microbiology and epidemiology disciplines have traditionally been used to quantify the risk posed by such hazards by statistical modelling based on historical data as the basis for calculating current risks. This approach might be sufficient when evaluating the strength of steel needed to construct a bridge to last beyond a century or the insurance premium for a house in a fire-prone area. However, from a food perspective, consumer choice is more likely to be influenced by social, cultural, religious and emotional interpretations of product attributes rather than the physical properties of the products themselves (Rozin *et al.* 1986).

Consequently, consumer evaluations of food safety risks are based more on social and cultural perceptions, and interpretations of food safety than technical evidence. As consumers' perceptions influence their attitudes and behaviour of what to consume, this collective knowledge guide their decisions in what food products they trust. Consumers judge their exposure to a risk situation with a focus on the *severity* of possible consequences rather than the *probability* of occurrence, while experts use a combination of the two, most often with a bias towards probability of occurrence. This divergence of perspective is at the root of the disparity between technical and social definitions of risk, and the reason why technical assessments of risk have proved to be an inadequate basis for the management of societal risks, including food safety issues (Yeung and Morris 2001a). The risk concept has progressed from covering only situations that can be calculated through a mathematical model, and extended to all other society risk areas interlinking different disciplines. The risk concept has become of particular significance within the area of food production, processing and food consumption, as these different food stages will ultimately influence the health and wellbeing of people.

The contrast between scientists' and consumers' views

In this book we explore the contradiction between experts' research and evidence-based advice and consumer perception of safe food. It is not sufficient merely to understand technical risks around food to explain consumers' perception of risk and the factors that influence their behaviour in selecting food for consumption. Risks need a social and cultural context as, '[n]othing is a risk in itself; there is no risk in reality' (Ewald 1991:199). Therefore, the government food safety experts' and the industry's communication of risk scenarios to consumers become misconstrued. The risks perceived by consumers as significant are often not acknowledged or given the expected importance by authorities and in expert assessments (Beck and Holzer 2007).

It is impossible to find a historical or modern period that has been free of any form of tangible or intangible risks or perceptions of risk. Protection against risks has been an issue, in one form or another, for all community settings since humans first established themselves (Vaughan 1997). Commercial assessments of risks and the possibility to get insurance against an emerging risk were first established in London, in 1667, when The Insurance Office opened in London as a response to the Great Fire of London in 1666 (Dickson 1960; Klein 2001). Risks that can be insured against and to which governments and businesses can take precautionary measures, are risks that are considered real and likely to happen sometime in the future. However, risks for which there is insurance have diversified from those mainly related to physical damage such as flood, fire, storm damage, earthquake, collapsing buildings and crimes like burglary and arson. In the twenty-first century, it is possible to gain insurance for almost any incident, such as retrenchment, bad health, income loss, personal or material accidents, life and liability, as well as livestock and pet insurance, with insurance premiums based on estimates of the likelihood of the risk eventuating.

Real and perceived risks can sometimes be difficult to separate as they both can produce adverse reactions. The anticipation of a risk situation can frighten people more than an actual event itself and elicit negative consequences. For example, the perceived risk of nutritional inadequacy of a normal diet has led to ever-increasing consumption of dietary supplements that in turn can have a negative health impact (see Chapter 6). Additionally, a risk situation might not be known to the individual or to anyone until long after the occurrence. This is especially the case in relation to consumption of food, where the effects of a carcinogen can take decades or more to be identified. An example is acrylamide, a carcinogen formed during heating of food. It has probably been around since the discovery of fire to cook food, but its negative health impact was not identified as an issue until 2002 (see Chapter 11).

Even after publicity in the popular press, the public appears to neglect these potential risks to their health. In reality, consumer choices related to diet and lifestyle can create relatively serious risks, but consumers often disregard such scientific findings, as the effects can be years away. At the same time, new and emerging food processing technologies, like irradiation or the use of synthetic chemicals like pesticides or additives, are examples of health threats that are often overestimated by the public, as in reality they pose only minimal actual risks to human health. It has been suggested that the contrast between consumer perception and scientific findings supports the view that the consumer's perception of risks involving food is more likely to be in the reverse order to the food safety ranking of risk as identified by experts (Slovic 2000; Verbeke *et al.* 2007). The difference between actual risk and the public perception of risk can partly be explained by difficulties in gaining a holistic perspective of the origin and history of individual food products.

To bridge the gap between real and perceived risk, mass media has a significant role to play in conveying information to the public about harmful products. News media is the central vehicle for disseminating information to the populace about everyday life, government policy and decisions, health warnings and product risks. The public would have little knowledge about situations and products classified by experts as 'risks', if not for mass media's news coverage (Kitzinger 1999). However, there is an imbalance in mass media reporting as catastrophes and disasters attract more attention than everyday news stories. An example from 2008 is the case of melamine added to infant milk formula in China, where six infants died and it was estimated that 54,000 babies in total were hospitalised (*The Guardian*, 2 December 2008). It was suggested that the chemical had been added to milk to make it appear to have higher protein content than what it actually had. This case has a parallel in a separate incident four years earlier with watered-down milk, which caused the death of thirteen infants from malnutrition (*BBC News*, 22 April 2004). Both events, although geographically limited, received worldwide coverage and had the potential to distort public opinion about the safety of infant formulae in unaffected countries. Hence, an uncritical consumption of news media reporting can portray the society as a more dangerous private and public space than the actual situation.

The current interest in the risk discourse and the perception of risk in our contemporary society has attracted researchers from diverse disciplines. It is puzzling that despite society's focus on the harmful impact of overweight and obesity on health (see Chapter 3), there is little change in our reliance on private transport rather than walking, an ever increasing sedentary lifestyle in urban living, as well as food servings exceeding personal needs. The sociological risk discourse is a useful strategy to better understand, analyse and organise social processes and experiences in an attempt to explain our dietary and lifestyle choices (Lupton 2006:3, 11; Taylor-Gooby and Zinn 2006). Within the sociological discipline the core risk discourse perspectives are the 'socio-cultural' or 'cultural-symbolic' perspective, the 'risk society' perspective and the 'governmentality' perspective. These risk discourse perspectives assist in exploring the role individuals, industry and government have in the food chain, in influencing food consumption choice, and the subsequent population health impact.

The nature of risk

In contemporary society, the word 'risk' is given a negative connotation denoting danger (Douglas 1992:24). However, as noted above, for an event to be classified and understood as a risk it needs to have happened previously or to be imagined as being possible to happen in the near future. Risks that have not yet happened and risks that are difficult to imagine as ever happening, might be risks, but they are problematic to perceive, plan for or know how to avoid. If people are aware of and anticipate possible dangers, they are more inclined to take the required precautions. Thus, reliable information and knowledge are essential precursors in prevention of risks. Ideally, risk situations and assessments of their danger and likelihood of materialising should be based on judgements of facts and objective evidences. The ambiguities of potential risks make them challenging to predict, but the portrayal of an event as a risk can become a useful tool in influencing people's behaviour in specific directions. Beck (1992) and Giddens (1994a) view risks in contemporary society as products of human action derived from human decision-making processes rather than being based on fate. Risks in relation to modern industrialisation logically should refer back to individuals or groups responsible for the decision leading up to the risk situation, whereas in relation to natural risks, humans cannot be blamed for natural disasters that 'could not be imputed to wrongful conduct' (Ewald 1993:226). Risks have become political and influenced by humans, rather than being a metaphysical phenomenon.

Furthermore, risks have moved from being a social issue to being an individual problem, where the individual is required to assess their own situation and be self-critical and self-reflexive, as modern society demands the individual to take a reflexive, accountable and responsible perspective on everyday life risk possibilities (Beck 1992:135). However, as Alexander (1996) notes, the lack of empirical research to evaluate the theories by both Beck and Giddens makes it difficult to be sure of the implications of the risk discourse. Alexander (1996:134) notes about Beck's risk society discourse: 'Broad tendential speculations are advanced about infrastructural and organizational processes that have little grounding in the actual processes of institutional and everyday life'. For example, the risk paradigm can be used for political purposes to increase or decrease the perception of the risk, such as emphasising acts of terrorism or migration overflow, while at the same time downplaying anticipated risks of climate change, environmental pollution, the danger of industrial waste, contamination of food or unhealthy food choice.

Hence, the application of a risk scenario can be used in a self-serving manner by an interest group, organisation or a government to gain a political or financial advantage, to create confusion, and to set community and population groups against each other. If the risk to the society construct is used in this manner, the risk situation can create trends of 'moral panic'. The risk discourse can have the same effect as Cohen's (2002) moral panic discourse, where the authorities and their representatives in power positions alert people to possible risks by creating a moral panic. Cohen focused on the threat to social order posed by new youth constellations, mods and rockers, if they were not 'controlled'. The risk discourse can be applied in a similar way to manipulate people, to frighten people to do the 'right thing' and to stay within the law, even if there are no real risks to societal order or societal wellbeing.

Governments' sentiments are augmented by mass media as it has the role as disseminator of the message to the general population. Nevertheless, independently of the seriousness of an anticipated risk event, any insufficient or excessive emphasis of the risk situation might be criticised, although less so when providing excessive warnings. Thus, overestimation is more likely than underestimation of the risk, except when it will reflect negatively on the government of the day or other organisations, business groups, social, legal or political interest groups.

The interconnection between nature-based and manufactured risks

Risks and adversity are interconnected, while not all risks lead to disasters, all adversities involve moments of risk. The modern risk and fear environment have created a milieu where everyone is expected to take on responsibilities for their everyday safety. It has become a personal duty to be vigilant against any unfamiliar activities, be careful with the unknown and be suspicious of strangers. These measures are presented as being good and sensible strategies to avoid future damage. Familiarity with the environment and the society are an advantage in any endeavour. To know where food products come from, how they have been grown, and how they have been handled throughout the process, gives people a feeling of security in knowing what they eat. A collective ideology of responsibility, assumed to have existed, at least among some societal groups, before the mid-twentieth century, has changed in the twenty-first century to a progressively global society with increasing individualism. Nonetheless, the anticipation of risk can unite people into collective action, such as engagement in environmental movements to create a sustainable coexistence between nature, people and industry as reflected in the opposition to genetically modified foods (see Chapter 8).

To identify changes and possible risks, people in the local area are the most important observers, as they can best recognise changes in their community. For example, the 11 September 2001 attacks on the World Trade Center in New York, USA, did not come completely unexpectedly. There were warning signs, such as a group of young men taking flying lessons with less focus on how to land the aircraft, which for most people is usually an essential skill. The American authorities were alerted to this (Bauman 2007:19–21), but if you do not know what to look for and do not freely share information between relevant local authorities, it is difficult to identify the possible risk scenario, to coordinate, and to find connections between diverse information sources, especially when the proposed scenario is unfamiliar or unimaginable. Thus, the enhanced focus on collecting information is mainly useful after the event, to understand how it could have happened, and to prevent it from happening again. This scenario is also applicable to food production and the way consumers engage with food.

However, in the world of expanding and increasing internet access there are serious issues around what information should be collected, how to store it and how and what should be shared between authorities and with the public to safeguard national security and protect intellectual property and commercial interests, while still upholding civil liberties. Personal engagement, from voicing concerns within the circle of family and friends, to protesting on the street or to a situation where a person or a group develop their protest into a violent act, is a protracted process. For most people the protest remains limited and non-violent, while for others civil disobedience becomes the only alternative when other options are seen as fruitless. Animal cruelty, genetically modified food, and the corporatisation of food, but also the use of productive agricultural land for mining purposes, are occurrences and issues that have incited protests in many countries. Increased knowledge about the food we eat, in the form of declarations of product origin, the use of genetically modified ingredients and the entire list of ingredients, are demands raised globally by more and more consumers, not just in the industrialised world.

Risks and dangers relevant to people's everyday life hinge little on possible terrorism attacks, as these are, in reality, only a risk to a small percentage of the population, despite extensive government and media exposure. More likely risks and dangers come from exposure to dubious chemicals, precarious work practices, contaminated food, and local air and soil pollution from modern industrialisation methods, rather than from terror attacks. Protest against polluting industrialisation might have less political power to sway voters, and it is thus less often classified as risky or seen as an anticipated risk (Beck 1999), but it is perhaps more important for the long term life and health of the general population. In the next sections, the socio-cultural, risk society and the governmentality risk discourses are set in a social and cultural context.

The socio-cultural perspective

The socio-cultural risk discourse is grounded within the sociology and anthropology disciplines. The discourse is concerned with the basic principles that determine how people see and understand themselves, and how this self-perception influences their behaviour and actions. Leading theorists within this discourse are the anthropologist Mary Douglas (Douglas 1969, 1985, 1992) and the political scientist Aaron Wildavsky (Douglas and Wildavsky 1982). Douglas and Wildavsky (1982) explored the socio-cultural risk discourse foremost in *Risk and Culture*, but they have also written extensively about societal risk and danger, in what way societies can unite to avert external danger and how the risk discourse can be applied to enforce community cohesion. Their central position is that danger and risk are social constructions, which causes different risk perceptions (Dake 1992). '[S]elective attention to risk, and preferences among different types of risk taking (or avoiding), correspond to cultural biases – that is, to worldviews or ideologies entailing deeply held values and beliefs defending different patterns of social relations.' (Wildavsky and Dake 1990:43)

The socio-cultural or cultural-symbolic discourse focuses on the fundamental rules for all societies' existence and social cohesion. It explores the distinction between 'self' and 'others'. The people who are defined as belonging to the 'self' group, are considered friends and trustworthy, while the people who are classified as 'others' (strangers) or outsiders, are treated with caution and suspicion (Becker 1963). The 'others' are not necessarily excluded from the 'self community', but they are not accepted and trusted to the same extent, as people who are identified as 'self people'. Hence, the 'others' are not given the same level of right to inclusiveness and belongingness, as the people classified as 'self people'. In a close community setting, the external boundary of accepted group behaviour is very clearly demarcated to separate between the 'self' and outsider members. Consequently, in the socio-cultural risk discourse, the wellbeing of the group is of greater importance than the interests of the individual member; therefore disloyalty to the group can be a reason for exclusion (Douglas 1982).

This approach, to differentiate between people defined as 'self' versus 'others', becomes the foundation for the creation of community identification, social cohesion and cooperative actions, and a way to recognise the characteristics that identify a 'self-person'. The emphasis on the differences between 'self' and 'other' people create social cohesion within a community, especially if the 'others' are defined in a negative and threatening manner. An identified outsider's threat can help to define and strengthen the 'self' group, its social network and social belonging (Becker 1963). The socio-cultural discourse can be applied to different functions and strategies within a society or a local community, but also in relation to food, as it can be applied to the way food is produced, which food is accepted to be cultivated and to be eaten. It can also classify food not grown in the 'accepted' place as inferior. In addition, different religious demands on dietary choices can be seen in this context as a uniting feature among devotees.

Douglas's (1969, 1985, 1992) socio-cultural approach to the risk perspective is grounded in her principal belief that ideas about risks are part of shared cultural understandings and practices. These cultural understandings stem from social expectations and responsibilities – from pre-established cultural beliefs that frame how people behave and how they are expected to react to potential risks within and against the community. The cultural understandings or the community's social and cultural capitals are developed within the community setting, thus creating an ambience that influences people's behavioural habitus in food preferences (Bourdieu 1984).

Douglas also emphasises that we need to understand the social, cultural and religious environment to comprehend the classification of risks:

> [I]t is implied that if we only knew all the circumstances we would find the rational basis of primitive ritual amply justified....The importance of incense is not that it symbolises the ascending smoke of sacrifice, but it is a means of making tolerable the smells of unwashed humanity. Jewish and Islamic avoidance of pork is explained as due to the dangers of eating pig in hot climates. (Douglas 1969:36)

The notions of risk are therefore not individualistic, but rather shared within a community. It is the community as a whole that identifies the risks and decides the potential threat the risk might impose on the community's social cohesion. The community represents the residents, but the community also represents the social and cultural environment that keeps all of them together (Durkheim 1933, 1951).

Douglas perceives risk as a cultural strategy whereby communities or subgroups identify real or anticipated dangers and threats against the community or the cultural group. These risks are mostly identified as coming from 'others', people or organisations outside the community, or people who proposes new ways of living. Risks directed towards the 'self' group can also come from people within the community or a group of community members who question the values, policy, beliefs and moral standing of the authority of the community or a distinct cultural group; an example is groups questioning the introduction of pesticides or acceptance of genetically modified crops. In these circumstances, risk beliefs and risk avoiding practices are ways to maintain social cohesion, stability and order within the community. It includes a strategy to deal with and to limit deviant behaviour and practices from what is expressed by community members as preferable.

Each community will label what is considered a risk or unacceptable behaviour and define what is threatening to the community's moral principles and social cohesion. However, the socio-cultural risk perspective also classifies what constitutes, for example, acceptable food based on their social, cultural and religious environment:

> There are two notable differences between our contemporary European ideas of defilement and those, say, of primitive cultures. One is that dirt avoidance for us is a matter of hygiene or aesthetics and is not related to our religion. ... The second difference is that our idea of dirt is dominated by the knowledge of pathogenic organisms. The bacterial transmission of disease was a great nineteenth-century discovery. It produced the most radical revolution in the history of medicine. So much has it transformed our lives that it is difficult to think of dirt except in the context of pathogenicity. (Douglas 1969:40)

Douglas's socio-cultural risk perspective is grounded in habitus and traditions, which are developed into moral and ethical norms, but the risk discourse also has a political purpose to maintain the community's unity and stability. It might be an ideology more suited for smaller communities, where social cohesion and social control can be maintained through close social networks and where shared majority agreements can be achieved (Lupton 2006; Renn 2005; Rohrmann 1999).

There are many examples in the area of food that are relevant to the socio-cultural perspective of the risk discourse. For almost as long as people have been eating, there have been socio-culturally derived rules about food that is off limits, some of them clearly emanating from a risk-based background. Jews who follow the laws of kashruth do not consume pork, shellfish, reptiles, amphibians and most kinds of insects. Islamic dietary law divides foods into halal, foods permitted under Islamic Shari'ah law, and haram, which forbids people following the law to eat meat from swine, dogs, cats and monkeys. Hindus do not eat beef, and many do not eat any meat products at all. The Moru of South Sudan allow only children and old people to eat chicken and eggs, and some groups of Cushitic people in northeast Africa avoid fish. The Yazidis in Iraq do not eat lettuce, and Jains do not eat onions or root vegetables (Kolbert 2014).

Although some religious prescriptions in relation to food consumption can clearly be linked to hygiene and health, there is a higher intended cultural goal for some other food handling practices. Shechita is the Jewish religious method of slaughtering permitted animals and poultry in the prescribed manner to make the food acceptable for human consumption. It is the only method of producing kosher meat and poultry allowed by Jewish law. The law describes the slaughter method in minute detail, any modification renders the meat forbidden for Jews to eat. The reason for use of shechita is said to be strictly spiritual as the Torah commands Jews to use the method in order to eat meat (Rosen 2004). All food, including plants and animals, are considered to carry a spiritual life force, with a crucial spiritual cycle that will be completed when eating the permitted foods, as it helps to perfect the universe.

Similarly, the vegan culture can be seen as a spiritual manifestation of the socio-cultural risk discourse. The social and cultural background to veganism involves compassion, empathy and reverence for all living beings inspired by the Vedic principle of Ahimsa, which aims not to harm any living being (Chapple 2011). The term 'vegan' is used to describe an individual who has chosen to abstain from using any product found to be derived from animals, including meat, dairy, fur, leather, gelatine, down feathers, and non-animal products manufactured by use of animals such as beer filtered with isinglass (fish bladder). While there are many reasons for abstaining from animal products, the most predominant reasons appear to be motivated by animal welfare and health. These modern categories have arisen from a greater historical diversity of vegan/vegetarian motivations such as religious restrictions and scarcity of animal-based foods (Guerin 2014).

Food taboos are known from virtually all human societies where the food prescriptions fulfil a fundamental human socio-cultural need (Meyer-Rochow 2009). The Paleolithic diet, also known as the paleo diet or caveman diet, is based on a set of food prohibitions adjusted to people living today. The diet claims to have its origin from ancient ancestors. The Paleolithic diet draws on an appeal to nature and a narrative of conspiracy theories about how nutritional research, which does not support the paleo diet, is controlled by a malign food industry (Hall 2014). It is a diet based on meat, nuts and berries. It excludes dairy and processed grains. Proponents of the diet posit that humans evolved nutritional needs specific to the foods available to our Paleolithic ancestors, and the contemporary paleo diet is adapted to the ancient diet. Modern humans are said to be maladapted to eating foods such as grain, legumes and dairy, and in particular, high energy processed foods that are staples of most modern diets. Proponents claim that the modern human being is not able to metabolise these comparatively new types of food properly, which has led to modern day problems such as obesity, heart disease and diabetes. They claim that followers of the paleo diet may enjoy a longer, a healthier and more active life.

The risk society perspective of modern industrialisation

There are similarities between the socio-cultural risk perspective and the risk society discourse in that they both focus on actual threats and not on perceptions of risk, however, the two discourses analyse risk from different standpoints.

The risk society discourse has its foundation in the risk concept of dangers and hazards that have proliferated throughout progressive modern industrialisation, urbanisation, globalisation of trade and commerce, and technological advances in communication within the networked society (Castells 2000, 2001; Castells *et al.* 2009). The risk society has become synonymous with the writings of Ulrich Beck (1992) with his book *The Risk Society*, and Anthony Giddens (2002) with *Modernity and Self-Identity*. Beck was especially influenced by Michel Foucault (1991) and his student François Ewald (1991). Ewald (1991:288) has described modern society as at its core an 'insurance society'. Before modern industrialisation, natural disasters such as floods, earthquakes, wildfires, storms, extreme cold, heat and prolonged droughts were the people's main risk concerns. With the introduction and expansion of modern industrialisation, manufactured goods and manipulation of food products, the food-producing environment has evolved to harbour fundamental risk factors.

Beck (1992) highlights the increasing complexity of contemporary society and the influence of multinational corporations on local and global food production, with mounting difficulties in identifying and singling out discrete organisations or fluid management teams responsible for the final outputs of multifaceted food chains. There are inherent short- and long-term risks within complex manufacturing processes that are not always fully recognised before the product is released to the public, and this can lead to a lack of appropriate safety considerations. Some products and processing procedures will not be exposed as dangerous until much later, when the operation might have changed ownership or been shut down and the people responsible have moved on. Such a scenario makes it increasingly difficult to rectify the process and to gain compensation through the justice system. People affected might even have died well before the problem is identified.

Asbestos production in Australia is one example where the fight for recognition of the disease caused by the asbestos fibres and the long-term effects of the disease have been hard fought by the sufferers and their supporters over a long time (Peacock 2009). The company involved even changed domicile to avoid prosecution.

There is no shortage of examples in the area of food, which could lead to future health issues. The use in some food packaging of bisphenol A, an endocrine disruptor with the potential to influence foetal development, has been questioned but is still allowed. The use in agricultural food production of cheap fertilisers, often with high cadmium content, could be responsible for kidney failure in the elderly, but cadmium in fertilisers is still common. Concerns have been raised in several countries about the health impact of so-called energy drinks with high levels of caffeine, often in combination with alcohol. Energy drinks are becoming increasingly popular among children and young people and are aggressively marketed to this group. Although health experts in the USA, the United Kingdom, Germany and France have warned about possible dangers, there has been little regulatory action so far to limit their use. As of 2014, Lithuania was the only country issuing a total ban, while Colombia and Latvia have introduced age restrictions.

The complexity and diversity of modern industrialisation, and the difficulty in realising the potential impact of all the elaborate aspects involved, can give rise to products and procedures that might be harmful to consumers as well as production staff. Innovation and evolution of processing technologies create a new risk environment that influences producers and consumers alike at all levels of society. From the risk society perspective, prospective and anticipated risks have changed from being identifiable and manageable at a local level to globally created risks. Consequently, it is increasingly difficult to recognise risk situations in such a global context, with raw material sourcing and food processing occurring at a multitude of geographically diverse places, making tracing of product origin almost impossible. Modern industrialisation has taken away people's control or feeling of control and their ability to influence their living environment and life choices (Beck 1992:35–36).

There has been a public backlash to the globalisation of the food chain, in that people have started to demand country of origin labelling. This was clearly manifested in early 2015 in Australia when a batch of berries imported from China caused an outbreak of hepatitis A across several states. In response, the Australian Federal Government has proposed the introduction of new labels showing the proportion of Australian content in mixed products, although the public would prefer a more detailed description of all countries supplying the ingredients (Lee 2015). In Europe, a 2011 outbreak of E. coli O104 in Northern Europe and a horsemeat scandal forced the European Commission to expand, from April 2015, decade-old country-of-origin labelling of beef to also require fresh, chilled and frozen meat from sheep, goats, pigs and poultry to state where the animal had been born, reared and slaughtered. This is similar to US legislation, introduced in 2002 after political pressure from the public, which requires cuts of meat to state on the label where the animal had been born, raised and slaughtered. Globalisation of the food supply chain has fostered a simmering conflict between the public's demands for transparency and the industry's reluctance to introduce such measures, which has repeatedly been manifested in legal challenges through the World Trade Organization (Food Safety News 2015).

Increased globalisation has been addressed by Anthony Giddens (2002, 1999) in framing a risk society discourse within a structuration paradigm. Giddens proposes that we live in a safer world today compared to our predecessors, and that the contemporary focus on societal risks are misconstrued, but he also points out that modern risks are different. Historical risks, such as lack of food or the danger posed by hunting for food, are very different from the risks presented when buying unhealthy and excessively processed food.

A safe world can be seen as an anomaly, as the risk society's focus on modern industrialisation and its implications have introduced new and different risk phenomena than the traditional nature-based risks. Giddens's (2002, 1999) risk discourse relates to the influence of cultural changes at the societal and the individual level. The move to an individualist society requires or forces individuals to become more conscious about their social context and their own role as actors within it. The change from collectivism to individualism has created a need for individuals to develop a reflexive approach to analyse everyday life situations, to manage risks and to develop resilient life strategies:

> Resilience implies a systematic, widespread, organizational, structural and personal strengthening of subjective and material arrangements so as to be better able to anticipate and tolerate disturbances in complex worlds without collapse, to withstand shocks, and to rebuild as necessary. … a logic of resilience would aspire to create a subjective and systematic state to enable each and all to live freely and with confidence in a world of potential risks. (Lentzos and Rose 2009:243; see O'Malley 2010 for a discussion of resilience)

Self-resilience and reliance on personal judgements to survive risks have also created scepticism about the objectivity of experts and uncertainty about whom to trust. Hence, a need has emerged for people to create their own biographies and continuously and reflectively assess changing situations they experience. Nonetheless, individualism from the risk society perspective is not seen as purely a negative aspect of life changes. Freedom of choice, the liberty to choose lifestyle and the experience of diverse cultural environments are positive aspects of an enhanced individualism. However, the ability to choose is not universal, but is predisposed towards people who are more culturally and socio-economically secure in the society (Bauman 1998:86).

The changing type of risk, from predictable nature-derived risks to more unpredictable modern industrialisation-derived risks has generated a kind of vacuum for experts, as their predictions become more unreliable and questioned by the general public. The uncertainty of experts' predictions is partly due to the complexity of assessing risks in the modern industrialised society. The danger can originate from long-ceased chemical production and disposal of dangerous chemicals with spill water pumped out into waterways. For example, in 2005, high levels of dioxin and dioxin-like polychlorinated biphenyls (PCBs) were found in fish and seafood in Sydney Harbour, New South Wales, in Australia. A factory for producing the herbicides 2,4-D and 2,4,5-T, the components of Agent Orange, had been situated in the inner part of Sydney Harbour, but had long since ceased production. Dioxin and dioxin-like PCBs, by-products of the herbicide production, had contaminated the factory soil that was later used for reclaiming land from the harbour. Contaminated fish and seafood from the harbour had been consumed for a long time and high levels of the contaminants were found especially in children of fishermen and recreational anglers. Commercial fishing was subsequently banned from a defined area of Sydney Harbour; however, it took considerable time to convince the state government minster to heed the scientific research and the experts' advice to ban fishing and consumption of fish caught in Sydney Harbour (NSW Food Authority 2006).

The complex production of goods today makes it difficult to assess the precise cause of a risk and to identify the point at which it materialises. The difficulty of identifying the direct cause leads to confusion and conflicting assessments among experts and politicians, and subsequently creates a politicisation of what is defined as a risk and what is not considered a risk (Beck and Holzer 2007; see The governmentality risk perspective, below). For Douglas, as for Beck and Giddens, risk is a concept with political implications. The risk construct is used to attribute blame and responsibility for adverse events. Douglas differs from Beck and Giddens, emphasising that contemporary responses to risk are not founded in distinctively new social, political or economic conditions, but they are rather continuous rejoinders of earlier Western society risk responses, which can also be found in traditional societies (Wilkinson 2001:3).

The risk society perspective is criticised both empirically and theoretically. It is criticised theoretically by Lash (1994), Boyne (2003), Elliott (2002) and Lupton (1999) and empirically by Tulloch and Lupton (2003:132). A more detailed critique of the risk society discourse is summarised by Sørensen and Christiansen (2013:123–39). The main critique relates to the status of risk in society and the uncertainties of the foundation of the theory. The critique also questions the processes of social change that create the proposed transformation to a new modernity – a modernity enforced by contemporary industrialisation and driven by multinational corporations, an industrialisation model that did not exist before the second modernity period (Beck, Bonß, and Lau 2003:1–2; Douglas 1992). The second modernity began, according to Beck, in the 1960s, and it is still continuing, being the consequence of the success of the first modernity. The second modernity is represented by a multidimensional process of globalisation, a radicalised individualisation, a third industrial revolution, a gender revolution and the global environmental crisis (Beck *et al.* 2003).

Theoretically, it is not obvious to what extent risks in society can be classified as real and external, and in what way risks enforce social change. Does a change shape social experience and consciousness, or is it merely a social construction that helps people make sense of and understand their social environment and their own position, within a transforming local and global society?

These two positions, of external forces of social change and culturally enforced change, appear to be supported by Beck and Giddens. However, Alexander (1996:134–35) recognises Beck's risk society thesis, especially in relation to modern industrialisation and its formal structure, as derived from Marx and Luhmann (1993). Nonetheless, Alexander challenges their neglect of culturally enforced change:

> [A] persistent materialism and atomism underlies Beck's entire approach. His independent variables are located in the material infrastructure, and his unproblematic understanding of the perception of risk is utilitarian

and objectivist. By ignoring the 'cultural turn' in social science that has gained increasing force over the last two decades. (Alexander 1996:135)

Alexander proposes, supported by Adams (2003:234–5), that 'it is necessary to explore alternative versions of self-identity which already and potentially exist' and that Beck has not considered this in the risk society discourse: 'Beck cuts himself off from the more sophisticated and symbolically mediated discussions of risks undertaken by thinkers like Mary Douglas and Aaron Wildavsky ... his theory reproduces the simplistic propositions about individual action and abstract collective order that inform the caricature of modernity and modernization theory of postmodern lore' (Alexander 1996:135).

In later writings, Beck's (2007:146) position is adjusted to a dual status of risk, and Beck agrees with Latour (1995), writing that: 'the hybrid world we live in and constantly produce is at the same time a matter of cultural perception, moral judgement, politics and technology, which have been constructed in actor-networks and have been made hard facts by "black boxing"' (Beck 2007:146) (Black boxing is the way scientific and technical work is made invisible by its own success, and when science and technology have succeeded it becomes more opaque and obscure (Latour 1999)).

However, in the same book Beck (2007:151–2) also disagrees with Latour:

> I disagree that 'We have never been modern'....If you take the issue of risk beyond its cultural definition and explore instead the details of the management of risks in modern *institutions,* the contemporary paradoxes and dilemmas come to the fore and it becomes apparent that the global risk society and its cultural and political contradictions cannot be understood and explained in terms of pre-modern management of dangers and threats. (emphasis in original)

The dangers in the world are real and there are real changes in the world that impact primarily through the ways in which social actors in networks construct them. The status of risk is thus interlinked to the way in which social actions are understood within the societal structure.

Giddens (1999:5) proposes that the development of the risk society and individual responsibility have given individuals freedom from traditional norms, and they are questioning their respect for government authorities and the acceptance of rules that govern everyday life. It has also changed people's acceptance of experts as the ultimate authority. This new freedom empowers individuals to question experts' advice at the same time as it imposes responsibility on them (Lash 1994:116).

> Inspired by Beck's conviction that the current crisis can lead to a more responsive and democratic way of life, Giddens turns Foucault on his head, suggesting that contemporary actors have gained enormous

control (reflexivity) over their selves and their environment by making use of various therapeutic techniques, including science, in the process often becoming experts themselves. (Alexander 1996:135)

This perspective might give a somewhat simplistic understanding of how people comprehend their public and private spheres, as tradition and cultural transformation will also play a part in acceptance of greater diversity and the ways in which their own current and future positions will develop in a changing society (Adams 2003:222; Giddens 1999:38–9). '[T]his newly gained reflexivity is deeply connected to meaning-making, and that critical action depends on a continued relation to relatively non-contingent, supra-individual cultural forms.' (Alexander 1996:138)

The question of periodization of social change is closely related to the above discussion and the suggestion by sociologists and other social scientists that the prevalence of the language of risk is a consequence of changes in the contemporary existential condition of humans and their world (Beck 1992). Nonetheless, Rose (1996:341) emphasises that the risk concept is not new: 'Most significant for present purposes have been genealogies of social insurance, that have traced the ways in which, over the course of the twentieth century, *security* against risk was socialized' (emphasis in original). However, the cultural centrality of the social construct of risk is more comprehensive than identifying possible risk events. Lash (2007), among others, has stressed the significance of culture and the emotional and aesthetic dimensions to life alongside the life choices individuals make. This is not to indicate that a unified response can be expected, as different groups may respond in various ways to the context of late modernity. It is likely that a particular privileged social stratum, rather than the society as a whole, can be classified as responsible, confident, self-creating individuals (Mythen 2005:129; Rose 1999).

An additional risk perspective associated with Giddens is the situation where self-confident and active people seek to interpret the views of different experts and then claim to have the knowledge to make decisions, whether or not they have the 'expert' knowledge (Wynne 1996, 1992).

The governmentality risk perspective

The third contemporary sociological risk perspective, which is applied in the analysis in this book, is the governmentality risk discourse. The governmentality risk theory draws initially from the work of Foucault (1991). Foucault's central position is that socio-cultural assumptions and the direct exertion of institutional authority or physical compulsion function as part of the apparatus by which power is exerted within a society (Rose 1990: ix). The society's culturally based power structure entails citizens' faith, gendered perceptions, employment relations, property, the rule of law, democratic traditions and political institutions. These cultural structures include citizens' position in society as well as the nation state's authority over its inhabitants.

Michel Foucault explored the governmentality perspective in his lectures in 1978 and 1979 at the Collège de France. The lectures focused on governmental rationalities and his analysis of imprisonment. Foucault's thoughts and lectures are analysed in *The Foucault Effect: Studies in Governmentality* (Burchell *et al.* 1991) and *Security, Territory, Population* (Senellart 1978). Foucault (2007:48) notes: 'The game of liberalism … basically and fundamentally means acting so that reality develops, goes its way, and follows its own course according to the laws, principles, and mechanisms of reality itself'. In the same text, Foucault later stresses that:

[T]his freedom, both ideology and technique of government, should in fact be understood within the mutations and transformations of technologies of power. More precisely and particularly, freedom is nothing else but the correlative of the deployment of apparatuses of security. An apparatus of security … cannot operate well except on condition that it is given freedom, in the modern sense [the word] acquired in the eighteenth century: no longer the exemptions and privileges attached to a person, but the possibility of movement, change of place, and processes of circulation of both people and things. (Foucault 2007:48–49)

Foucault's writings about security and the disciplinary powers where states and their apparatuses regulate citizens, have contributed to an intense debate. Castel (1991), Ewald (1991) and Dean (1999) have furthered the discussion of the power of governments and the governmentality risk perspective. The governmentality risk discourse is closely associated with neo-liberal ideology, which adheres to a free market philosophy, individual freedom and liberty from excessive interventions by the state (Foucault 2007:48). Ewald (1991:199) notes that if manufactured risks are a product of the society's modernisation process and are based on a governmentality-derived perspective of risks, then '[n]othing is a risk in itself; there is no risk in reality. But on the other hand, anything can be a risk; it all depends on how one analyses the danger, considers the event'.

The governmentality risk perspective persuades citizens voluntarily to adopt practices and behaviours that are classified as 'good citizen' conduct. To become a good citizen is in the person's own interest as well as in the interest of the nation state. Citizens are encouraged to accept the government's laws and norms and through self-regulation of their behaviour, they will become good citizens.

A capital at the end of an elongated and irregular territory would not be able to exercise all its necessary functions … [it] must be the ornament of the territory. But this must also be a political relationship in that the decrees and laws must be implanted in the territory [in such a way] that no tiny corner of the realm escapes this general network of the sovereign's orders and laws. The capital must also have a moral role, and diffuse throughout the territory all that is necessary to command people with regard to their conduct and ways of doing things. The capital must give the example of good morals. (Senellart 1978:28)

In the governmentality discourse, expert knowledge becomes 'central to neo-liberal government, providing the guidelines whereby citizens are assessed, compared against norms and rendered productive' (Lupton 2006:13). Nonetheless, it can be a major apparatus to encourage and to enforce individuals to engage in self-regulation. Thus, it becomes a necessity within the neo-liberal risk discourse that the issues encircling the risk concept and the construction of risk, the organised ways of talking about risks and acting upon risks, are shared within the social group. Foucault did not consider it necessary for people to be overly regulated by oppressive governments, as it is more a moral obligation to be a good citizen, to accept and to follow governments' laws and regulations in contemporary societies.

For the governmentality perspective, risk avoidance is a moral enterprise derived from the traits of self-control, self-knowledge and self-improvement. It is the person's responsibility to take note of and understand risk warnings, and to act on them in the right precautionary manner (Lentzos and Rose 2009; O'Malley 2010). Those who do not conform to the good citizen scenario will be stigmatised and in danger of subjection to moral judgements. The governmentality perspective on risks is concerned, like Douglas's and Wildavsky's socio-cultural risk discourse, with moral meanings that underpin the risk discourse, with the way that risk discourses and strategies are used to deal with social disorder and with regulating and demanding community members to internalise self-control (Douglas 1969, 1985, 1992; Douglas and Wildavsky 1982). Governments are increasingly devolving the responsibilities for protection against risks upon the individual, a process that also influences how people view others and themselves.

Although initial US government meat inspection legislation dates from 1890, the continuous presence of government inspectors in all meat establishments was made compulsory in 1906 following a public furore after the publication of the novel *The Jungle* by Upton Sinclair in 1905. It described in nauseating detail the filthy conditions existing in Chicago meatpacking houses and the threat they posed to consumers. Official government meat inspection has existed to this day in most countries. However, industry-devolved product safety is the norm in most other parts of the food industry, recently including a preventive system called Hazard Analysis Critical Control Point (HAACP). An example of the evolution of the government risk discourse is when responsibility to deliver safe meat to consumers was entrusted to the Australian meat industry in the 1990s. With the introduction of the HAACP framework, only intermittent oversight by government remained (Fabiansson 1998), but such a strategy has proved to be difficult in most other countries, as there is a lingering mistrust that the meat industry can embrace such governing modernity.

More recently, risk society theorists analysing the governmentality perspective have highlighted the disparity in nation state's responses to modernity. The erosion of the official system of nation state management requires a new governmentality approach: externally, an ability to secure a stable and competitive position and, internally, to manage rising living standards. Notably pinpointed by Rose (1996:328) as 'the death of the social', the current governmentality approach emphasises the limitations of official arrangements and the importance of citizens' self-activity in managing their own careers, training and health (Dean 1999, 2009). Furthermore, Rose (1996) and Lentzos and Rose (2009) argue that the current analysis is concentrated on an individual level rather than attempting to capture cultural shifts in societies.

The societal risk discourses tend to take a reasonably realistic approach to risk, in their emphasis on how risks have proliferated in modern Western societies. From their perspective, risks are objective and real, although how we respond to them is always mediated through social and cultural processes. While the socio-cultural or symbolic perspective takes a social constructionist approach in identifying what is risk, and emphasises the role played by social and cultural processes, the governmentality perspective adopts the strongest social constructionist approach of the three perspectives. Nothing is seen to be a risk in itself; rather, events are constructed as risks through discourses. While there are all sorts of potential dangers or hazards that exist in global and local environments, only a small number of them are singled out and dealt with as 'risks'. This risk approach is significant in determining how the society differentiates between whether or not certain foods, food production methods and consumption of food poses a risk.

Conclusion

The three sociological risk discourses demonstrate commonalities, although their core starting points differ and they situate risk on different societal levels. On the individual level, individuals' socio-cultural place within the community influences their level of belonging and their gained position within the community setting. The organisational level focuses on modern industrialisation, where individuals are separated from the decision-making processes and influences within globalised multinational corporations and have no control over possible risk scenarios. The state level, where governments' devolution of individualised responsibilities put the onus on the citizen to adhere to government-imposed regulation and become a moral citizen. Irrespective of starting point, when the risk discourse is analysed from a sociological perspective it is understandable that the individual's notion of and response to risk depends on their social and cultural environment.

Perception of risk is based on shared understandings that emerge from membership of and adjustments to social and cultural groups. From the sociological discipline perspective, it can be argued that risks cannot be separated from the social and cultural lens through which we view and understand the society. Thus, from this perspective, experts' views cannot be isolated from the wider social and cultural milieu in which people construct their own judgements about potential risk events. Both experts' and laypeople's knowledge about risk are products of pre-established beliefs and assumptions that individuals bring with them in making their judgements of risks (Lupton 2006:14–15).

A question that the discussed risk discourses augment is how we can gain sufficient and reliable knowledge about potential risks, and whether it is possible for experts and non-experts ever to gain enough knowledge to manage risks created within the modern industrialisation era. Is it possible that comprehensive information and knowledge have grown beyond individual capacity to disseminate, that we are deemed to only understand small fractions of the current society and, even with technological capacities, that we cannot connect the different segments to gain a holistic understanding and assess when the risks are imminent or not?

The sociological perspective provides an account of the universality of risks and the extensive disjunction between expert and non-expert understanding of what constitutes a risk, especially in relation to the ability of trusting experts' advice and assessments. Additionally, the greater emphasis on social regulation, through life expectations, moral expectations, and assumptions about people behaving according to the societal social norms, is a shift in official approaches to regulate citizens, thus not seen as governmentally over-regulating people, but relying on self-government. From this follows the development of a more sophisticated comprehension of how social and cultural contexts influence the understanding, identification and response to risk. The societal risk discourse also explores social changes and the way in which these changes shape both the understanding of risk, and uncertainty, the social actors' awareness of themselves and their position, and how they should react towards the impending risk situation.

It is often assumed that there is an observable shift towards increasing possibilities of risk events and a concern for being exposed to risks in the future (Lupton 1999:8ff). Nonetheless, there is no systematic current or historical analysis of a change in the usage of the risk discourse, and as Giddens (1994b) notes, we live in a safer world today than the one our predecessors knew; but the risks have different origins. From this follows the question of by whom and how a risk should be defined and identified: 'Risk refers to uncertainty about and severity of the events and consequences (or outcomes) of an activity with respect to something that humans value' (Aven and Renn 2009:6; see Aven and Renn 2010).

Hamilton *et al.* (2007:165) highlight the lack of clear definitions of the meaning of 'risk'. They question Lupton's (1999:8–9) assessment that 'in everyday laypeople's language, risk tends to be used to refer almost exclusively to a threat, hazard, danger or harm'. Even if a risk assessment in relation to health and illness mainly constitutes a negative connotation, it does not have a negative outcome in other areas of everyday life, politics or economics (Zinn 2010:109). Risk can have a neutral or a partly positive connotation; 'a risk worth taking' (Hamilton *et al.* 2007). Thus, as long as the risk and the risk taking have a positive conclusion, the risk has an affirmative connotation, while if the outcome of the risk taking strategy results in a negative outcome it is defined as having an undesirable connotation.

A definition based on the conclusion of the action or strategy gives the risk concept contradictory connotations; it is defined more by its outcome than by the action taking. This definition of risk takes it away from the anticipation and the assessment of an expectation of a future event, where the possible future event can only be classified or needs to be re-classified after the event.

The following chapters are structured into the three risk discourse perspectives: the Socio-cultural Risk Perspective, the Risk Society Perspective of Modern Industrialisation and the Governmentality Risk Perspective. Even if there are no ultimate boundaries between food, food production and consumption, as aspects of and perceptions of risk are all related to all three different perspectives of risk, the classification is based on each chapter's topic analysed from mainly one of the discourse's perspective. This structure aims to highlight each topic's position within the respective risk perspective and to give the reader a logical structure for understanding how food, food production and consumption can be analysed from these risk perspectives.

Since the topics overlap, each area can be analysed within any of the three risk discourses, but the main characteristic is the area of food, how consumers view each aspect of food consumption, and how they select the food they eat are assumed to be more relevant to the risk discourse it is structured under.

Part II

The socio-cultural risk perspective

Food consumption and food attitudes are developed within a social and cultural milieu, where the habits around eating and traditional acceptance of food items are established. An individual's family culture, tradition, religion, social setting and physical environment are all factors that influence habitual food consumption.

Bourdieu (1984) researched taste and how it is grounded in the society's cultural and social capital. People develop preferences for certain food based on their social and cultural environment, but also according to how the natural environment and climate conditions support a food production that can sustain the population group. Hence, people's food consumption is based not only on social and cultural traditions, but also on the natural physical environment and climate conditions.

Risks in food production and consumption have been experienced and managed throughout history. Populations have gained knowledge of crops suitable to growth in different environments and of food preservation methods appropriate for different conditions. This knowledge has often been developed through trial and error and passed on through generations; consequently, citizens develop preferences and adjust to special food groups dependent on what nature and the local weather can produce.

Douglas (1969) explored, through the socio-cultural discourse, how food has become accepted as fit for consumption or considered unacceptable within historic cultural and religious teachings (see Chapters 1 and 2). She emphasised that restrictions around food should be understood from a safety perspective, with climatic conditions determining how long food can be kept safe for human consumption. According to Douglas, pork is one example of meat that will deteriorate more quickly than other meats in warm climates without access to preservation techniques or refrigeration. This amassed knowledge within the social and cultural context helps in preventing illness, and similarly, in adjusting storage conditions to be better suitable for seasonal crops, such as fruit and vegetables, which normally have a short shelf life and easily spoil.

Food knowledge has evolved within the society's social and cultural environment over a long time, to help guide people to what food is safe to eat and does not pose a risk to their health. Today, science has superseded local knowledge and tradition in defining what is safe and hygienic food; however, cultural traditions and social perceptions are still driving people's consumption more than science-based guides, as will be explored in this section.

In the past, when food had a short shelf life and conservation of food was uncommon, access to a variety of fresh food items were limited to some periods of the year, hence the food needed to be consumed when available, which encouraged overeating when food was abundant and compelled fasting when it was not. To follow the changing weather and plant-growing seasons became a necessity, and was the prevailing strategy for how people sustained their life throughout the year. The same patterns seem still to be present in current food consumption behaviour, except that, in the twenty-first century, food preservation techniques and the availability of crops out of season through the global food chain have ensured ample food supply. The risk of going hungry has mostly faded for people in the developed world, and this is increasingly the case for a rising middle class in developing countries; however, some people still eat as if there would be no food on the table the next day.

The obesity epidemic (see Chapter 3) should be seen from this socio-cultural risk perspective, where the quality and availability of food has increased immensely, but energy-dense food has become commonplace. Little consideration seems to be given to the reduced physical activity of today's urban populations compared to the manual and physically hard work carried out by people in the past. Social and cultural traditions can also be a factor driving overeating; in some Pacific Island societies, for example, a large body is seen as demonstrating power and wealth.

On the contrary, in Western cultures it is fashionable to be thin. Unfortunately, this has not curbed the increases in body weight seen in so many countries. This is not simply an individual problem, but a growing societal issue in a progressively modernised society. Workplaces have been moved far away from residential areas, making it impossible to walk or ride a bicycle to work and forcing a reliance on private and public transport. Risks involved in walking or running in the urban environment are highlighted by mass media reporting of gruesome crimes directed at people being out late in the city. Crime reports create fear about using the urban neighbourhood for exercise. Modern work practices with increasingly sedentary deskwork and easy accesses to food through fast food outlets in the surrounding precinct also contribute to surges in body weight.

Availability of stimulating or intoxicating beverages and food supplements affects the body in different ways. Coffee, tea and energy drinks have an impact on alertness, but can contain high sugar levels, thus unnecessarily increasing energy intake (see Chapter 4). Alcoholic beverages also provide ample calories (see Chapter 5). Increased access to a diverse range of high-quality foods has not diminished the perceived need of taking dietary supplements. These are marketed as supplementing assumed deficiencies in natural food composition to sport and health conscious people who can afford to buy supplements but commonly already eat healthy food (see Chapter 6).

Fashion is for the young and beautiful, the people who can fit into a size 10 or smaller, despite a growing group of people requiring larger sizes. The majority of the female populations in Australia and the USA wear a size 12 or larger (see Chapter 7). The numerous slimming diets presented in mass media are a further indication that obesity is not favoured by the Western culture. The risks to personal health posed by some of the diets are well documented, especially in that they rarely include a balanced healthy diet that can be sustained over many years.

The socio-cultural risk discourse focuses on social, cultural and diverse religious traditions developed over many decades and centuries. These ingrained customs are difficult to modify based on scientific knowledge, as the science competes with social, cultural and religious based traditions, and with perceptions of what kind of food is safe or should be avoided. In situations where scientific advice contradicts existing perceptions, inherent traditions are likely to have much more influence on how people choose and consume their food.

In the following chapters, food production, processing and consumption are analysed from the socio-cultural risk discourse perspective.

3 Obesity

The new normal

Introduction

People's individual wellbeing and health might not be considered an area of societal risk, but rather a personal issue. However, collective trends that influence the general health of the population have implication for the whole society, the work force, transport, health services and the sustainability of the society. The socio-cultural risk discourse provides a framework for understanding how an increase in overweight and obese individuals influences a society on all levels: the government level, the organisational level and the individual level. The unrestrained growth in obesity, evident in both developed and developing societies, has become a societal threat that affects more people globally than any other known natural or anthropogenic risk factor. It is a socio-cultural risk issue, as it cannot easily be reversed by government intervention or experts' advice, as history demonstrates (Lindsay 2010).

The rising number of overweight and obese individuals, amid concomitant threats to public health and mounting pressures on health care costs, has become a serious global issue with public health officials devoting increasing attention to prevention strategies (O'Hara and Gregg 2010). It is also within this food area that the diversity in approach and understanding between public policy and advocacy on the one side and individual behaviour on the other show the widest gaps. This discrepancy is particularly worrying as obesity is linked to numerous social, physical and medical problems, including hypertension, high cholesterol, diabetes, cardiovascular diseases, asthma, arthritis and some forms of cancer. Mortality also increases sharply once the threshold to being overweight is crossed (Sassi 2010).

There is no shortage of publicity around issues associated with being overweight, as is demonstrated by the popularity of almost daily advice in mass media about how to lose weight and attain an ideal body image (Hogan and Strasburger 2008). Public health campaigns have long warned against carrying excess body fat with messages highlighting the importance of healthy eating and regular exercise. However, health messages compete with strong and aggressive advertising campaigns for a range of convenient high-energy-dense food products, which are formulated and presented to fit an increasingly hectic public and private life (Budd and Peterson 2014). Marketing messages promote 'lifestyle choices' for good looking, healthy and active young adults who enjoy outdoor life and sport. The advertisements aim to appeal to people identifying with such portrayals. However, this positive and encouraging atmosphere is often far from reality, with time-poor people increasingly adopting a sedentary lifestyle. Few consumers practice this ideal healthy living paradigm, but many still embrace the promoted food products, and this leads to an excessive energy intake exceeding their energy expenditure. This is the basic tenet for the soaring accumulation of body fat, although additional factors are at play that will be discussed in detail later in this chapter.

The food industry has acknowledged the increasingly serious health situation, and has responded by introducing 'lite' food alternatives and conveying the risk of overeating by giving serving size suggestions (Gasparro and Jargon 2014). Although, 'lite' products might be low in fat, they are not necessarily low in total energy. Further, one-person food containers often contain a slightly larger amount than the recommended serving size. This forces the consumer 'on the run' to either eat more than intended or reluctantly throw away part of the food (Rolls *et al.* 2004).

Even if official strategies and numerous campaigns with the message of healthy eating have been communicated and understood by adult populations, this message has not necessarily been accompanied by social, cultural and behavioural change. Personality traits play an important role both for risk taking as well as protective behaviour in the development of being overweight and obese (Gerlach *et al.* 2015). Acquiring the knowledge is not the same as acknowledging that it refers to 'me' personally, since individual perceptions of body weight might not necessarily concur with scientific definitions of being overweight or obese. The difficulties in controlling body weight are closely entangled with a perceived lack of control over time at both collective and individual levels (Felt *et al.* 2014). Additionally, to become overweight is a protracted process where a few kilograms are piled on every year, and where the overweight or obesity stage is reached well before the individual realises the unhealthy weight calamity.

The obesity 'epidemic'

Overweight and obese populations are without question a growing global problem. Between 1980 and 2013, the prevalence of worldwide obesity increased substantially, from around 29 to 37 per cent in adult males and from 30 to 38 per cent in adult females. In 2013, it was thought to affect over 2.1 billion adults, 20 years and older (Ng *et al.* 2014), and in 2012 approximately 40 million children under five years of age were overweight or obese (World Health Organization 2014a). In the USA, the prevalence of obesity increased rapidly during the two last decades of the twentieth century. National data on obesity prevalence among US adults, adolescents and children shows that more than one-third of adults and almost 17 per cent of children and adolescents were obese in 2009–2010 (Ogden *et al.* 2012), with a later analysis adding the years 2011–2012 to the study population confirming a similar prevalence of overweight subjects (Yang and Colditz 2015). A decade after the USA, the obesity rate in Europe is following the same trend, with the incidence almost doubled in many European countries over the last 20 years. Recent data from Europe shows that 17 per cent of the adult population were obese in 2010, varying from a minimum of around eight per cent in Romania and Switzerland to a maximum of about 25 per cent in Hungary and the United Kingdom (Organisation for Economic Co-operation and Development 2012). Nearly 13 per cent of children across the developing world are now overweight or obese, with particularly high rates among girls in North Africa and the Middle East. There are several countries, including Kuwait, Libya, Qatar and Samoa, where more than half of the female population is obese. In Tonga, half of both the male and female populations are obese. In South Africa, 42 per cent of females are obese (Ng *et al.* 2014).

Extra fat has not always been a challenging issue, as throughout most of human history temporary weight gain and added fat storage were necessities during the short periods of abundant food supply. Thus, in times of frequent food shortages, securing an adequate energy intake to meet requirements for intensive work or to survive in cold climates posed major challenges. However, this is not the situation any longer for most parts of the population of the developed world.

Weight gain and obesity in contemporary society is very different from historical survival demands, as people's energy intake is no longer exposed to seasonal availability of food. Instead, permanent excessive weight gains pose a growing health threat in countries all over the world. The current situation is quite often referred to as an obesity epidemic, although obesity might be better understood as an unintended consequence of affluence, sedentary life styles, and easy access to affordable food high in fat and sugar, than labelled as an epidemic (Lee 2013). Instead of regarding obesity as a disease or a risk that has an individual solution, it makes much more sense to view obesity as a societal problem. A context that involves the interaction between the individual and the society, where the socio-cultural risk discourse is well placed to analyse what has been called the 'obesogenic society' (Swinburn and Egger 2004).

Multifactorial causes behind increases in obesity

The World Health Organization (WHO) concurs that the causal pathways driving the increase in obesity prevalence involve societal, cultural and environmental changes positioned onto the underlying, but relatively stable, individual genetic and behavioural susceptibility to overindulge in food when available. In 2007, WHO, reporting on obesity in the European region, stated that 'excess body weight poses one of the most serious public health challenges of the twenty-first century' (Branca *et al.* 2007). The report highlighted the European region's challenge in coming to grips with an already established overweight and obesity trend among a growing number of people. Previous research had demonstrated that there were major differences in the prevalence of overweight and obesity between countries and between different socio-economic groups within those countries. These variations pointed to the importance of environmental and socio-cultural determinants of diet and physical activity in governing bodyweight (Branca *et al.* 2007:1). Similarly, the United States Department of Health and Human Services (2002:15) considers being overweight and obese to be multifactorial, including contributions of inherited, metabolic, behavioural, environmental, cultural and socio-economic components. Although it is understandable that remedies will need to involve policies and programmes that change the relevant societal and environmental drivers in a direction that promotes healthy population weights, the methods to do this are not straightforward. The processes influencing food intake and physical activity are fundamental, complex and dynamic; this makes a change very difficult (Swinburn *et al.* 2005). In addition, food and food consumption encompass social and cultural traditions with the well-ingrained past perception of possible food shortages difficult to eradicate, while access to food has changed dramatically for a sizeable part of the world population. The risk of going hungry has been surpassed by the risk of excess food consumption.

The number of overweight and obese individuals has increased since the late twentieth century and continues to rise into the twenty-first century, but it is not only people's weight that has increased. It is believed that improved diets initially caused a gradual growth in height over many decades. The average height of European males increased by an unprecedented eleven centimetres between 1950 and 1980 (Hatton 2014). This trend is now surpassed by increases in individual's weight. People are carrying more excess body weight than ever before, and the prevalence of being overweight and obese is still growing. Currently, there is little indication that this trend is plateauing or decreasing (Martin-Gronert and Ozanne 2013). It is spreading, if not to whole countries, at least to sections of the population, such as middle class groups within countries. An example is India, where obesity is growing among specific population groups, such as the urban middle class, while other groups, such as the rural poor, remain underweight. The outcome is a higher prevalence of obesity in urban areas of developing countries believed to be associated with the change from a rural to an urban lifestyle that requires less physical activity. Developing countries also have a growing middle class that can afford to buy fast food, which is more energy dense than food products prepared in the home (Ramachandran and Snehalatha 2010).

In the twenty-first century, being overweight and obese have become synonymous with the fast-moving contemporary society, where the whole life is fast paced, with expanding affluent populations sidestepping potential risks in adopting new food consumption habits. Lack of time becomes the norm, and excess money drives developments, not careful assessment of short-term and long-term risk factors. Contemporary food consumption is embroiled in risk, as complex and secret or difficult to assess food production systems have flourished and become the norm (Beck 1992). This is a society where it has become increasingly difficult for the individual, but also for many experts, to gain a comprehensive knowledge and understanding of modern food manufacturing processes and the composition of the presented food. This includes details about the origin of ingredients used, especially for fast food restaurants and for precooked ready-to-eat meals.

The twenty-first century is a fast moving society where multitasking and food convenience are promoted. Walking and eating simultaneously, food that saves time while rushing from one meeting to the next, but also the convenience of picking up something to eat on the way home (Jabs and Devine 2006). Food that is ready-made to heat and eat in front of the computer or the television is now common, and these settings distract our inherent mechanisms for controlling the amount of food consumed (Blass *et al.* 2006).

The causes behind people becoming overweight and obese are complex, and it is clearly a health issue for many sufferers. The medical profession and other health experts agree that accumulation of excess body fat amplifies an individual's health problems and that the healthcare sector needs to plan accordingly by allocating scarce recourses to meet increasing demands (Wang *et al.* 2011). However, being overweight or obese has gone beyond being only a health issue, it has also social, cultural and economic implications for the society and for an individual's everyday activities (Yates and Murphy 2006). To carry excess body fat makes it more difficult to move around, catch public transport, exercise or play sport. In a society not yet adjusted to large increases in body size, it is also a burden on the individual by making everyday life more expensive (Colagiuri *et al.* 2010). For example, the obese person might not be able to buy ready-made clothes without the need for adjustments, the person might need to buy an extra seat when flying and retrofitting of buildings might be necessary to accommodate larger people. The health service sector has already made some adjustments to facilitate the handling of obese people with larger beds to accommodate heavier people. Hospitals have also been forced to have more staff or new equipment to lift and carry patients, but they are still facing difficulties in moving extremely obese people from the home to the hospital for treatment (Polley 2006). While newer medical facilities incorporate measures for obese patients within their design budgets, it has been estimated that an older facility starting from scratch might face a median retrofitting cost of US$1.2 million to accommodate morbidly obese patients (Rice 2014).

A new and growing sector of medical procedures focus on restricting food intake to manage the increasing number of obese people. These procedures are also used on young people in their early teens (Wang *et al.* 2009). In 2005, the USA spent an estimated US$190 billion a year on treating obesity related health conditions, corresponding to 21 per cent of the medical spending that year (Cawley and Meyerhoefer 2012). It is anticipated that this allocation of money to combat health issues in relation to overweight and obesity will continue to increase putting further pressure on the whole health system (Wang *et al.* 2008).

The worldwide increase in body mass

From a historical perspective, overweight and obesity were rarely seen before the middle of the twentieth century, except in some minority cultures (Haslam 2007). However, the last 30 years has seen a dramatic increase in its prevalence in both adults and children to the extent that it is now a leading preventable cause of death worldwide. WHO has assessed that being overweight and obese is the fifth leading cause of global deaths. Research undertaken by WHO estimates that at least 2.8 million adults die each year because of being overweight or obese. In addition, the organisation states that 44 per cent of the diabetes burden, 23 per cent of the coronary heart disease burden and between 7 per cent and 41 per cent of certain cancer types could be attributable to being overweight or obese (World Health Organization 2014a).

As can be seen in Figure 3.1, the WHO indicated in 2009 that being overweight and obese had replaced more traditional public health concerns, except for the impact of tobacco use (World Health Organization 2009). Over time, major risks to health have shifted from traditional risks, for example inadequate nutrition or unsafe water and lacking sanitation, to modern health risks triggered by overweight and obesity. However, modern risks may take different trajectories in different countries, depending on the risk scenario and its social and cultural context.

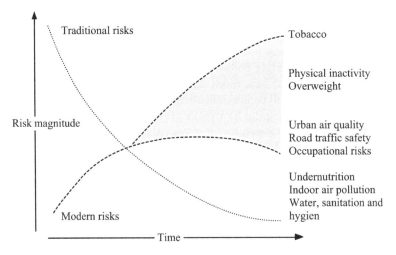

Figure 3.1 The risk transition, modified from World Health Organization (World Health Organization 2009:3)

Public health guidelines and campaigns in many countries seek to prevent and minimise the factors most commonly considered responsible for the increasing prevalence of obesity. These include guidelines about how to maintain healthy eating habits, a better understanding of suitable portion sizes, and promotion of increased exercise routines, but also how to change the physical environment to make it easier to walk or ride a bicycle to work. However, so far the effects of these campaigns are modest, as demonstrated by the increase in the overall population weight, which has not yet slowed down (Martin-Gronert and Ozanne 2013).

The state of being overweight: 1980 and 2014

Obesity is not only a health issue, as it also affects diverse circumstances of an individual's private and public life. To understand the obesity trend and the reasons for its development, explanations need to be sought outside the medical and health context. Overweight and obesity are significant societal problems with underlying social, cultural as well as socio-economic causes (Branca *et al.* 2007:1; Swinburn *et al.* 2005). The growth in obesity can be seen as a product of decades of changing social and physical environments, food production innovation and increases in people's disposable incomes. There is also a change in the public perception of being overweight or obese. Historically, an overweight person was seen as having power and wealth, an opinion still prevailing in some parts of the world including Tonga and some other Pacific Islands, while more recently overweight and obese people have been stigmatised in much of the Western world (Puhl and Heuer 2010). Whereas being overweight and obese were once considered a problem only for high income countries, obesity rates are now rising worldwide. The only remaining region of the world where obesity is not common is in sub-Saharan Africa (Haslam and James 2005).

Being overweight and obese are labels for ranges of weight that are greater than what is generally considered healthy for a given height. For adults, overweight and obesity ranges are determined by calculating a person's body mass index (BMI), a measurement obtained by dividing a person's weight in kilograms by the square of the person's height in metres. According to definitions established by the World Health Organization (2000:9), people are considered overweight when their BMI equals or exceeds 25 kg/m^2 and obese when it equals or exceeds 30 kg/m^2. Severe obesity is defined as a BMI of more than 40 kg/m^2.

The BMI was developed as an index of overall body size by removing the influence of body height on body weight, but it has been criticised as an inaccurate index of body fat. In addition to BMI, other measurements of body fat percentage are available, such as skinfold measurement with callipers or the use of bioelectrical impedance measurements (Durnin and Womersley 2007; Kyle *et al.* 2004). However, epidemiological studies of BMI and per cent body fat in relation to death rates and risk factors have shown that in no instance is

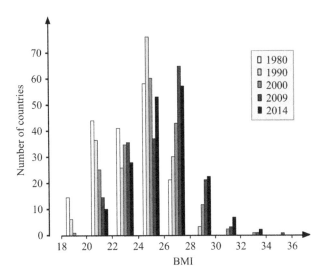

Figure 3.2 Female average BMI in 1980, 1990, 2000, 2009 and 2014 in 179 countries (World Health Organization 2014b, 2015)

per cent body fat superior to BMI in predicting health risk factors. The BMI
measurement is more closely related to health risk factors than what direct
body fatness measurements predict, hence the continued use of BMI is justified (Ernsberger 2012).

Using BMI measures, the World Health Organization (2014a) estimated
that in 2009 at least 500 million adults in the world were obese, with higher
rates among females than males. Thus, more than ten per cent of the world's
adult population were considered obese at that time. Figures 3.2 and 3.3 show
average changes in BMI for women and men respectively between 1980 and
2014. It can be seen that in 1980, none of the countries had an average female
BMI over 27.8 kg/m^2 or an average male BMI over 26.6 kg/m^2, while females
in 41 countries and males in 43 countries had a BMI of 21 kg/m^2 or less. In
2014, the average BMI for both females and males had increased; the highest average BMI was 33.5 kg/m^2 for females and 30.4 kg/m^2 for males (in
Tonga, it was slightly higher in 2009). For females in 2014, Eritrea, Ethiopia
and Timor-Leste were the only countries with a BMI of 21 kg/m^2 or less.
For males in 2014, Eritrea, Ethiopia, Burundi, Bangladesh, Madagascar and
Uganda all had a BMI of 21 kg/m^2 or less, with Eritrea having the lowest at
20.1 kg/m^2. The weight increase has continued across the board, as can be
seen in the 2014 figures (Figures 3.2 and 3.3).

The averages give a general estimate only, and it is important to acknowledge, as pointed out by Swinburn *et al.* (2005) and Branca *et al.* (2007), that
there are large variations between urban and rural areas and between social

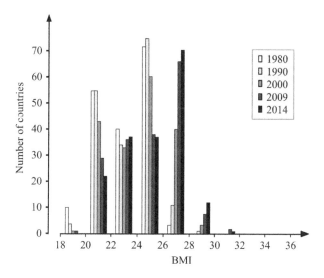

Figure 3.3 Male average BMI in 1980, 1990, 2000, 2009 and 2014 in 179 countries
(World Health Organization 2014b, 2015)

classes within countries. In general terms, in less industrialised societies the urban population and the middle class are more likely to be in the over-weight or obese categories than poorer people and people living in rural areas (McLaren 2007; Wang *et al.* 2009). India is an example where the middle and upper classes are increasingly becoming overweight and obese, but the coun-try's average BMI does not reflect this, with a low BMI of 21.3 kg/m² in 2009 (Unnikrishnan *et al.* 2012). Similarly, in Sri Lanka, there is a social gradient with higher prevalence of overweight and obese individuals observed in the more educated, urban, high income and high social status segments of the society (de Silva *et al.* 2015). The situation is reversed in Western countries with more people carrying higher weights in semi-urban and rural areas, and among the working class (McLaren 2007).

Is obesity a risk to society or is the twenty-first century society creating an obese environment?

While genetic and cultural influences are important for understanding obes-ity, they cannot fully explain the current increase seen within the global society. In countries with a previously small middle class, higher disposable incomes for private consumption have encouraged adoption of western-ised diets, including an increased use of processed and ready-to-eat food. Globally, the availability of energy-dense food products – foods high in fat and sugar – has increased, with an abundance of such processed foods on the market (Swinburn *et al.* 2011). Furthermore, the twenty-first century work environment has created a new habit, making eating and working at the same time an accepted practice.

Creation of convenience food

One aspect of the resistance to change of behaviour to a healthier lifestyle is the social narrative created around new convenience food products, which are first fashioning a need and then filling the generated need. In this respect, it is useful to take a closer look at an early example of the ability to combine eating dinner and viewing television simultaneously. Although there had been previous attempts, the first successful frozen dinner meal or 'TV Dinner' was produced in 1953 by C.A. Swanson & Sons in the USA and called the TV Brand Frozen Dinner (Phipps 1977). It consisted of a Thanksgiving meal of turkey, cornbread dressing, frozen peas and sweet potatoes packaged in a tray like those used at the time for airline food service. Each item was placed in its own compartment and the aluminium tray could be heated directly in the oven without any extra crockery. The meal could be eaten directly from the tray. The company had expected to sell about 5,000 dinners for the first year, but with a few meal varieties, they soon ended up selling more than ten million dinners. Part of the success was because it opened the door to the combination of activities that before were separate events: eating dinner or viewing television, became dinner and television viewing combined into one joint activity. People could enjoy dinner without missing their favourite television programme and still having a family dinner together at the end of the day.

The new habit came with several caveats. A focus on television viewing reduced attention given to the food and the amount consumed creating a tendency to increase food intake (Jeffery and French 1998). The combination of eating and entertainment had previously been restricted to watching movies at the movie theatre and buying popcorn, ice cream and a soft drink. This was a special and occasional activity and not an everyday occurrence, as became the case for regularly combining television viewing and a quick dinner in the private home. Further, the freezing process of TV Dinners tended to degrade the taste of food and the meals thus had to be heavily processed with extra salt and fat to enhance the flavour of the food. In addition, stabilising the product for a long period usually meant that companies had to use partially hydrogenated vegetable oils high in trans fats for some items (Singh and Wang 1977). Trans fat, rare in nature but formed during partial hydrogenation of unsaturated fat, both raises LDL or 'bad' cholesterol and lowers HDL or 'good' cholesterol, thus increasing the risk of coronary heart disease. Such dinners are frequently less nutritious than fresh food and TV Dinners can significantly contribute to weight gain.

Fast food is another example of the convenience concept. Fast food is the term given to food that can be prepared and served very quickly. The fast food concept has loosely been defined as food purchased in self-service or take away restaurants without waiter service (French *et al.* 2001). From its inception, fast food was designed to be eaten when in a hurry, and it often does not require traditional cutlery.

About the same time as TV dinners were introduced, an attempt to create a fast food franchised restaurant chain was launched by Czech-American businessman Ray Kroc in Des Plaines, Illinois, on 15 April 1955, building on the initial work of Richard and Maurice McDonald in San Bernardino, California, USA. Their introduction of the 'Speedee Service System' in 1948 furthered the principles of the modern fast food restaurant that the White Castle hamburger chain had already put into practice more than two decades earlier (Hess 1986). The McDonald's Corporation has since evolved into the world's largest chain of hamburger fast food restaurants, serving around 70 million customers daily in more than 100 countries across 35,000 outlets in 2013 (McDonald's Corporation 2014).

Fast food meals have been criticised and food chains have come under fire over issues such as energy content, trans fats and portion sizes of the meals. Their food encourages people to eat while working at their desk, driving to work or walking between appointments, which have become common features of modern life. The need to have access to packaged food alternatives that are easy to handle with one hand, taste good, and are affordable, thus likely to be higher in fat and sugar, has created a demand for these convenience products.

A study of children who ate fast food, compared to those who did not, showed that the former group of children tended to consume more total fat, carbohydrates and sugar-sweetened beverages. These children also tended to eat less fibre, fruits, non-starchy vegetables and drink less milk. After reviewing these test results, the researchers concluded that consumption of fast food by children seems to have a negative effect on an individual's diet in ways that could significantly increase the risk for obesity (Bowman *et al.* 2004).

Another concept initially targeting sport people is the energy drink, which is designed to replenish quickly energy lost during strenuous exercise. Among the first drinks on the market was Lucozade, developed in the UK in 1928 to aid in the recovery of people sick with everyday illnesses, like the common cold or influenza. In 1983, Lucozade was rebranded as an energy drink to shift the brand's associations away from illness. The slogan 'Lucozade aids recovery' was replaced by 'Lucozade replaces lost energy' (BrandRepublic 2005). Initially, energy drinks for sport people only contained sugar and electrolytes to support recovery. With a broadening marketing concept, stimulant substances like caffeine, guarana, taurine and ginseng were added to provide mental and physical stimulation, although there is little or no evidence that any of the ingredients found in energy drinks apart from caffeine or sugar have significant physiological effects. However, the energy drinks quickly appealed to a larger group of people and became popular not only among young sport people, but also among more sedentary people adding to energy intake not disposed of by physical activity. With mounting popularity of energy drinks, particularly among young people, they increasingly contribute to weight gain and the risk of becoming obese (Duchan *et al.* 2010; McLellan and Lieberman 2012).

Public perception through mass media

Even if a person can decide how much and what to eat and drink, and be responsible for excessive intake or an unbalanced diet profile, this would not explain the general attribution of weight gain. The choice of food also depends on tradition, culture, social and financial circumstances. Furthermore, it is governed by ease of access to basic ingredients and cooking facilities, and availability of nearby fast food restaurants (Boone-Heinonen *et al.* 2011). To better understand the issues involved, the pervading view of reasons for undue weight gain needs to change from a simplistic sole focus on individual behaviour to also include the impact of societal circumstances.

In the 1990s, the mass media conveyed overweight and rising obesity levels as linked to individual conduct. This changed by the early 2000s, when obesity became associated also with influential societal factors. Common promotion of the ultrathin 'waif' or 'heroin chic'; fashion model ideals that did not represent the shape of the main population, and the message it sent to young people started to be questioned (Featherstone 2010). A better understanding evolved about socially induced dieting attempts and related weight increases caused by so called 'yo-yo dieting' (see Chapter 7) or disturbances like anorexia nervosa, at the dangerous end of healthy eating and wellbeing.

Lawrence (2004:57) stated that the more an issue is framed in terms of involuntary or universal risks outside of personal agency, the more likely it is that community opinion becomes conducive to public policy solutions, 'and hold political institutions responsible for addressing the problem'. Defining 'a problem in individualized terms limits governmental responsibility for addressing it, while systemic frames invite governmental action' (Lawrence 2004:57). Although clearly of multifaceted origin, the closer the overall pattern of public discourse moves toward the societal end of the continuum, the more conducive the environment will be for public policies to combat the growing obesity prevalence.

In summary, while environmental and genetic influences are important to understand obesity, they cannot alone explain the current dramatic increases in being overweight and obese seen within individual countries and globally. Although energy consumption in excess of energy expenditure is an important and accepted factor that leads to obesity at a personal level, what causes the shift in energy balance on the societal scale is still uncertain. There are a number of theories as to the cause of obesity and an overweight population, but most believe that it is a combination of environmental, behavioural and genetic factors interacting to cause the high prevalence of obesity. Although genetic factors are important in determining individual susceptibility to becoming overweight, broadly defined environmental factors, such as changes in agriculture, food processing, marketing, transportation, physical demands of work, and the contextual effect of residential areas must also be considered. All these factors create the milieu that facilitates the conditions for obesity. The structure of the built environment affects obesity through its effect on physical activity and diet. Inverse relationships of weight with indices suggesting higher walkability were most consistently found to be significant, while weight was positively related to spatial accessibility to convenience stores, and inversely related to the spatial accessibility to recreational physical activity facilities (Casey *et al*. 2014; Huang *et al*. 2014).

The risk scenarios of overweight and obesity

Energy-dense food

Technical advancements in food production, improved food preservation techniques and the availability of energy-dense and refined food for easy consumption have created a culture supporting excessive energy intake. These advancements, in combination with a population who can increasingly afford to buy commercially prepared food and ready-to-eat meals, facilitate an environment of overconsumption (Sturm 2008; Rosin 2008; Putnam *et al*. 2002; Kant 2000; Cavadini *et al*. 2000). Mass production of energy-dense food has made it cheaper and thus accessible to diverse population groups. Ready-to-eat food is now available in fast food outlets in countries that were not seen as economically viable markets a decade ago, such as Russia, China and India (French 2003; Putnam *et al*. 2002; Drewnowski and Specter 2004).

Intensive promotions of ready-to-eat energy-dense food and drink to children and adults have created a new model of convenience, especially attractive to small households and time-poor families with fewer incentives to prepare elaborate meals (Burnett 2007). In 2010, for example, pre-schoolers viewed an average of 213 advertisements for sugary drinks and energy drinks, while older children and teenagers watched an average of 277 and 406 advertisements respectively (Harris and Graff 2011; Harris *et al*. 2013). Hence, the concept of fast food has become well established and it has managed to win over large population groups of children and young people through enticing advertisements.

Today, fast food has become synonymous with unhealthy food, being high in sugar and fat. However, food that is quick to prepare, such as a salad, does not need to be low in nutrition or high in fat and sugar. Fast food relates more to the type of food that has a short span between being ordered and delivered and food that is easy to eat with one hand when doing something else. In the late twentieth and early twenty-first centuries, fast food has become embodied in a rushed existence with shorter attention spans. Time has become increasingly busy, and fast food – food that can provide satisfaction in the shortest time possible – has become the norm in an increasing number of societies. In 1970, Americans spent about US$6 billion on fast food; in 2000, they spent more than US$110 billion (Schlosser 2001). With people on the run, an increasing number of single-family households, single parents or couples trying to split time between work and the demands of a busy family schedule, fast food restaurants can offer a quick, often cheap and filling meal.

Studies have shown that it is not just the energy-dense food as such, but also the larger portions of the food that augment obesity (Nielsen and Popkin 2003). Studies that have examined possible contributions to the obesity epidemic have pointed the finger at several factors, such as dietary sugars and fats (Harnack *et al.* 1999; Bray and Popkin 1998) and larger portion sizes (Young and Nestle 2002). Furthermore, fast food eaten away from home often has lower nutrient density (McCrory *et al.* 1999). This was found to be true when scrutinising the content of school lunches (Chapman *et al.* 1995), and even food assistance programmes have come under attack for their alleged role in 'fattening the poor' (Besharov 2002; O'Beirne 2003).

Mass production is central to fast food, but the composition of the food is different from home-cooked food in order to appeal to mass consumption. Overall, fast food is higher in fat, sugar and salt, but lower in fibre. According to McDonald's nutrition charts, a Big Mac, a large order of fries, a baked apple pie, and a large soft drink provide 1,701 kcal or 7,116 kJ, 72 grams of fat, and 1,630 milligrams of sodium. This is in comparison to the 2005 United States Department of Agriculture Food Guide that recommends that most adults limit their daily consumption to about 2,000 kcal or 8,368 kJ, 65 grams of fat, and 1,779 milligrams of sodium. That means that one McDonald's meal in itself closely provides or exceeds the recommended daily limits for all three categories (Britten *et al.* 2006; Nefer Ra Barber 2014). Although it would be possible to limit the size of the meal, studies suggest that the size of the portions and the fact that the next larger size only costs a little more, encourage people to eat a lot more than they normally would.

A changing food environment from fat to sugar

It is perplexing that the last 30 years have seen a decrease in the consumption of total fat and saturated fat, due in part to an increased focus on low-fat products, but this has not resulted in a reduced intake of energy. Replacing fat, consumption of carbohydrates has increased considerably according to the Centers for Disease Control and Prevention (2004). Largely, this has been caused by the boosted consumption of soft drinks and other sugary foods (Popkin *et al.* 2014). Some researchers believe that excessive carbohydrate consumption, as opposed to fat consumption, is responsible for the current obesity escalation. This argument rests on the observation that the percentage of energy from fat decreased from 38 per cent in 1976–1980 to 34 per cent in 1988–1991 in the USA, whereas the prevalence of obesity continued to increase (Willett 1998; Willett and Leibel 2002).

Sugary drink portion sizes have risen consistently over the past 40 years. Children and adults drink more soft drinks than ever. Over the past decades, an increase in the consumption of sugar-sweetened soft drinks has paralleled the increase in obesity (Gaby 2005). Mean per capita sugar-sweetened soft drink consumption in the USA now averages approximately 350 mL per day, a three-fold increase over the past three decades. About 73 per cent of adolescent boys and 62 per cent of adolescent girls consume carbonated soft drinks (mostly sweetened with sugar) on any given day (French *et al.* 2003). For each additional serving of sugar-sweetened drink consumed, both BMI and the frequency of obesity increased after adjustment for anthropometric, demographic, dietary and lifestyle variables (Ludwig *et al.* 2001). It was found that for each additional 350 mL soft drink can children consumed each day, the odds of becoming obese increased by 60 per cent during the 1.5 years the children were followed (Ludwig *et al.* 2001).

A review of research on soft drink consumption and obesity showed that the majority of the 15 selected cross-sectional studies and ten selected prospective cohort studies identified as relevant, showed an adverse association between sugar-sweetened soft drink consumption and body weight (Malik *et al.* 2006). In adolescents, two clinical trials have indicated that efforts to replace sugar-sweetened soft drinks with non-caloric beverages slowed weight gain (Ebbeling *et al.* 2006; James *et al.* 2004). Further proof of this association was obtained in two randomised control trials (de Ruyter *et al.* 2012; Tate *et al.* 2012) and one longitudinal study (Ebbeling *et al.* 2012). The trials all strongly suggested that energy from sugar-sweetened beverages contributes to weight gain.

Between 1977 and 2001, Americans increased total energy intake from soft drinks from three to seven per cent of energy, which translates into an almost tripling of calories per day, from 50 kcal to 144 kcal (Nielsen and Popkin 2004). Children and young people obtained nearly 11 per cent of their daily energy intake from sugary beverages in 1999 to 2004 (Wang *et al.* 2008). During this period, soft drink intake also increased to ten per cent of energy for the 19 to 39 age group (Nielsen and Popkin 2004). However, lately there has been a gradual shift to marketing low calorie or diet beverages in high-income countries, while sugar-sweetened beverages continue to be heavily promoted in low and middle-income countries like Brazil and China (Kleiman *et al.* 2011).

A strategy promoted by public health authorities to halt the increase in obesity, uses as its basis the World Health Organization (2003:70) recommendation to restrict consumption of energy-dense snacks and sugar-sweetened soft drinks and to increase the consumption of whole grains or energy dilute vegetables and fruit. However, an inverse relationship between energy density and cost suggests that obesity-promoting foods are simply those that offer the highest dietary energy at the lowest cost. Given the difference in costs between energy-dense and energy-dilute foods, the advice to replace fats and sweets with fresh vegetables and fruit may have unintended economic consequences for the consumer, as fresh vegetables and fruit are more expensive overall (Drenowski *et al.* 2004).

Physiological factors

Environmental factors, together with physiological factors, have shown in studies using laboratory animals that sugar and fat are powerful sources of neurobiological rewards (Yeomans and Gray 2002; Levine *et al.* 2003). Energy-dense foods provide more sensory enjoyment and more pleasure than do foods that are less energy dense (Drewnowski 1997; Mela 1999; Drewnowski 1999). Clinical studies suggest that those foods that contain fat, sugar or both have the strongest influences on food cravings (Yanovski 2003), and, historically, humans have sought energy-dense foods to enhance survival in times of food scarcity (Drewnowski 1995).

Human tastes are either innate or acquired very early in the life cycle. A growing contemporary supply of convenience food, which is habitually high in sugar and fat, has made young people accustomed to a diet high in sugar and fat (Birch 1999). Studies with children have consistently shown that food familiarity, sweetness and energy density are the main preference determinants in food choice (Birch 1992).

Ghrelin, the only known appetite-stimulating hormone in humans, may be one factor involved in increased appetite, special food cravings and food intake during attempts to lose weight. Innovative strategies for suppressing ghrelin and maintaining a decreased appetite for weight loss would help people to keep a healthy weight. Recent research has highlighted relationships between ghrelin, stress and lifestyle factors. A review of the relationships between ghrelin, stress, exercise and sleep found that ghrelin levels were positively related to stress hormones, and that stress management interventions including exercise and sleep might help to reduce ghrelin and corresponding appetite (Adams *et al.* 2011).

Malnutrition in early life is believed to play a role in the rising rates of obesity in the developing world. Hormone changes that occur during periods of malnutrition may promote the storage of fat once more food energy becomes available (Caballero 2001). Endocrine disrupting chemicals mimic hormones in the human body and have the capacity to interfere with organ development and function. This effect might alter susceptibility to different types of diseases throughout life. There might be links with pregnancy complications, cancers, thyroid disorders and metabolic problems in adults. In infants and young children, the impact of such chemicals can be more severe because their bodies and brains are developing more quickly and their endocrine disturbances will have a disproportionate impact (Diamanti-Kandarakis *et al.* 2009).

In the early years of the twenty-first century, international organisations had a rather cavalier attitude to endocrine disrupting chemicals. However, scientists have started to sound warning bells, but there is still no critical mass of information available. Henceforth, a report published by the International Programme on Chemical Safety (2002), which is a joint programme of the World Health Organization, the United Nations Environment Programme and the International Labour Organization, raised the issue. Overall, they found no evidence of causal links between observed changes and actual levels for many of the chemicals, but for a few examples where sufficient evidence for endocrine mediated effects warranted concern.

The understanding of endocrine disruptors has increased and, in a new report published in 2012, their effects have been emphasised. In the intervening period the Endocrine Society, the European Commission and the European Environment Agency have published scientific reviews drawing renewed attention to concerns about public and wildlife health (Diamanti-Kandarakis *et al.* 2009; European Commission 2011; European Environment Agency 2012). Furthermore, the European Society for Paediatric Endocrinology, and the Paediatric Endocrine Society have called for action on endocrine disruptors and their effects (Skakkebaek *et al.* 2011). In an update of the initial International Programme on Chemical Safety report, under the auspices of the Inter-Organisation Programme for the Sound Management of Chemicals, it is now claimed that increasing scientific evidence proposes that endocrine disrupting chemicals are a cause for global concern. Hence, more research is critically needed to understand these chemicals and their human health effects in more depth (Bergman *et al.* 2013).

Potential endocrine disrupting chemicals can be found in a range of consumer products. They can be pesticides, herbicides, industrial pollution or other chemicals. Close to 800 chemicals are known or suspected to be capable of interfering with hormone receptors, hormone synthesis or hormone conversion. However, only a small fraction of these chemicals has been investigated in tests capable of identifying overt endocrine effects in intact organisms (Bergman *et al.* 2013).

Bisphenol A is mainly used in combination with other chemicals to manufacture polycarbonate plastics and resins used for canned food, but it can also be found in carbonless copy paper and thermal point-of-sale receipt paper. It is clear that bisphenol A is an endocrine disruptor at high doses, but there are some indications that it might be equally disrupting at very low doses. It has been speculated, and even proposed, that very low doses of endocrine disruptors might be one explanation of many to the obesity situation. According to this theory, exposure to bisphenol A might induce epigenetic changes turning on obesity genes (Kundakovic and Champagne 2011).

Epigenetics is the study, not of changes in the underlying DNA sequence, but the activation or inhibition of genetic switches. Methylation (the addition of methyl groups to the DNA) switches genes off and acetylation (the addition of acetyl groups to the histones; the proteins in which DNA is wrapped) switches them on (Dolinoy 2008). Since all cells in a multicellular organism have the same 23 chromosome pairs with their 25–30,000 genes, and different cells will need different genes to be active, depending on their particular functions, the on and off switching is crucial for proper function (Alberts *et al.* 2015:399).

New findings show that epigenetic changes can remain through cell divisions for the remainder of the cell line's life and may last for multiple generations if it occurs in a sperm or egg cell. Reprogramming resets the epigenome of the early embryo so that it can form every type of cell in the body. In order to pass to the next generation, epigenetic tags must avoid being erased during reprogramming. In mammals, about one per cent of genes escape reprogramming, and this is sufficient to take epigenetic impact seriously as an evolutionary tool (Migicovsky and Kovalchuk 2011).

To summarise, epigenetics suggests that the choices individuals make with their diet selection and lifestyle can possibly lead to changes in how cells express their genes. This will have implications for their children and further descendants. New characteristics can be generated and passed on via epigenetics, which are subject to the same mechanisms of evolution as those with a purely genetic origin.

Societal factors

As discussed above, the changing rates of obesity can be related to a number of societal factors, including social class, socio-economic status, culture and social traditions, smoking status and acceptance of smoking, general health status, exercise, and the physical environment as a facilitator to promote or restrict physical activity. Additionally, weight status is associated with aspects of the food environment: easy accessibility to supermarkets or less access to take away outlets are both associated with a lower BMI and thus a lower prevalence of being overweight and obese. However, research indicates that obesogenic dietary habits do not consistently mirror these associations, as there are other links between the environment and societal factors. Living in a socio-economically deprived residential area is the only environmental factor consistently associated with obesogenic behaviour. Associations between the environment and weight status are more consistent than that seen between the environment and dietary habits. This suggests that the environment may play an important role in weight gain in restricting physical activity (Giskes *et al.* 2011).

The rates of obesity and type 2 diabetes in the US follow a socio-economic gradient, with the burden of disease falling disproportionately on people with limited resources and ethnic minorities (Adler and Newman 2002). The highest obesity rates have been associated with sections of the population with the lowest income and educational levels (Schoenborn *et al.* 2002). However, the disparity in obesity prevalence decreased over the years 1970 to 2000 from as much as a 50 per cent between the lowest and highest socio-economic status groups in 1970 to 14 per cent in 2000. This trend was more pronounced for females. At the same time overall prevalence of obesity increased dramatically in the United States with considerable variations in the changes of socio-economic association across gender and ethnic groups, suggesting that individual characteristics are less influential than socio-environmental factors (Zhang and Wang 2004).

Increased access to motor vehicles, mechanisation of work and sedentary lifestyles are all factors that reduce energy expenditure. Ultimately, energy intake in excess of caloric expenditure causes obesity, but external factors alone cannot explain why this occurs in some but not all individuals (Rosengren and Lissner 2008).

The correlation between social class and BMI varies globally. A review in 1989 found that in developed countries females of a high socio-economic status were less likely to be obese. No significant differences were seen among males of different social classes. In the developing world, females, males and children from upper social classes had greater rates of obesity (Sobal and Stunkard 1989). An update of this review carried out in 2007 found the same relationships, but the association was weaker. The decrease in the strength of correlation was not uniform, as healthy eating is continuing to be a social class issue, where sections of the population who can afford to eat plenty of fruits and vegetables and can take advantage of global food markets show a decrease in obesity, but this is not the case for less well-off groups (McLaren 2007:37). Among developed countries, levels of adult obesity, and percentage of teenage children who are overweight, indicate a correlation with income inequality. A similar relationship is seen among US states: more adults, even in higher social classes, are obese in states that have an unequal socio-economic structure (Wilkinson and Pickett 2009).

Figure 3.4 shows an Index of Health and Social Problems in relation to income inequality in wealthy countries. Income inequality is measured by the ratio of incomes among the 20 per cent wealthiest compared with the poorest 20

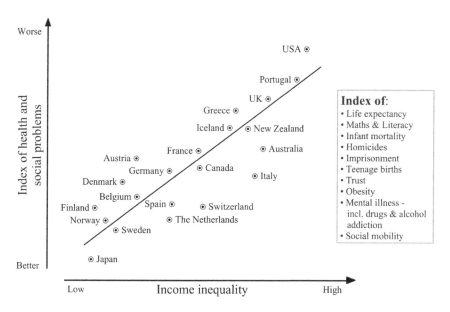

Figure 3.4 Correlation between inequality and an index of health and social problems (modified from Wilkinson and Pickett 2009:498)

per cent in each country. Raw scores for each variable were converted to z-scores and each country given its average z-score (Wilkinson and Pickett 2009:498).

Even if the obesity score in Figure 3.4 is not presented separately, but based on a score among other factors that influence a person's wellbeing, what is undoubtedly demonstrated is the inverse relationship between high-income inequality, better health and fewer social problems.

Smoking has a significant effect on an individual's weight (Friel 2009), as those who quit smoking gain an average of 4.4 kilograms for males and 5.0 kilograms for females over a ten-year period (Flegal *et al.* 1995). However, changing rates of smoking, with lower rates of smoking among higher socio-economic status groups, has had little effect on the overall rates of obesity.

In the US, it has been noted that the number of children a female carries is related to her risk of developing obesity. A female's obesity risk increases by seven per cent per child, while a male's risk increases by four per cent per child. This could be partly explained by the fact that having young children and children close in age decreases recovery time between the children and restricts the female's ability, in particular, to participate in physical activity (Weng *et al.* 2004; Bellows-Riecken and Rhodes 2008). Working outside the home might also have an impact, where the temptation to snack or to eat the children's leftovers may be more limited.

Consistent with cognitive epidemiological research, obesity is associated with cognitive deficits (Smith *et al.* 2011). Investigations suggest that weight gain can result, at least in part, from a neurological predisposition characterised by reduced executive function, and in turn, obesity itself has a compounding negative impact on the brain via mechanisms currently attributed to low-grade systemic inflammation, elevated lipids and/or insulin resistance (Smith *et al.* 2011). Whether obesity causes cognitive deficits or vice versa is unclear at present.

Dieticians note that, despite an abundance of healthy food choices in the developed world, many are not eating well (Rowe *et al.* 2011). Information advising people to follow restrictive diets – ranging from raw food, low fat or low carbohydrate food, low GI food, vegan diets, high protein diets, paleo food or even eating for your specific blood type – surrounds and possibly overwhelms people on a daily basis. Claims that specific nutrients or foods are responsible for weight gain or weight loss, or cause chronic diseases such as diabetes and heart disease, may be creating confusion among the public, while also making them more susceptible to food industry marketing. The focus on nutrients within nutrition science and dietary advice may have been counterproductive. Studying single nutrients in isolation and out of any food or dietary context has led to some fairly exaggerated and simplified claims about the role of these nutrients in the body rather, than considering the overall quality of whole food.

The intense focus on low-fat food is a good example of a single nutrient focus. Food manufacturers have responded by successfully engineering the nutrient profile of foods to reflect nutritional trends, but without producing particularly healthy food. It sounds plausible that a high fat intake will lead to an increase in the fat deposition of consumers. This perception of the danger with fat has allowed the food industry to appropriate the low-fat discourse and reformulate their products accordingly. However, there are still no comprehensive and convincing scientific findings to support the purported multiple health benefits of low-fat foods and diets. The low fat discourse led to the very simplified idea that the definition of a good or bad food was its fat content, rather than overall energy levels, nutritional value or the percentage of highly processed ingredients the product contained. In many cases, fat has simply been replaced with sugar or refined and modified starches. Counter trends in diets are the recommendation to restrict severely the intake of carbohydrates, while indulging in fatty foods to lose weight. Such diets have proved at least partly successful in lowering an individual's weight, but the long term effects of the diet have not been scientifically verified (Astrup *et al.* 2004).

The focus on 'good' or 'bad' nutrients by experts in nutrition and food marketers has accentuated the nutritional anxieties of the public (Scrinis 2008). A fear of bad nutrients dominated the second half of the twentieth century, but this has now been joined by anxieties about not getting enough of some of the good and supposedly health-enhancing nutrients and food components, such as omega-3 fats, antioxidants or plant sterols. This has led to an increase in the consumption of nutritional supplements and nutrient fortified processed foods (Gahche *et al.* 2011).

Being overweight and obese has gone beyond being an individual problem to become a societal issue in a growing number of countries. Diet trends and fashion driven diets will not change the overall trajectory of a population's steady increase in body weight. It has become, in addition to an individual issue, a productivity issue, a transport and service issue, and especially a medical issue. Excessive weight might not be the primary medical problem, but it can affect the whole person and augment or lead to other medical conditions. Overweight and obesity have become medicalised, thus taken beyond the individual's responsibility (Blackburn 2011). Medicalisation of obesity might mitigate the stigmatisation of obesity and gradually change public perception to normalise obesity and making it the new normal – to the frustration of medical experts.

Conclusion

In this chapter, the focus has been on risks in relation to an increasing obese and overweight global population. It has developed from an individual risk issue to a societal health issue, where social, cultural and economic problems interlink, and at this stage does not have a local or global socio-cultural risk management solution. If some parts of the world have stopped the steep increase in the incidence of obesity, others have just started the risk trajectory.

As excess body weight is a major individual, societal and economic problem of global significance, it is a highly relevant socio-cultural risk issue. Excessive weight gain has increased rapidly over the last 30 years and, as noted, it can have diverse and multifactorial health consequences. In its more severe form, obesity places huge financial burdens on governments and individuals. It has been reported to account for up to 21 per cent of the total health care costs in some developed countries (Cawley and Meyerhoefer 2012).

Although knowledge and awareness about health risks associated with consuming high-energy-dense food and living a sedentary life are common, the knowledge is not always acted upon. Excessive weight is accompanied by a negative stigma, initiated by and reflected in a wealth of weight loss advice provided on an almost daily basis in the mass media. Public health campaigns have long warned against excess body fat and promoted messages highlighting the importance of a healthy diet and moderate exercise. Yet it is a conundrum of the modern risk society that many of current prevention strategies for limiting weight gain seem to be simply ignored by individuals and society alike. Individuals continuously make choices in their everyday life to evade a multitude of risks, but advice to avoid risks associated with excess weight gain seems to be more difficult to follow. Society continues to provide tempting food choices and facilitates sedentary lifestyles. Intensive promotions of energy-dense food and drink to children and adults have created a new food model of convenience, especially attractive to small households and time poor families. The structure of the built environment in itself affects obesity by not facilitating physical activity, such as walking, bike riding or running, but also through people's fear of being a victim of crime.

In its simplest form, it is unambiguous that excess weight gain is caused by an imbalance between an individual's energy consumed and energy spent. Obesity could be seen as an unintended consequence of affluence leading to overindulgence, a sedentary lifestyle and bad food choices. However, it is now commonly agreed that the reasons for the growth in overweight and obesity are multifactorial, including contributions of inherited, metabolic, behavioural, environmental, social, cultural and socio-economic components. Instead of seeing it as a weakness of the individual, it makes much more sense to view obesity as a societal problem involving an interaction between the individual with what, in line with the socio-cultural risk discourse, has been called the 'obesogenic' society.

The twenty-first century is a fast moving society where multitasking and food convenience are promoted. Leisure time has become increasingly scarce and fast food that can provide satiety in the shortest time possible has become the norm in an increasing number of societies. Globally, the availability of energy-dense and refined foods for easy consumption, foods often high in fat and sugar, has created a milieu of excessive energy intake. Sugar and fat are powerful sources of neurobiological rewards. Energy-dense foods provide more sensory enjoyment and more pleasure than do foods that are less energy dense. The most likely targets of food cravings are those foods that contain fat, sugar or both.

Food that is readymade to heat and eat in front of the computer or the television is now common, and this distracts our inherent mechanisms to control the amount of food consumed. Furthermore, fast food has become synonymous with time efficiency. Because of its success, fast food has become low in price and thus easily affordable. It has evolved into a middle-class status symbol of efficiency in developing countries, while in developed countries it has become affordable food for people on low income and the disadvantaged people in society.

From a socio-cultural risk discourse perspective, it is proposed that we need an overall system change. We need to rethink the way we design cities, to make them conducive to a healthy lifestyle, and our healthcare system needs to focus on prevention and primary care. We need to reconnect with food and teach food skills to young people. We need to take back our social and physical urban environment and take responsibility for how advertising space is used to promote unhealthy food choices. Without decisive action, being overweight and obese might become the new normal.

4   Caffeine – a common psychoactive stimulant – from a socio-cultural perspective

Introduction

The socio-cultural risk discourse is grounded within social and cultural tradition, developed social cohesion and societal belonging. Its established way of living and social order aim to keep people united against outside danger and to reduce risks by minimising external influences that might unsettle the societal environment. Douglas (1992, 1982), and Douglas and Wildavsky (1982) emphasise that the behaviour of people is informally monitored to make sure the society members follow the customs and traditions of the society, but the society also creates an ambience of belonging among the members, especially around food and drink traditions.

An example of a uniting socio-cultural activity is to consume beverages containing caffeine with friends, a pursuit that in contemporary society is perceived as a harmless social activity. However, this has not always been the case, as throughout history these beverages were occasionally classified as dangerous, not necessarily for the effects of caffeine as a psychoactive stimulant, but rather for the socio-cultural context in which they were enjoyed. Although drinking coffee, tea or cocoa are social activities, they can also be seen as activities that can be interpreted as taking people away from essential tasks, and giving people an opportunity to conspire against the social order. In contemporary society, however, caffeine beverages serve a purely social purpose; they are enjoyed by millions of people, and few would see their consumption as causing any risk to personal health or to societal order if savoured in moderation.

There are good reasons for consuming caffeinated beverages as well as a few risks. Since caffeine is a psychoactive stimulant (Nehlig *et al.* 1992), it has become a common practice to start the day with a caffeinated beverage to face the challenges of a new day. Thus, on the benefit side, caffeine enhances alertness and mood, and increases performance (McKim and Hancock 2012). Further, it is legal, easy to obtain, and socially acceptable to consume. Moderate use is generally considered to be safe (Temple 2009). However, there are also risks with drinking such beverages. Caffeine may aggravate pre-existing health conditions such as migraines and arrhythmias, and cause sleep disturbances. Caffeine can also promote anxiety and panic attacks, especially in high doses and in those with pre-existing anxiety disorders (Lara 2010). In a contemporary fast-moving society, there is rarely time to consider the benefits or risks associated with the food and beverages consumed, with potential risks posed by excessive caffeine consumption usually neglected.

Typically, the perception and understanding of a risk is based on the individual's scientific knowledge, the social and cultural traditions in which the food product is used, and the individual's awareness of the danger or hazard the item might pose to them or the wider society (Yeung and Morris 2001a). In relation to coffee, the socio-cultural influences are so deeply entrenched that potential risks are rarely considered. However, the perception of a food product as a public health threat is not static, as it will change according to new knowledge, food trends and the official declaration of the product as a risk or a non-risk to human health. Additionally, the perception of risk will depend on how the new knowledge is communicated, how it is accepted as significant, and if it is seen to merit behavioural change. The current knowledge might be challenged if new information and scientific discoveries question the traditionally accepted perception of the food item. In society, there are few certainties in relation to the ultimate safety of food; there are always risks involved, but some of the risks associated with food are less serious than others. Thus, the proven risks associated with excessive caffeine consumption appear to be mostly ignored, so far, by the general public. Even if excessive coffee drinking can cause some obvious discomforts like an upset stomach and heartburn, coffee is not perceived as a serious risk to our health at such a level that we are prepared to reduce consumption or give it up.

From a governmentality risk context, there are certain worrying trends around some novel drinks/beverages containing caffeine, as well as caffeinated beverages mixed with alcohol. Although once mostly restricted to use among adults, children now regularly consume beverages containing caffeine. This is particularly true for caffeinated soft drinks, and 'energy drinks'. Energy drinks are the perceived provinces of young people (Babu *et al.* 2008) and these energy drink brands align themselves with an alternative cultural attitude, allowing young people to embrace the artificial sweetness of mixed alcoholic drinks. Energy drink companies are deliberately focusing on contemporary youth cultures. Compounding the potential negative effects of caffeine itself, excessive sugar-sweetened soft drink and energy drink consumption have also been associated with overweight and obesity, as discussed in the previous chapter. For governments, the introduction of energy drinks pre-mixed with alcohol has become a serious issue, as they are attractive to young people below the legal drinking age. Hence, these energy drinks pre-mixed with alcohol might introduce young people to alcoholic drinks earlier than what they would otherwise be, as the sweetness helps to mask the strong taste of alcohol.

Caffeine is regularly added to many beverages, and through dependence effects, it has the potential to promote excessive consumption of drinks containing caffeine. In a human trial, Keast *et al.* (2015) showed that young adults offered unlimited access to a caffeinated beverage, consumed 419 mL daily during a 28 day period, while participants offered the non-caffeinated beverage only consumed 273 mL a day. They concluded that the addition of even low concentrations of caffeine to a beverage significantly increased consumption. Unfortunately, our knowledge of the effects of caffeine use on behaviour and physiology of children remains poorly understood (Temple 2009). Hering-Hanit and Gadoth (2003) showed, based on a number of children and adolescents visiting their clinic, that complaints about daily headaches could be traced back to a high daily caffeine consumption in the form of cola drinks. In addition, case studies of caffeine toxicity and deaths among adolescents and adults following extreme energy drink consumption highlights the potential dangers of excessive caffeine exposure (Seifert *et al.* 2011; Meier 2012).

Socio-cultural context to caffeine consumption

There is a long socio-cultural tradition associated with consuming caffeine-containing beverages all across the world (Ashihara and Suzuki 2004). It has been suggested that caffeine was first consumed as far back as 2737 BC, when the Chinese Emperor Shen Nung boiled drinking water and leaves from a nearby bush, creating a pleasant aroma and the first recorded pot of tea (Arab and Blumberg 2008). The widespread natural occurrence of caffeine in a variety of plants undoubtedly played a major role in the long-standing popularity of products containing caffeine, especially beverages.

It has been estimated that approximately 80 per cent of the world's population consume a caffeinated product every day (James 1997). From a socio-cultural risk perspective, the pendulum has swung considerably over the years between the positive and negative side of caffeine use. Caffeinated beverages all have very different flavours and modes of consumption, but all are intrinsically linked in the cultural psyche to positive properties like alertness, vitality, enhanced physical ability and social engagement. Concurrently, throughout history, there have been perceived threats of political upheaval linked to coffee's social aspects of creating a social networking environment, as well as concerns about the toxic effects of overconsumption.

Caffeine-containing beverages, and coffee in particular, are consumed in socio-cultural contexts. Coffee has been described as a 'practical experience of socialization beatified with chat' by cultural historians (Argan *et al.* 2015:28). Coffee can serve as a work break, a casual meeting starter, or an introduction to a longer conversation. A coffee break is a routine social gathering involving a short downtime from work relished by employees in many countries. Business meetings often start with the ritual serving of a cup of coffee as a courteous offering to the participants. Coffee get-togethers have long been a popular form of social contact and conversation especially in several northern European countries. Tea, another caffeine-containing beverage, has served the same socio-cultural purpose in countries like the United Kingdom and India, to name just two. Coffee is also important in Austrian and French culture. Coffeehouses are prominent in Vienna and well known internationally, while Paris was instrumental in the development of a new style of fashionable cafés. The formation of culture around coffeehouses dates back further to sixteenth-century Turkey, where they were traditional social hubs as well as artistic and intellectual centres (Oral 1997). In seventeenth- and eighteenth-century Britain, there were venues associated with reading newspapers, playing games and smoking tobacco, as well as drinking tea and coffee (Cowan 2001). In addition, they were venues for political and religious debates, hence were a potential risk to the social order.

Looking through history, coffee drinking seems to have had a more troubled journey than tea and cocoa. Tea was seen as a healthy drink and, in a secular society focused on herbal remedies, it rapidly grew from medicinal use to daily consumption. Cocoa, a spiritual drink of the Mayans and Aztecs, became a favoured drink of the Catholic aristocracy in Spain during the early sixteenth century, and it soon was devoured as a nourishing drink for the clergy and the wealthy across Europe on fast days, as the devout could not consume food, but liquids were allowed. Coffee, on the other hand, in spreading from Africa to the Middle East initially appealed to a Muslim majority as being non-alcoholic and was not condemned by the Koran. As the Muslim faithful spent more and more time in coffeehouses, the first backlash against coffee began. It was thought that an invigorating beverage consumed by the 'chattering classes' could lead to discussion of politics that could create dissent, inspire uprisings and instigate revolutions. This enabled the religious advocates to challenge coffee drinking. In 1570, imams called for Muslims to renounce the drink, as coffeehouses were full and the mosques were almost empty (Ukers 1922). Restrictions spread, with Turkey being among the sternest, banning coffee around 1656: the first offence was punished with a beating and the second offence with drowning (Roden 1981).

On the contrary, when introduced to Europe coffee became a favoured drink, together with tea, as a replacement for beer. Beer had been the earlier beverage of choice, contributing to the liquid intake of the urban and rural poor as a ready form of energy. It served as an alternative to both untreated water, a common instigator of disease, as well as easily spoiled milk. Beer was consumed at breakfast and as beer soup mixed with eggs, which was served warm during the day, often eight to nine litres per day (Roden 1981; Bond 2011). The boiled water used for making coffee and tea was less dangerous to health, and less contaminated than unboiled water. Furthermore, coffee and tea became popular during the industrial revolution, as they were much safer to drink than alcohol for people operating complex machinery (Macfarlane and Macfarlane 2009). Unlike Far Eastern cultures, the West did not view bitterness as a positive feature of food and beverage items, so sugar played a role in the increasingly widespread acceptance of tea and coffee (Bond 2011).

During the seventeenth century, coffee drinking was spread amongst the upper class in Europe, but the habit quickly trickled down to the lower classes who drank coffee for its invigorating qualities and as a cure for hangovers and flatulence. However, there were further reactions. The wine dealers in France and Italy resisted the incursion of coffee, as it competed with their livelihood. Coffee met with similar opposition from alehouse keepers in Germany.

Throughout a lifelong campaign against coffee, Frederick the Great of Prussia promulgated bans and taxes, and introduced a special police squad to keep his subjects safe from the coffee's threats to their health; he also imposed a state monopoly on coffee imports. In 1777, he issued a manifesto claiming beer's superiority over coffee. The king argued that coffee interfered with the country's beer consumption, apparently hoping a royal statement would make Prussians prefer beer. His efforts were partially successful for a short period, but, as it had elsewhere, coffee's progress ultimately proved inevitable (Weinberg and Bealer 2001; Kjeldgaard and Ostberg 2007).

In Sweden, the situation was initially somewhat different, with coffee placed on the pharmacy list of approved drugs in 1687 and recommended for overall strengthening of stamina. However, coffee, as well as tea, quickly gained popularity outside its use as medicine, and it finally became so popular in Sweden that the state saw no other solution than to levy heavy taxes on coffee and tea consumption. Coffee and tea imports caused too much money to pour out of the country, and the state aimed to stop this outflow. When the taxation was unsuccessful, coffee drinking was totally banned, in the summer of 1794, to save the state finances. A special police force was designated to patrol the cities, and those caught in the act of drinking coffee were sent to prison (Weinberg and Bealer 2001; Kjeldgaard and Ostberg 2007). The ban, which was renewed multiple times until the 1820s, was never successful in stamping out coffee drinking. Once the ban was lifted, coffee became the dominant beverage in Sweden.

Today, consumption of coffee and tea occupies a significant place in the national cultures of most nations of the world and government bans have long been discontinued. Taken in moderation, caffeine seems to present little general risk. But traditions and customs in many countries, to drink coffee as a social activity and to meet for coffee, can lead to more than moderate consumption, and the recent appearance of caffeinated energy drinks has increased intake, especially among young people. The combination of energy drinks with alcohol by young people is especially worrying.

While authorities have long given up on any prospects of limiting consumption of naturally caffeinated beverages, the situation is different for some other products. Thus, several regulatory agencies around the world have reviewed, regulated and authorised the addition of caffeine to specific beverages where caffeine does not occur naturally. Australia and New Zealand, the United States and Canada regulate caffeine as a food additive. In the European Union, it is specifically identified and regulated as a flavouring. Approved levels of caffeine in such beverages are generally below 350 mg/L. Labelling requirements vary internationally, with the European Union requiring caffeine to be mentioned by name in the list of ingredients, with the quantity of caffeine specified for beverages (other than tea and coffee) that contain more than 150 mg/L of caffeine.

Canadian legislation requires caffeine to be listed as an ingredient if it has been added separately to the product as a 'pure' ingredient. In the United States, any food product that contains added caffeine must list caffeine as an ingredient, but the actual quantity of caffeine does not have to be stated on the label.

Although the overall access to caffeinated beverages is not regulated, some official agencies have set guidelines on caffeine daily intakes recommending a maximum of about 400 mg per day for adults. Recommendations have been issued for pregnant females by Australia, the United Kingdom, Ireland and other countries including limits of 200 mg of caffeine per day.

Despite some early attempts to discourage caffeine use, it is clear that caffeine consumption in its different forms will continue unabated throughout the world, while total daily intake and the major sources of caffeine will vary according to custom and age group. Despite recommendations to limit caffeine intake, the public do not seem to heed that advice, since worldwide coffee consumption comprise of approximately 500 billion cups annually (Aluko 2012).

Apart from the socio-cultural aspects, the sensory milieu is also a significant part of the positive perceptions associated with the consumption of caffeine-containing beverages. Bangcuyo *et al.* (2015) showed the importance of the contextual – visual, auditory and olfactory – environment in forming consumer perceptions, penchants and behaviours when testing coffee preferences. Their results suggest that extrinsic contextual information is processed simultaneously with the intrinsic product attributes to influence hedonic assessments and to shape reward outcomes. This is particularly true for coffee, which is consumed in a café environment with a lingering coffee smell, the sound of coffee grinding, and the view of shiny equipment. As a further affirmation of the olfactory sense, in some countries a variety of flavours are added to the coffee to mask its bitter taste and make it more appealing to an even wider audience.

Coffee culture has recently been affected by a hegemonic influence of large corporate coffee chains threatening to overpower local coffee cultures all over the globe. However, in parallel, a coffee connoisseurship culture has evolved as a counter trend with the coffee consumption landscape showing a plurality of cultural styles along differing types of coffee establishments (Kjeldgaard and Ostberg 2007). Over the years, the focus of coffee drinking also seems to have partly moved away from being a social activity. While people still commonly visit cafés they are far more likely to be working on laptops or reading, than socialising. A current trend is the Internet café where social contact is conducted via the Internet, with or without a cup of coffee. Coffee on the run has become a common feature of today's fast-paced society.

Caffeine and other methylxanthines

The caffeine in coffee and tea and in some other food products is the most well known member of a family of chemical compounds known as the methylxanthines. There are many methylxanthines besides caffeine, but only an additional two are found naturally in food. These are theophylline and theobromine, most commonly found in cocoa. Theophylline and theobromine are also formed when caffeine is metabolised by the liver (Thorn *et al.* 2012). All three substances have similar structures and similar behavioural and physiological effects, although caffeine and an additional metabolite, called paraxanthine, has more pronounced effects compared to the other two (Orrú *et al.* 2013). The three methylxanthines can be found naturally in the leaves, seeds and fruits of more than 60 plants, including coffee beans, tealeaves, kola nuts, guarana and cocoa beans. Caffeine is regularly added to cola-type soft drinks and more recently to energy drinks. Caffeine is also found in hundreds of prescription and over-the-counter drugs, including analgesics, weight control aids, allergy relief compounds and stimulants. Theophylline and caffeine are sometimes used as respiratory stimulants for newborn babies.

Two main raw plant ingredients, coffee beans and tea leaves, provide 71 per cent and 12 per cent of the caffeine consumed, respectively, with the remaining 17 per cent coming from soft drink, energy drink and cocoa consumption (Anon 2008). Coffee is the major source of caffeine in the diets of adults, whereas soft drinks are the primary source for children and adolescents (Frary *et al.* 2005). However, this varies by country, for example, considerably fewer Canadian than American children consume caffeinated beverages: 36 per cent and 56 per cent, respectively (Knight *et al.* 2006).

In the following, naturally or artificially caffeinated products and their usage are discussed in more detail. From a socio-cultural risk perspective, it is worth noting that, in 2015, the European Food Safety Authority (2015a) concluded that single doses of caffeine up to 200 mg, and daily intakes of 400 mg, did not raise safety concerns for the general adult population. However, single doses of 100 mg of caffeine may increase sleep latency and reduce sleep duration in some adults, particularly when consumed close to bedtime. It was recommended that pregnant females should limit daily intake to 200 mg. For children and adolescents, the information available was insufficient on which to base a safe level of caffeine intake, but it was proposed that the pregnant female adult level of 3 mg/kg body weight may be used also for children. The estimated proportion of the adult population in 13 European countries exceeding daily intakes of 400 mg ranged from about 6 to 33 per cent. The proportion of adolescents exceeding that amount ranged from 5 to 10 per cent and for children it ranged from 6 to 13 per cent.

Coffee – a source of methylxanthines

Coffee is the third most consumed global beverage after water and , and is the richest source of caffeine; it makes caffeine the most commonly consumed psychoactive drug in the world (Butt and Sultan 2011). Although coffee and tea are both everyday beverages that contain caffeine, an ordinary cup of tea will not give the same effect as coffee, as it provides only half the amount of caffeine found in a cup of coffee. While tea leaves contain more caffeine than coffee beans weight for weight, fewer tea leaves are used to make a cup of tea, hence giving a lower caffeine level in the final brew. This makes coffee the most common source of dietary methylxanthine intake across the world with a coffee bean production of about 8.8 million tonnes in 2012 (FAOSTAT 2014). Coffee is made from the fruit of a bush or small tree of the genus *Coffea*. Two varieties in particular, *arabica* and *robusta*, account for close to 99 per cent of the world's coffee production. Although initially native to Ethiopia, they are now grown in about 70 countries in Africa, South America, and in many other tropical areas of the world (Butt and Sultan 2011).

The caffeine content of coffee beans varies with the plant species and the local environment in which the plant is grown. *Arabica* coffee, grown mostly in Central and South America, contains about 1.1 per cent caffeine, while beans of *Robusta* coffee, grown mostly in Indonesia and Africa, contain about 2.2 per cent caffeine. The caffeine content in coffee beans also depends on the length of the growing season, time of harvest, the method of processing and subspecies. In analysing 28 coffee bean samples, Fox *et al.* (2013) found that the majority of samples had caffeine levels of around 10–12 mg/g with an upper level of 19.9 mg/g. The average caffeine content of instant coffee, the freeze- or spray-dried granules of pre-brewed coffee, can be estimated at 31.4 mg/g (United States Department of Agriculture 2013).

The amount of caffeine extracted during beverage preparation is dependent on the method used. Coffee can be brewed in several different ways, with the methods falling into four main groups depending on how the water is introduced to the coffee grounds: boiling, percolating, filtering or pressurised extraction in espresso machines. A Canadian study attempted to quantify the amount of caffeine extracted using different brewing procedures (Stavric *et al.* 1988). They found great variations in the amount of caffeine extracted, even between people using the same brewing method. Several studies have looked at average caffeine content of the finished brew and found variations between 386 to 652 mg/L for percolated coffee; 555 to 845 mg/L for filtered coffee; and 1,691 to 2,254 mg/L for coffee from an espresso coffee machine (Barone and Roberts 1996; Gilbert 1976; Heckman *et al.* 2010). The caffeine content for instant coffee would vary between 119 to 763 mg/L (Heckman *et al.* 2010). Because of the great variation in caffeine content of the coffee beans and the differing extraction efficiency of the brewing methods used, it is difficult to calculate accurately how much caffeine is consumed in a regular cup of coffee. In addition, cup sizes differ widely between countries. For instance, in the USA, coffee is typically served in a 240 mL cup, which is twice the amount of a typical European serving, while an espresso cup would contain only 30–40 mL. A standard recipe when calculating exposure is to use the caffeine amount of seven grams of ground coffee beans diluted in 120 mL of boiling water, which would result in close to 80 mg of caffeine in the cup assuming complete extraction. A restaurant style serving of an espresso would contain from 40 to 75 mg of caffeine. Even a 'decaffeinated' espresso can contain up to 15 mg of caffeine. On the other hand, a 240 mL cup of generic instant coffee can contain any amount from 27 to 173 mg of caffeine depending on the dilution used, while a Starbucks Pike Place 480 mL cup of brewed coffee contains 330 mg of caffeine (United States Department of Agriculture 2013). A moderate intake of caffeine is approximately 300 mg per day, which is roughly three to four cups extracted from ground-roasted coffee beans or five cups of instant coffee.

The people of Finland are among the biggest coffee consumers in the world. Finns consume an average of 12 kg of coffee per capita annually or four to five large cups of coffee a day, which is over twice the amount of what most other Europeans drink. It might have been expected that countries like Italy and France would be at the top of the coffee consumption charts with their legendary high quality coffee. However, the French and the Italians only consume an average of between 5 and 6 kg of coffee per year, slightly higher than the 4 kg drunk in the USA (ChartsBin 2011).

Tea – a source of methylxanthines

Tea is the second most consumed beverage on earth after water. In 2012, the global tealeaf production reached over 4.8 million tonnes (FAOSTAT 2014). Tea is grown in about 30 countries but is consumed worldwide, although at greatly varying levels. The largest producers of tea are China, India, Kenya, Sri Lanka and Turkey. India is the world's largest tea-drinking nation counting the total volume, although annual per capita consumption of tea remains a modest 0.52 kg per person. Turkey, with 6.87 kg of tea consumed per person per year, is the world's greatest per capita consumer, followed by Morocco with 4.34 kg and Ireland with 3.22 kg (FAOSTAT 2014).

Tea is made from the leaves of *Camellia sinensis*, which is a bush in its commercial form. For the best quality tea, only the bud and the first two leaves of each twig are picked. After picking, the tealeaves will quickly wilt and oxidise unless they are immediately dried (McKim and Hancock 2012). The leaves turn progressively darker as their chlorophyll breaks down and tannins are released. The plant's intracellular enzymes cause this enzymatic oxidation process, also called fermentation. In tea processing, the darkening is stopped at a predetermined stage by heating, which deactivates the enzymes involved. Tea is manufactured in three basic forms. In green tea production, the leaves are steamed soon after picking to completely prevent oxidation. For oolong tea, roasting the leaves before the oxidation is fully completed stops the oxidation process. In the production of black tea, the halting of oxidation by heating is carried out at the end of fermentation simultaneously with drying. Black tea dominates the world market, with only 20 per cent being green tea and two per cent oolong tea (Graham 1992).

Caffeine is present in tea at an average level of 3 per cent along with very small amounts of the other common methylxanthines, theobromine and theophylline. A study was undertaken to measure the methylxanthine contents in the three different types of tea to determine the actual amounts present. On a dry leaf weight basis, total caffeine content was highest in green (36.6 mg/g) and black (32.8 mg/g) tealeaves and lowest in oolong tea (23.8 mg/g). Total theobromine was highest in black tea (1.64 mg/g) and least in oolong tea (0.65 mg/g). Theophylline was not detected in any tea tested (Hicks *et al.* 1996). The brewing method used to produce the tea beverage can significantly influence the methylxanthine content of the final brew (Hicks *et al.* 1996). As a rule of thumb, after a steeping time of five minutes the caffeine content is estimated to be 27 mg in an average cup of tea of about 150 mL or 180 mg/L. However, this will vary considerably with steeping time. A one-minute steep can be expected to extract about 15 mg in an average cup and a three-minute steep about 23 mg (Gilbert *et al.* 1976; Graham 1984; Chin *et al.* 2008).

Although excessive consumption of tea might have a negative health impact due to the caffeine content, health benefits have been attributed to tea, especially green tea consumption. In vitro and animal studies provide strong evidence that polyphenols derived from tea, particularly epigallocatechin-3-gallate, may affect the pathogenesis of several chronic diseases, including inhibition of tumorigenesis in a variety of animal models of carcinogenesis.

Cocoa – a source of methylxanthines

The fourth most common global drink is cocoa (Pipitone 2012). There were about five million tonnes of cocoa beans produced in 2012 (FAOSTAT 2014). Cocoa is made from beans extracted from the seedpods of the cacao tree, *Theobroma cacao*. It is a tree originally native to the tropical Amazon rain forest, but now cultivated in Central and South America, the West Indies and West Africa (McKim and Hancock 2012). The seedpods are picked and left to ferment for five to six days before the cocoa beans can be removed. The beans are dried before shipping to processing plants where they are roasted to enhance the flavour.

Cocoa beans are used to produce cocoa powder and cocoa butter that in turn are used to make cocoa beverages, chocolate or as flavouring in a range of food applications. The diversity in use of cocoa beans makes it very difficult to calculate total consumption of different cocoa products, with chocolate being an exception. Although the earliest recorded reference to cocoa was in 1502, it was not until 1876 that milk chocolate was invented, an event that formed the backbone of the chocolate industry of today (Shively and Tarka 1984). To make one kg of chocolate, about 300 to 600 beans are processed, depending on the desired cocoa content.

The largest total consumption of cocoa in metric tonnes is in the United States, although the highest per capita consumer can be found in Switzerland. According to numbers provided by Leatherhead Food Research as cited by

Nieburg (2013), Switzerland has an annual per capita consumption of 11.9 kg, followed by Ireland at 9.9 kg and the United Kingdom at 9.5 kg.

Cocoa is the major natural source of theobromine. Small amounts of caffeine are present in the bean along with traceable amounts of theophylline. The methylxanthine content of beans depend on the varietal type, and it is influenced by the fermentation process. Cocoa powder contains about 1.9 per cent theobromine and 0.21 per cent caffeine. A 125 mL cup of cocoa was estimated to provide between 40 and 80 mg of theobromine and between 1 and 7.8 mg of caffeine when prepared from commercial instant mixes (Blauch and Tarka 1983). This would equate to an average of 480 mg/L of theobromine and 32 mg/L of caffeine. The methylxanthine content of sweet chocolate ranges from 3,590 to 6,280 mg/kg for theobromine and 170 to 1,250 mg/kg for caffeine (Shively and Tarka 1984).

Currently, there is limited market survey data available for the consumption of methylxanthines in chocolate foods and beverages, although cocoa rank the lowest of the three main plant sources in providing caffeine, it constitutes the major source of dietary theobromine (Shively and Tarka 1984). In general, the amount of theobromine found in chocolate is small enough that humans can safely consume chocolate. However, occasional serious side effects may result from the consumption of large quantities, especially in the elderly, including sweating, trembling and severe headaches (Cady and Durham 2010). Serious poisoning happens more frequently in domestic animals, which metabolise theobromine much more slowly than humans, and can easily consume enough chocolate to cause theobromine poisoning (Stidworthy *et al.* 1997).

Energy drinks – a source of methylxanthines

Energy drinks are beverages containing stimulants and marketed as providing mental and physical stimulation. Global energy drink consumption climbed by 14 per cent in the 2011 year, according to the latest report from food and drink consultancy Zenith International, reaching 4.8 billion litres. North America was the leading region, with 36 per cent of global volume in 2011, followed by the Asia Pacific with 22 per cent and Western Europe with 17 per cent (Zenith International 2012).

Energy drinks may or may not be carbonated, and generally contain large amounts of caffeine and other stimulants. They may also contain sugar or artificial sweeteners, herbal extracts and amino acids. Energy drinks, with added caffeine, vitamins, taurine, guarana, kola nut, yerba mate and herbal supplements, are sold to improve drinkers' performance and alertness. The additional ingredients may act in synergy to provide a stimulant effect greater than that provided by caffeine alone (Miller 2008; O'Brien *et al.* 2008).

Energy drinks have been around for some time, but their popularity did not take off until the introduction of Red Bull in 1987. Since then, the energy drink market has grown extensively, with hundreds of different brands with varying caffeine content now available (Reissig *et al.* 2009). While caffeinated soft drinks regularly contain around 80–120 mg caffeine/L, energy drinks often contain three times this amount or more than 300 mg/L. Energy shots are a specialised kind of energy drink usually sold in small bottles of around 60 mL. They contain the same amount of caffeine as a 250 mL energy drink bottle or more than 1,300 mg/L. Energy shots are the fastest growing part of the energy drink category. Energy drinks are targeted at young active people. Approximately 66 per cent of its drinkers are between the ages of 13 and 35 years old, with males making up approximately 65 per cent of the market (Malinauskas *et al.* 2007; Heckman *et al.* 2010).

Although healthy people can tolerate caffeine in moderation, heavy caffeine consumption through energy drinks has been associated with serious health effects such as seizures, mania, stroke and sudden death. It has been suggested that both the known and unknown pharmacology of various ingredients in energy drinks, combined with reports of toxicity, may put some children at risk for serious adverse health effects (Seifert *et al.* 2011).

Caffeine metabolism and physiological effects

Irrespective of its source, caffeine is absorbed rapidly into the bloodstream from the gastro-intestinal tract. Caffeine reaches maximum concentration within less than one hour. It is distributed throughout the body, even crossing the blood-brain and placental barriers without difficulty due to its hydrophobic properties (Tanaka *et al.* 1984; Kimmel *et al.* 1984). About 10 to 30 per cent of caffeine in the blood becomes bound to protein and trapped in the circulatory system (Arnaud 1993; Axelrod and Reisenthal 1953). The half-life of caffeine in the human body varies between three to five hours, but it is up to seven hours for theophylline and theobromine (Arnaud 2011). Females metabolise caffeine 20 to 30 per cent more quickly than males, but the rate will vary according to the menstrual cycle (Arnaud 1993). Some people are slow metabolisers of caffeine depending on their genetic makeup and the same amount of caffeine will therefore have a greater effect in such individuals (McKim and Hancock 2012).

It is clear that caffeine, theophylline and theobromine are psychoactive stimulant drugs that influence brain chemistry (McKim and Hancock 2012). They mimic adenosine by binding to adenosine receptors and thus blocking the effects of adenosine. Adenosine has many functions in the body. In general, its effect is to inhibit neurotransmission in specific synapses in the brain, which slows down nerve impulses and cause drowsiness. The methylxanthines will thus have the opposite effect and improve alertness (Fissone *et al.* 2004). As a secondary reaction, blocking adenosine also increase the levels of dopamine in the brain. The increase in dopamine is responsible for most of the behavioural and reinforcing effects of the methylxanthines (McKim and Hancock 2012). There is ample evidence that these effects are induced through a different set of brain receptors compared to the action of most other centrally stimulating drugs like cocaine and amphetamine (Fredholm *et al*. 1999).

Early experiments show that low concentrations of caffeine may produce small decreases in heart rates, whereas higher concentrations may make the heart beat abnormally fast. In the brain, it constricts the cerebral blood vessels, while it dilates blood vessels in other parts of the body. By constricting blood flow to the brain, caffeine is able to reduce headaches caused by high blood pressure. However, if a person is used to drinking several cups of coffee a day but then quits, the blood vessels in the brain will dilate, sometimes enough to give a powerful headache. This is one of the most common withdrawal symptoms from caffeine (McKim and Hancock 2012).

Caffeine can also contribute to insomnia – delaying the onset of sleep and reducing total sleeping time. It has a small effect on respiration by increasing blood flow through the lungs and increasing the supply of air by relaxing bronchiolar and alveolar smooth muscle. That is why it is proving effective in treating the breathing problems of some prematurely born infants (McKim and Hancock 2012). Additionally, some people experience tremors after drinking coffee and tea. That is thought to be due to over activation of the central nervous system (Shirlow and Mathers 1985).

Beneficial health effects of caffeine

Global consumption of caffeine is estimated to be 120,000 tonnes per annum. This is the approximate equivalent of one caffeinated beverage per day for each person in the world. With such volumes of caffeine consumed, it would be reasonable to expect that the effects of caffeine and related methylxanthine compounds on human health would be clear. Extensive scientific research has been conducted to examine the relationship between caffeine consumption and a range of harmful medical conditions, but there are still conflicting opinions in the literature.

From reporting of mainly negative health effects like gastric ulcers and cardiovascular disease in the past, the situation changed when, in 2008, a Harvard-led study reported finding no detrimental effects of consuming up to six cups of coffee a day based on results from 130,000 participants (Lopez-Garcia *et al*. 2008). This was further supported by a 2012 meta-analysis concluding that people who drank moderate amounts of coffee had a lower rate of heart failure, with the strongest inverse association seen for four cups a day, but a potentially higher risk at higher levels of consumption (Mostofski *et al*. 2012).

Thus, caffeine in moderate amounts is no longer considered a significant risk factor for coronary heart disease, while other detrimental health effects of excessive caffeine consumption remain to be resolved. Hence, findings are contradictory as to whether caffeine has any specific health benefits. However, over a long time, caffeine has been associated with improvements in cognitive functions. It improves mood, the feeling of wellbeing, and makes pending tasks seem easier (Fredholm *et al.* 1999). Caffeine has been found to reverse decreases in performance due to boredom, fatigue and the common cold (Lara 2010). It improves attention, speeds up reaction times and is capable of improving performance in normally alert individuals (Smith 2009).

Encouraging effects of caffeine intake on memory have been found for especially older people. Commonly, the memory will decline with age, and people's memory performance will be influenced by the time of day, with the performance being optimal early in the morning and declining during the late afternoon. However, in a trial, participants who consumed decaffeinated coffee showed a significant decline in memory performance from morning to afternoon, while those who consumed caffeine showed no such decline (Ryan *et al.* 2002).

Epidemiological and animal experimental studies of the development of Alzheimer's disease have found indications that moderate daily consumption of coffee over decades could reduce the risk of developing the disease (Arendash *et al.* 2006; Arendash *et al.* 2010; Eskelinen and Kivipelto 2010). Researchers in Finland reported findings from a study that followed the coffee drinking habits of over 1,400 people over 20 years. They found that those who drank three to five cups of coffee a day in their midlife years had a 65 per cent lower chance of developing dementia and Alzheimer's disease compared with those who reported drinking no coffee at all or only occasionally (Eskelinen *et al.* 2009).

For Parkinson's disease, another neurodegenerative disorder, it appears that there is a link between higher coffee consumption and a decreased risk of developing the disease. Since the cause of Parkinson's disease is multidimensional, it is not clear exactly how caffeine exerts its effects. However, a deficiency of dopamine producing cells is central to the development of the disease and since caffeine increases dopamine activity by blocking adenosine receptors, this could partly explain its benefits (McKim and Hancock 2012). Epidemiological studies have consistently demonstrated an inverse association between coffee consumption and the development of Parkinson's disease (Cavin *et al.* 2008; Joghataie *et al.* 2004). Additionally, there are also studies indicating that caffeine can reduce some symptoms of Parkinson's disease, such as tremors and deterioration of motor skills (Trevitt *et al.* 2009).

Several studies have looked at caffeine's inhibitory effect on some cancers. The role of caffeine in the progress of liver cancer has generated considerable interest (Montella *et al.* 2007; Cadden *et al.* 2007). Coffee consumption may protect against the development of liver cancer as its consumption has been shown to be inversely associated with the disease (Gelatti *et al.* 2005). Inoue *et al.* (2005) arrived at the same conclusion for the Japanese population. However, these findings need to be further explored and ideally be addressed in well-planned studies to corroborate the findings (Tanaka *et al.* 2007; Shimazu *et al.* 2005). Additionally, Hussain and El-Serag (2009) have highlighted the positive role of coffee and its active ingredient caffeine for the control of liver cancer.

Although promising, the influence of caffeine and related compounds in slowing down progression of a disease or increase human alertness should be understood from the scientific perspective of the early part of the twenty-first century. New discoveries will confirm or reattribute the existing findings and there will be new discoveries and new risk scenarios. Human history is littered with discoveries and health advice that have later been questioned, refuted, but still later re-evaluated. Thus, it is essential to think of caffeine and related compounds not as a cure or a medication, but as contributing factors that might benefit some people, but can also be a risk to others affected by certain health conditions as will be discussed in the following section.

Adverse health effects of caffeine

Excessive amounts of caffeine can cause very unpleasant and even life-threatening adverse effects. Although it is possible to die by consuming too much caffeine, it is unlikely. The lethal dose has been estimated to be between 3,000–8,000 mg, which is roughly equivalent to 30 to 80 cups of coffee in a day, but such doses are more likely to be the result of excessive intake of pills designed to keep one awake. Death results from convulsion and respiratory collapse (McKim and Hancock 2012). The American Association of Poison Control Centers received reports of around 46,000 cases of caffeine poisoning between 2006 and 2008, of which 45 had life-threatening symptoms and three people died (Seifert *et al.* 2011). There have also been reports of hospitalisations after excessive consumption of chocolate. Despite these reports, most symptoms of excessive caffeine intake from coffee, tea and chocolate consumption are less severe.

If the risks in relation to coffee, tea and cocoa consumption are minimal, the same cannot be said about energy drinks. There are several reports of harmful effects of excessive consumption of these drinks and anecdotal suspected deaths due to extreme caffeine intakes. In fact, the number of emergency department visits involving energy drinks among patients 12 years of age and older increased from 10,068 to 20,783 between 2007 and 2011 in the USA (Center for Behavioral Health Statistics and Quality 2013). Caffeine's harmful effects can be exacerbated by simultaneous consumption of alcohol, pointing to a particular problem for drinks combining caffeine and alcohol, a drink that is gaining in popularity (Rath 2012; Wolk *et al.* 2012). The Adverse Event Reporting System (CAERS) run by the Center for Food Safety and Applied Nutrition of the United States Food and Drug Administration collects information about adverse health events and product complaints. This includes complaints for energy drinks classified as dietary supplements. A summary of adverse effects for products under the brand names 5 Hour Energy and Monster Energy, an energy shot and an energy drink, respectively, lists 13 deaths linked to 5 Hour Energy consumption and five deaths linked to Monster Energy consumption between 1st of January 2004 and 23rd of October 2012 (Center for Food Safety and Applied Nutrition Adverse Event Reporting System 2012).

In 2008, energy drinks were granted marketing authorisation in France. In 2009, this was accompanied by a national nutritional surveillance scheme, which required national health agencies and regional centres to send information on spontaneously reported adverse events to the French agency for food safety. During the 2009 to 2011 period, 257 cases were reported to the agency, of which 212 provided sufficient information for food and drug safety evaluation. The experts found that 95 of the reported adverse events had cardiovascular, 74 psychiatric and 57 neurological symptoms. The adverse events did overlap with cardiac arrests and sudden or unexplained deaths occurring in at least eight cases, while 46 people had heart rhythm disorders, 13 had angina and three had hypertension (Drici 2014).

The coroner's report on a New Zealand woman who died by cardiac arrhythmia, stated that she reportedly consumed up to nine litres of Coca Cola per day, and suggested that consumption of the caffeine containing cola drink could have contributed to her death (Crerar 2013).

As an example of mild effects of excessive caffeine intake, a review of the available literature suggests that acute consumption of 250–300 mg of caffeine, or two to three cups of coffee, results in a short-term stimulation of urine output in individuals who have been deprived of caffeine for a period of days or weeks. However, regular coffee consumption quickly leads to a tolerance and the diuretic effect is diminished. Caffeine also has an effect on the detrusor muscles in the bladder that helps determine capacity limits and can cause an urgency to urinate. This indirectly compounds the diuretic effects of caffeine (Maughan and Griffin 2003; Arya *et al.* 2000).

Although caffeine alleviates headaches and is used medically for this purpose, generally in combination with a painkiller such as ibuprofen, excessive caffeine use as well as withdrawal from caffeine can on the contrary cause headaches. Research has consistently linked caffeine withdrawal to headaches even in those who, before the withdrawal, drank coffee in moderation. Additionally, studies have suggested that those who consume excessive amounts of caffeine also can experience headaches (McKim and Hancock 2012; Hering-Hanit and Gadoth 2003).

Caffeine may aggravate pre-existing conditions such as migraines and arrhythmias, and can cause sleep disturbances. Caffeine can also contribute to anxiety and panic attacks, especially in high doses and in those with pre-existing anxiety disorders. This ability seems to be associated with a particular phenotype of the adenosine receptor (Lara 2010), but it does not seem to have this effect in healthy individuals unless used excessively (Carroll 1998).

There are signs that females' caffeine consumption can have a detrimental effect on human reproduction and retard foetal growth (CARE Study Group 2008), although others point to confounding factors like morning sickness (Peck *et al.* 2010). As noted above, based on available evidence, there are suggestions that reproductive-age females should not consume more than 300 mg caffeine per day while children should not exceed 2.5 mg/kg bodyweight and day (Nawrot *et al.* 2003). This is slightly contrary to the European Food

Safety Authority (2015a) recommendations mentioned earlier. Studies have indicated that elderly people with a depleted enzymatic system do not tolerate coffee with caffeine well, while moderate amounts of caffeine of 50–100 mg a day are most often tolerated (Zivković 2000).

The negative effects of caffeine tend to emerge after excessive drinking and not when used in moderation. There are caveats, in that most studies about the health benefits and risks of caffeine are from prospective studies in which self-reported consumption of beverages and foods are linked to health outcomes. Such studies make it difficult to identify caffeine itself as the causative agent and to exclude residual confounding by other compounds in the food or beverage.

Some people are more sensitive to caffeine than others are, and even small amounts may prompt unwanted effects, such as restlessness and sleep disturbances. People who do not regularly drink caffeine tend to be more sensitive to its negative effects. There are some specific health concerns related to high caffeine consumption in children and pregnant females. Energy drinks pose a particular problem in that they are targeting young people and, especially when combined with alcohol, can exacerbate the harmful effects.

Concordance in risk opinion between experts and the public

As one of the most researched substances in the food supply, caffeine has a long history of safe use, and overwhelming scientific evidence maintains that when consumed in moderation, caffeine has few adverse health effects. Serious harm due to a caffeine overdose from consumption of traditional beverages is extremely rare, with only a few reported fatalities known globally. As a result, conflict between the expert view and public perception of risks posed by ingestion of traditional caffeinated food and beverages seems to be less pronounced than for many other substances covered in this book. Some debate persists as to whether the contemporary coffee culture is solely beneficial or somewhat troublesome for human health. Health-related news headlines often try to sensationalise coffee as either a caffeinated curse or a cure-all (Mizen 2014), but most consumers take little notice of warnings as evidenced by the continued popularity of coffee.

Even if governments would like to limit excessive caffeine consumption, they face a serious hurdle to do so. Since caffeine occurs naturally in two commonly consumed beverages – coffee and tea – it is exceedingly difficult to regulate their labelling or their permissible maximum levels. In addition, the regulation of caffeine has become difficult because coffee and tea are not always consumed on their own as they have been incorporated into hundreds of new food and beverage items. In addition, because of the varying amounts of caffeine consumed in each country, it is difficult to set an international standard.

The use of caffeine as a food ingredient has been approved, within certain limits, by numerous regulatory agencies around the world, as a safe dietary ingredient for use mainly in carbonated beverages and dietary supplements. Energy drinks have been treated as a special case. The known and unknown pharmacology of agents included in such drinks, combined with reports of toxicity, raises concern for potentially serious adverse effects in association with energy drink use. Several countries and states have debated or restricted energy drink sales and advertising based on expert opinions of their potential for harm. Several experts assessing the possible health risks of energy drinks have concluded that harm can result from high consumption, especially if the products are consumed in conjunction with strenuous physical activity, such as sport or all-night dancing, or together with alcoholic drinks (Lindtner *et al.* 2013; Breda *et al.* 2014). The warnings are not reflected in the public perception among young people, as energy drinks have quickly become a central part of dance subcultures. The full impact of the rise in popularity of energy drinks has not yet been quantified, but the aggressive marketing of energy drinks targeted at young people combined with limited and varied regulation have created an environment where energy drinks could pose a significant threat to public health.

Conclusion

There is a long history of use of caffeine-containing beverages, with caffeine being the most commonly ingested psychoactive stimulant in the world. Its widespread natural occurrence in a variety of plants undeniably plays a major role in its recognition. The most commonly consumed caffeinated beverages, coffee and tea, are often consumed in a socio-cultural context. Coffeehouses served as social gathering points that in the past were seen as threatening the political power base and were even banned in some countries. However, most attempts to limit the consumption of caffeine-containing beverages failed, and coffee and tea now occupy a significant place in the national cultures of most nations of the world.

There are good reasons to consume caffeinated beverages, and there are a few reasons not to. From reporting of mainly negative health effects in the past, new findings point to potential beneficial effects of moderate coffee consumption. On the beneficial side, caffeine enhances alertness and mood, and increases performance. It has even been suggested that caffeine consumption could help ease cognitive decline, lower the risk of developing Alzheimer's disease and ease symptoms of Parkinson's disease. On the downside, caffeine may aggravate pre-existing conditions such as migraine, heart arrhythmias and cause sleep disturbances. It can also contribute to anxiety and panic attacks, especially in high doses and in those with pre-existing anxiety disorder. Concerned about potential side effects of caffeine, official authorities in several countries recommend that daily consumption should be limited to 400 mg for adults and 200 mg for pregnant females, equivalent to four to five cups of coffee for adults in general and half that for pregnant females. However, in contemporary fast-moving society there is rarely time to consider the benefits and risks associated with the food and beverages consumed, with potential risks posed by excessive caffeine consumption usually neglected.

Although science seems to point to individual sensitivities and little general societal risk, the custom and tradition in many countries to drink coffee as a social activity – to meet for coffee – encourages increased caffeine intake. Similarly, from a socio-cultural risk discourse perspective, young people might incite friends to consume energy drinks with added alcohol during parties. The appearance of soft drinks and energy drinks with added caffeine is a relatively new phenomenon. It is of particular concern to official authorities, since the effects of caffeine use on behaviour and the physiology of young people remain poorly understood. Reports of caffeine toxicity and deaths among young people and adults following extreme energy drink consumption reflect the potential dangers of excess caffeine exposure.

Overall, in trying to determine the balance between risks and benefits of caffeine intake, a consensus in the medical community seems to be that moderate regular consumption in healthy individuals is essentially benign or mildly beneficial. Nonetheless, the findings about caffeine's influence on human beings are not agreed and are still under discussion, with research continuing to explore concerns with high consumption in particular.

5   Alcohol consumption and the socio-cultural risk discourse

Introduction

The socio-cultural risk discourse focuses on social, cultural and religious traditions developed over many centuries, giving beverages, such as caffeinated and alcoholic drinks, individual significance in diverse societal settings and historical periods (Douglas 1966; Douglas and Wildavsky 1982). The nomination of caffeinated drinks as a low risk beverage, in the previous chapter, does not pertain to alcoholic drinks, which have a much higher risk profile, except when consumed in low volumes. The use of alcoholic drinks has a long tradition within numerous societies' socio-cultural environment and has an equally long history of being linked to health concerns within the public health domain. Alcohol is a social drink enjoyed during cultural, festive and social settings, but it is also a powerful poison if consumed in large quantities.

Alcohol is a psychoactive substance with dependence-producing properties that, at moderate consumption levels, can be beneficial to health but is harmful at higher levels. For a liquid to be classified as an alcoholic beverage it should typically contain between 3 per cent and 60 per cent ethanol, commonly known as ethyl alcohol or simply alcohol. Traditionally, alcoholic beverages are divided into three drink classes: beers, wines and spirits (distilled beverages), each with its own socio-cultural customs and social status. The different classes of drink are more or less widely consumed by adults' worldwide. Historically alcohol has been prescribed medicinally, as is documented in texts throughout the written history. For example, alcohol's medicinal properties are mentioned 191 times in the Old and New Testaments (Ford 1988).

The adult population commonly drink alcoholic drinks at low risk levels most of the time or abstain altogether, but there is a broad range of alcohol consumption patterns, with extremes of daily heavy drinking or occasional risky drinking causing significant risks to public health and safety. Harmful effects caused by alcohol consumption include toxic effects on organs and tissues, intoxication leading to impairment of physical coordination, consciousness, cognition and perception, and behavioural changes. In addition to physical and mental harm, alcohol consumption can also have socio-economic consequences (World Health Organization 2014c).

However, in a report to the European Commission, the authors pointed out that the dominance of problem-oriented perspectives has led to a serious imbalance in the study of alcohol, whereby problems affecting only a small minority of drinkers have received disproportionate attention, while the study of normal drinking has been neglected (The Social Issues Research Centre 1998). It is documented that, historically, alcohol consumption was most commonly associated with cultural celebrations and festive occasions, and as such had, and still has, a significant social and cultural role in contemporary society. Indulgences of alcoholic beverages have a long human history, and in the main they provide vital opportunities for social bonding (Becker 1963). Alcohol consumption is possibly inspired by the observation of animals becoming drunk when gorging on fermented fruits and becoming docile.

Next to breathing, drinking is more important than ingestion of food, as we will die of thirst long before we perish from starvation. Access to liquids played a major role when our ancestors ventured across the globe by following rivers and lakes. Finding a water source in times of drought was an occasion for celebration, and social drinking rituals were born (The Social Issues Research Centre 1998). Although water could be made special by incantations that converted it into a sacred liquid, it was still just water. Until the invention of alcoholic drinks through fermentation of fruit juices, the only alternatives to water were milk, fresh plant juices and blood (The Social Issues Research Centre 1998).

Alcohol has played a central role as an intoxicating substance in almost all human cultures since Neolithic times, the last stage of the Stone Age some 10,000 years ago at the dawn of agriculture. The oldest kinds of alcoholic drinks were beer and wine, with beverage residues on drinking implements found in tombs and settlements of early civilisations (Patrick 1952). It is commonly argued that the introduction of cereal agriculture made it possible to invent beer (Katz and Voigt 1987). Figs, dates and grapes were used to make wine (Cavalieri *et al.* 2003). Chemical analyses of ancient organic material absorbed into pottery jars from the early Neolithic village of Jiahu in Henan province in China revealed that a mixed fermented beverage of rice, honey and fruit was being produced as early as 6500–7000 BC (McGovern *et al.* 2004).

Humans have consumed alcoholic beverages since prehistoric times for a variety of hygienic, dietary, medicinal, religious and recreational reasons (Lucia 1963). It seems to be general agreement that the conditions for refining the fermentation process existed mainly in the southerly regions of the Northern Hemisphere between the eighth and fourth millennia BC, hence among the very early Bronze Age cultures of the Eastern Mediterranean and Mesopotamian societies. Based on artefacts from this period, there is a consensus that it was beer production, rather than wine or other beverages, which provided the earliest source of freely available alcoholic drinks (Rudgley 1994). There is evidence that ancient Egyptians brewed beer from cereals, but also made different varieties of wine from pomegranates about

5,000 years ago. They made at least 17 types of beer and 24 varieties of wine (Ghaliouqui 1979).

The first documentary evidence of alcoholic beverages, written in Sumerian around 3200 BC, describes beer rather than wine production, as evidenced by an outline of a clay vessel marked with short, diagonal lines symbolising beer. While wine production dates back to about 3000 BC, it seems clear that beer remained the most popular drink and featured centrally in temple rituals for nearly 2,000 years (Mandelbaum 1965). However, wine was the favourite alcoholic drink in what are now Italy, Spain and France. It became the primary alcoholic beverage in much of Europe from the first century AD. Alcohol was also central to Viking culture and their heaven was conceived as a place where they could drink endless quantities of mead, a drink made from honey and water, which is regarded as the ancestor of all fermented beverages. Mead, beer and wild fruit wines became increasingly popular, especially among Celts, Anglo-Saxons, Germans and Scandinavians (Babor 1986).

Monasteries developed as the central place for maintaining and advancing the knowledge of brewing and winemaking techniques, and monks carefully guarded their knowledge. Monks brewed virtually all beer of good quality until the twelfth century (Cherrington 1925–1930). Although the Alexandrian Greeks knew how to make distilled spirits at the beginning of the Christian era, production of such beverages did not occur to any significant extent in Europe until the twelfth century. Knowledge of the process of distillation began to spread slowly among monks, physicians and alchemists, who were interested in distilled alcohol as a cure for ailments (Hanson 1995). Many legendary distilled spirits still carry the name of the monasteries, where the spirits were developed.

Alcohol as an enabler of social interaction

In societies where alcoholic drinks are part of the social and cultural environment, reciprocal giving of alcohol is at the heart of the process by which essential social, economic and political networks are constructed and maintained. Cross-cultural research indicates that alcohol was frequently used as an important social artefact, and alcoholic drinks play an integral part in creating social relationships, which are presented or demonstrated during social events and through hospitality during business meetings (Dietler 1990). Drinking in the twenty-first century meets largely similar individual, collective and cultural needs to those experienced in ancient times. Since the earliest use of alcohol, drinking has been a social act together with friends, and used to manifest partnership and business transactions. Research indicates the early use of alcohol consumption and its integration into the core systems of myths and ritual practices within emergent cultures. These cultural traditions and rules prescribed the use of alcohol for social and ceremonial functions and proscribed continuous or excessive inebriation (The Social Issues Research Centre 1998).

Alcohol is a substance that is habitually shared, as almost all drinking rituals and etiquettes involve communal consumption. In contrast, solitary drinking is frowned upon and seen as an indication of an individual having a problem with alcohol. Mandelbaum (1965:282) stated that: 'Drinking together generally symbolizes durable social solidarity – or at least amity – among those who share a drink'. In the past, people not only drank together, but also often drank from the same vessel. Ancient Egyptian pictures show a single pot with long straws for communal drinking. In Bolivia, the practice of the Camba tribe is drinking from the same glass, as it is in the Republic of Georgia where it is called 'megobarebi', which is translated as 'close friends' (Heath 1958; Mars and Altman 1987). Even where separate cups are used, sharing is prescribed. Among the Lele people of Zaire, drunkenness is disapproved of because it indicates drinking alone and too much, without sharing. Virtually all of the known ritual practices and etiquettes associated with drinking are specifically designed to promote social interaction and social bonding (Ngokwey 1987).

In many cultures, alcohol is shared not only with fellow drinkers, but also with the gods and with the dead. A typical example is the Christian tradition of communion, where wine is symbolising the blood of Christ. At Navajo Indian gatherings, drinking begins when one of the older men produces a bottle of wine and pours the first drop as an offering to Mother Earth, before taking a drink and passing the bottle on. The drinking is brought to a close when the last drop is again presented to Mother Earth (Topper 1985). Hispanic youth gangs in New York pour a drop from their bottles on the ground before drinking, to honour their dead 'Brothers', while Hungarian Roma gather around family graves on All Souls' Day to share drinks with the departed (Stewart 1992).

Social and cultural customs regulate drinking of alcohol in most societies. Informal rules governing drinking stipulate not only that alcohol should be consumed in a social context and shared, but that this sharing should be conducted in a friendly manner, with frequent expressions of goodwill and amity between participants. The practice of toasting is observed in some form in most cultures, from a simple salute at the start of drinking to settings where any sip of a drink is done only after elaborate and inventive toasts (The Social Issues Research Centre 1998).

Alcoholic beverages as a means to classify a social class or occasion

As humans, we feel comfortable following known customs and rituals. Almost every event of any significance in our lives is marked with some sort of ceremony or celebration with many of these rituals involving alcohol. Major life cycle events such as birth, coming-of-age, graduation, marriage, retirement and death all require ritual endorsements. The events serve to facilitate and enhance the change from one social, cultural, religious, physical and economic stage to the next. Alcohol or a festive drink is in most cultures a central element of such rituals.

In American as well as in the Australian culture, alcohol is commonly served as a transition from work to free time (Gusfield 1987; Fabiansson 2010). However, such a symbolic meaning of alcohol can vary and can traditionally even serve the opposite purpose, as in some cultures the stop off at the pub on the way to work, home, or to 're-fuel' at lunchtime, is just as common. The stop at the bar, café or pub for a glass of wine on the way to work is a longstanding tradition in France; it is also widely practised in Spain (Rooney 1991). In Andalucía, it can include having an anisette or a cognac with a cup of coffee (Driessen 1992) and in Denmark a Gammel Dansk to the breakfast meal. In Peru, alcohol is consumed before any work requiring strength or energy, such as roofing, sowing and other tasks that are seen to require particular collaboration or supernatural intervention and thus use alcohol to get invigorated (Harvey, 1994). The symbolic meaning of these pre- and post-work drinking rituals may be quite explicitly ingrained into people's everyday behaviour.

The social and cultural settings of alcohol drinking are further structured in accordance with the type of alcohol served, especially when more than one type of alcoholic beverage is available. Alcoholic beverages are classified in terms of their social meaning, and the type of drink indicates the drinker's social status and professional position in the social world. Few alcoholic beverages are socially neutral, as serving alcohol is traditionally a symbolic vehicle for identifying, describing, constructing and manipulating cultural systems, values, interpersonal relationships, behavioural norms and expectations. In this respect, each individual alcoholic beverage serves a particular purpose.

An American survey examined perceptions of the appropriate setting for various types of alcoholic beverages. The researchers found that wine, but not spirits or beer, was considered an appropriate accompaniment to a meal, while wine and spirits, but not beer, were suitable for celebratory events, and finally beer was the most proper drink for informal occasions designed for relaxation (Klein 1991). In France, with the more established heritage of traditional practices, an aperitif is drunk before the meal, white wine is served before red, and brandy is served only at the end of the meal (Nahoum-Grappe 1995). Among Hungarian Roma, equally strict rules apply to brandy as it may only be consumed first thing in the morning, during the middle of the night at a wake, or by females prior to going on a rubbish scavenging trip. It would be regarded as highly inappropriate to serve or drink brandy outside any of these specific situational contexts (Stewart 1992).

Traditionally, the choice of beverage has become a significant indicator of social status. In general terms, beverages imported to the country have a higher status than local varieties. Preference for high-status beverages may also be a manifestation of aspiration, rather than a reflection of actual position in the social hierarchy. In Poland, wine is regarded as a high status, middle class beverage, while native beer and vodka belong to the working class. Consequently, Polish university students have been found to drink eight times as much wine as their American counterparts, hence reinforcing their university status as distinctive (Engs *et al.* 1991). In France, by contrast, where wine drinking is commonplace and confers no special status, the young elite is turning to imported beers (Nahoum-Grappe 1995).

Furthermore, the choice of beverage may also be a statement of affiliation, a declaration of belonging to a particular group, class, tribe or nation and its associated values, attitudes and beliefs with certain drinks becoming symbols of national identity (Douglas 1966; Douglas and Wildavsky 1982). Guinness is indispensable for the Irish, tequila for Mexicans, vodka for Russians and ouzo for Greeks. These symbols are often linked to idealised or romanticised images of the national character, culture and way of life. For Scottish Highlanders, whisky represents traditional values of egalitarianism, generosity and virility, and to refuse a dram may be seen as a rejection of these values (Macdonald 1994).

Beneficial or harmful effects of individual alcohol consumption

Worldwide per capita consumption of alcoholic beverages in 2010 equalled 6.2 litres of pure alcohol consumed by every person aged 15 years or older, which is equivalent to 13.5 grams of pure alcohol per day (World Health Organization 2014c). Almost a quarter of the alcohol consumed across the world, or 1.5 litres per capita, has been estimated by the WHO to comprise of homemade or unlawfully produced alcohol, hence mainly unrecorded alcohol. The consumption of homemade or unregulated produced alcohol may be associated with an increased risk of harm, because of unknown and potentially dangerous impurities or contaminants in these beverages (Ostapenko and Elkis 2010).

As expected, there exists a large variation in adult per capita consumption. Almost half of the global adult population has never consumed alcohol. The highest consumption levels can be found in the developed world, mostly the Northern Hemisphere, but also in Argentina, Australia and New Zealand. Moderate consumption levels can be found in southern Africa, with Namibia and South Africa having the highest levels, and in North and South America. Low consumption levels can be found in the countries of North Africa and sub-Saharan Africa, the Eastern Mediterranean, southern Asia and the Indian Ocean (WHO 2014c). These latter regions represent large populations of the Islamic faith, which have very high rates of abstention.

Some religions prohibit, discourage, or restrict the production, sale and consumption of alcoholic beverages for various reasons, including Buddhism, Islam, Jainism, the Rastafari movement, the Bahá'í Faith, and various branches of Christianity, such as the Baptists, the Church of God in Christ, Methodists, the Latter-day Saints, Seventh Day Adventists and the Iglesia ni Cristo (Gudorf 2013). Thus a number of abstemious Christian denominations and sects, especially in the United States, have made abstinence a fundamental tenet for their followers. Jews disapprove of alcoholic beverages, but do not totally forbid them. In reality, wine is a very important element in their ceremonial celebrations and feasts, leading to an interesting socio-cultural phenomenon in which people with the highest proportion of drinkers exhibits one of the lowest rates of alcoholism or other alcohol related problems. The historical encouragement of abstinence in Islamic culture is based in the belief that central Muslim values and ideas of community negate the grounds for a requirement to use alcohol (European Parliament 1996).

Although forbidden to everybody in many Muslim countries, irrespective of personal faith, particularly in the societies of Iran, Saudi Arabia, Libya and Pakistan, where alcohol consumption is legally banned, drinking still occurs. Here, alcoholic beverage consumption consists almost exclusively of what the WHO classifies as unrecorded alcohol (World Health Organization 2014c). In the societies of Lebanon, Turkey, Indonesia, Malaysia and Egypt, it is legal to consume alcohol in both the private and public sphere.

Recorded alcohol consumption is augmenting worldwide. This trend is mainly driven by an increased consumption in China and India, which could potentially be linked to active marketing by the alcohol industry, but also to a growing middle class with increased income in these countries to spend on nonessential items. In most other societies, alcohol consumption is stable or decreasing slightly (World Health Organization 2014c).

Research demonstrates a link between excessive alcohol consumption and an increase in global mortality and morbidity. Alcohol has neurotoxic, hepatotoxic and carcinogenic properties, which makes it a potent risk factor for a variety of diseases. The effect on the human body and mind is significant, even at relatively low doses that are not necessarily harmful (Eckardt *et al.* 1998). Overall, about 3.3 million deaths in 2012 were estimated to have been caused by alcohol consumption. This corresponds to 5.9 per cent of all deaths caused by an identifiable cause, excluding natural and old age deaths. The highest numbers of deaths were from cardiovascular diseases, followed by injuries, liver cirrhosis and cancers (World Health Organization 2014c). However, alcohol consumption is not only a personal health, social and cultural problem, but a serious societal and economic issue, where heavy drinking is related to lost working hours, family violence, criminal behaviour, brawls in public places and dangerous driving (Leonard 2001).

Although public health messages most often focus on the hazards of consuming alcoholic beverages, there are both good and bad sides to this as the issue is not black and white. Alcohol consumption at the low-risk levels practiced by adults in most countries can actually be beneficial to health and, as a cultural facilitator, improve human interaction and social wellbeing. Much discussion has revolved around the diverse findings on the complex relationship between alcohol consumption and ischemic heart disease, the leading cause of death and disability. Research indicates that some alcoholic beverages consumed in moderation can actually protect against heart disease and obesity, increase the beneficial high-density lipoprotein (HDL) cholesterol and lower the detrimental low-density lipoprotein (LDL) cholesterol, and help reverse cellular damage and thus help reduce cancer risks (Saremi and Arora 2008).

Research demonstrates strong and consistent relationships between moderate alcohol consumption and reduction in cardiovascular disease in general, and coronary artery disease in particular (Moore and Pearson 1986; Roerecke and Rehm 2014). Substantial evidence has shown that alcohol consumption as such in moderation can lower the levels of fibrinogen and other prothrombotic factors, as well as lowering fibrinolytic potential and antiplatelet activity. Thus, studies have found that survivors of acute myocardial infarction who drink moderately have a risk of death approximately 20–30 per cent lower than abstainers or rare drinkers (Mukamal 2003). There is also evidence that low to moderate alcohol consumption is associated with decreased mortality compared to those who either abstain or drink heavily (Bellavia *et al.* 2014). However, for a minority of the population daily heavy drinking or occasional hazardous drinking or binge drinking can create significant public health and safety issues. Hazardous drinking can increase, for example, the risk of stroke and high blood pressure, while heavy drinking can trigger malnutrition, chronic pancreatitis, liver disease, cancer and damage to the central and peripheral nervous system (Cargiulo 2007; Rehm *et al.* 2009).

Even if only a minority drink heavily, it is nonetheless perturbing to see parts of the world population ignore explicit warnings about the dangers of high alcohol consumption. This situation is particularly related to young people, but it might not be because of lack of information, as there are multitudes of warnings easily available. The message is not getting through within the social and cultural environment young people at risk occupy. The scientific information is not communicated in a manner that makes young people take notice of the warnings. Binge drinking is more or less a youth tradition in some Western societies and a common growing up phase among partying young people, despite the concomitant risks to their health, and the alcohol-fuelled violence that threatens to damage friends, innocent bystanders and themselves.

Messages that moderate alcohol consumption in itself can benefit health and that some alcoholic beverages might even contain other substances beneficial to health seems to have become more widely acknowledged. Wine contains various polyphenolic substances, which may be beneficial to health and resveratrol, in particular, seems to have a positive effect on longevity (Giacosa *et al.* 2014). Beer contains numerous nutrients and polyphenolic antioxidants, which help reverse cellular damage and thus help reduce cancer risks. Whisky contains more beneficial ellagic acid, a natural phenol antioxidant, than any other type of alcohol. On the other hand, some fruit brandies in particular might contain high levels of ethyl carbamate, a genotoxic and carcinogenic compound, in addition to the ethanol itself. The following sections will discuss in more detail beneficial and harmful substances in alcoholic beverages.

Beneficial compounds in red wine

Beneficial effects of moderate alcohol intake against atherosclerosis have been attributed to its antioxidant and anti-inflammatory effects, as well as to its actions on vascular function. In this framework, part of these effects may be attributed to polyphenols mainly contained in wine and beer, as these compounds exhibit antioxidant (Vinson *et al* 2003), anti-carcinogenic (Ramos 2008), anti-inflammatory (Palmieri *et al.* 2011), hypotensive (Bhatt *et al.* 2011) and possibly anti-coagulant properties (Crescente *et al.* 2009).

The search for an understanding of health benefits of alcohol, paradoxically began in relation to French food habits. Despite a relatively high intake of saturated fats in parts of France, in an apparent contradiction to the widely held belief that high consumption of saturated fats is a risk factor for coronary heart disease, unexpectedly epidemiological results showed that in the wine districts of France, the population presented a relatively low incidence of cardiovascular disease and mortality. The 'French paradox' was a phrase coined in the late 1980s to summarise this apparently contradictory epidemiological observation (Simini 2000). If the link between saturated fats and coronary heart disease is valid, an additional factor or factors in the French diet or lifestyle must be responsible for mitigating this risk. It has been suggested that France's high red wine consumption could be the primary protective factor. In a seminal publication, researchers at Bordeaux University, in the middle of the famous wine district, compared age standardised annual mortality from coronary heart disease and related risk factors in some selected populations, including the French. The mean serum total cholesterol concentrations were similar in France, the USA and the UK. After further examination and statistical regression analysis between death rate from coronary heart disease and consumption of dairy fat and wine, the authors concluded that the French paradox might be caused by a high consumption of red wine (Renaud and de Lorgeril 1992).

Alcoholic beverages, specifically red wine, have since been shown to play a key role in the prevention of cardiovascular disease and other chronic pathologies, including cancer. Its regular and moderate consumption has been found in numerous epidemiological studies to correlate inversely with vascular disease and mortality, despite the presence of risk factors such as high consumption of saturated fats, elevated smoking and low physical activity. This phenomenon could possibly be explained by the high levels of phenolic compounds present in red wine, making it more advantageous than beer, spirits and even white wine. It has even been suggested that the habit of having one or two drinks of red wine every day with meals may translate to a longer, healthier and better quality of life (Cordova and Sumpio 2009).

Wine contains several hundred phenolic compounds that affect the taste, colour and mouth feel of wine. These compounds include phenolic acids, stilbenoids, flavonols, dihydroflavonols, anthocyanins, catechins and proanthocyanidins. Phenolic acids are largely present in the pulp, anthocyanins and stilbenoids in the skin, and catechins, proanthocyanidins and flavonols in the skin and the seeds of the grape (Kennedy *et al.* 2002). In searching for compounds that could explain the red wine paradox, scientists initially focused on a stilbenoid called resveratrol (Liu *et al.* 2007). Red wine contains between 0.2 and 5.8 mg/L of resveratrol, depending on the grape variety, while white wine has much less. This is because red wine is fermented with the skin, allowing the wine to extract the resveratrol, while white wine is fermented after the skin has been removed. The skin itself contains 50–100 mg/kg of resveratrol (Gu *et al.* 1999).

Research now suggests that resveratrol may possess a range of health benefits including anti-cancer effects, anti-inflammatory effects, cardiovascular benefits, anti-diabetes potential, energy endurance enhancement and protection against Alzheimer's disease (Guerrero *et al.* 2009; Li *et al.* 2012). Although moderate alcohol consumption has been consistently associated with 20–30 per cent reductions in coronary heart disease risk, it is not yet clear whether the amounts of resveratrol in red wine is sufficiently high to provide any further risk reduction. It is true that resveratrol can inhibit growth of cancer cells in a culture and in some animal models, but it is not known whether it can prevent cancer in humans (Latruffe and Rifler 2013). Whereas resveratrol administration has increased the life span of yeast, worms, fruit flies, fish and mice fed a high calorie diet, currently, relatively little is known about the actual effects of resveratrol in humans. Although research continues on resveratrol, the concentration in wine seems too low to alone account for the French paradox (Tomé-Carneiro *et al.* 2013).

Unlike resveratrol, another group of polyphenols called procyanidins are present in wine in quantities that seem to be high enough to be significant. They are the most abundant flavonoid polyphenols in red wine with around 260 mg/L found in some traditional style red wines (Hammerstone *et al.* 2000). It is believed that they offer the greatest degree of protection to human blood vessel cells. Tests with 165 wines showed that the highest concentration of procyanidins are found in red wines from the Tannat grape, grown in the Gers area of southwest France, which correlates with longevity in those regions (Corder *et al.* 2006). However, the exact mechanism responsible for the beneficial health effects of moderate red wine consumption is still elusive. The health benefits may be attributed to the overall mix of the different components and not to a specific effect of one. It might also be plausible that the versatile bioactivities exhibited by polyphenols, beyond being mere antioxidant substances, contribute to the health benefits (Arranz 2012).

Beneficial compounds in beer

Beer, a beverage with a low alcohol level, is the most consumed type of alcoholic beverage in the world (Kondo 2004). Beer drinking in moderation can be a healthier beverage choice than soft drinks or sugary fruit cocktails as beer is produced with ingredients like hops, brewer's yeast, barley and malt.

Beer is thus a source of numerous nutrients (Kratky and Buiatti 2008). It has a high concentration of B vitamins like niacin, pantothenic acid, folate, riboflavin, pyridoxine and cyanocobolamin, although bioavailability might be low for some as the alcohol inhibits their absorption. The folate found in beer may help to reduce homocysteine in the blood, hence create a lower risk of cardiovascular disease (Mayer *et al.* 2001).

Beer, depending on country and brand, can contain 200–450 mg/L of potassium, 25–120 mg/L of calcium and 90–400 mg/L of phosphorus, all minerals that are essential to a healthy diet (Buiatti 2009). It is also rich in silicon, an important nutrient for bone growth and development. A 2010 study by scientists at the University of California's Department of Food Science and Technology suggested that drinking beer moderately might ward off osteoporosis due to the beneficial impact of the silicon nutrient (Casey and Bamforth 2010).

One of the most effective forms of soluble fibre for lowering cholesterol is betaglucan, which is the predominant form of fibre in beer. Beer contains around 2 g/L of soluble fibre. A bottle containing 350 mL of beer is equivalent to approximately 10 per cent of the recommended daily fibre intake (Goñi *et al.* 2009). Beers with high malt content like craft beers may even provide up to 30 per cent of the recommended daily fibre intake.

Research suggests that some specific components in beer may play a role in fending off disease. Beer contains polyphenolic antioxidants, mainly from hops, which help reverse cellular damage and thus help reduce cancer risks. Dark beers tend to have the most antioxidants. Most of the hops' polyphenols are made up of higher molecular weight compounds, such as tannins. Only about 20 per cent of the hops' polyphenols consist of low molecular substances like catechin or proanthocyanidins, phenolic carbon acids and flavonols. Even resveratrol can be detected in hops, but at very low concentrations. Hops prove to be a rich source of prenylated polyphenols of which xanthohumol is the most important at concentrations of 0.1–1.1 per cent dry weight. Studies suggest that xanthohumol may be one of the more important compounds that help prevent cancer (Goto *et al.* 2005). Unfortunately, during wort boiling, much of this is converted to isoxanthohumol, a less biologically active compound, leaving 0.15 mg/L of xanthohumol in conventional pale beers versus up to 3.44 mg/L of isoxanthohumol (Stevens *et al.* 1999). This is not a sufficiently high level of xanthohumol to be pharmacologically active (Liu *et al.* 2015). However, a high xanthohumol level of 10 mg/L or more can be found in microbrews made with more hops and dark roasted malts and there are attempts to increase the xanthohumol levels in beer even further (Wunderlich *et al.* 2005). As with wine, the overall mix of polyphenolic antioxidants found in beer might be responsible for the beneficial health effects identified in the studies referred to below and not to the specific action of one.

In a meta-study published in 2011, researchers at Italy's Fondazione di Ricerca e Cura reviewed 16 previous studies, which involved more than 200,000 participants. They found that people who drank about 500 mL of beer a day had a 31 per cent reduced risk of heart disease. However, consuming a larger quantity of alcohol from beer, wine or liquor reversed the benefit (Costanzo *et al.* 2011).

A 2011 Harvard study of 38,000 middle-aged males showed that consuming one or two glasses of beer a day reduced the risk of developing type 2 diabetes by 25 per cent. There was, however, no noted benefit from drinking more than two beers a day (Joosten *et al.* 2011).

A 2005 study involving 11,000 mature-aged females showed that those who had one beer a day had better mental function than those who did not drink beer. The beer drinkers reduced their risk of mental decline by as much as 20 per cent (Stampfer *et al.* 2005). Additionally, an Emory University study published in 2001 involving over 2,200 senior males and females discovered that those who consumed at least 1.5 drinks daily had up to a 50 per cent lesser risk of suffering from heart failure (Abramson *et al.* 2001). The studies indicate that one beer per day could be beneficial; however, drinking a week's supply of seven beers in one day would not.

Beneficial effects of spirits

In research on the health benefits of spirits, the concentrations of 11 phenolic compounds and the total antioxidant status were measured in 12 types of distilled spirits (Goldberg *et al.* 1999). Ellagic acid was the polyphenol that was present in the highest concentration in all beverages. Moderate amounts of syringaldehyde, syringic acid and gallic acid, as well as lesser amounts of vanillin and vanillic acid, were measurable in most samples of whisky, brandy and rum, but were largely undetectable in gin, vodka, liqueurs and some less common spirits. The highest total antioxidant activities were found in armagnac, cognac and bourbon, all three of which tended toward the highest concentrations of phenolic compounds.

Ellagic acid is a natural phenolic antioxidant found in numerous fruits and vegetables. It is believed that phytochemicals such as ellagic acid function either by countering the negative effects of oxidative stress by directly acting as an antioxidant or by activating/inducing cellular antioxidant enzyme systems (Vattem and Shetty 2005). The highest levels of ellagic acid are found in blackberries, cranberries, pecans, pomegranates, raspberries, strawberries, walnuts, wolfberries and grapes. Ellagic acid is also found in oak species, like the North American white oak and European red oak. Wood aging is the most likely source of phenolic compounds in distilled spirits. Those beverages exposed to this treatment contain significant antioxidant activity, which are between the ranges for white and red wines. Armagnac contained 30.7 mg/L of ellagic acid, cognac 14.8 mg/L, American bourbon 11.6 mg/L and Scotch whisky between 5 and 10 mg/L (Goldberg *et al.* 1999).

Ellagic acid has been shown to have anti-proliferative and antioxidant properties in a number of in vitro and small animal models (Devipriya *et al.* 2007). The anti-proliferative properties of ellagic acid may be due to its ability directly to inhibit the DNA-binding of certain carcinogens, including nitrosamines and polycyclic aromatic hydrocarbons (Mandal and Stoner 1990). As with other polyphenol antioxidants, ellagic acid has a chemoprotective effect in cellular models by reducing oxidative stress. However, since the high alcoholic content of distilled spirits by itself can generate free radicals, cause severe membrane damage and affect almost all organs of the human body, the antioxidant and cytoprotective properties of ellagic acid in combination with the mix of antioxidants in the spirits might not be sufficient to counterbalance the oxidative stress induced by the alcohol. The question of whether or not distilled spirits are harmful is still to be resolved.

Ethyl carbamate

Not all substances found in alcoholic beverages have beneficial effects. Ethyl carbamate is a chemical formed naturally during fermentation of food and beverages. It is commonly found in stone fruit brandies, but also at much lower levels in other spirits, wine and beer, as well as in bread, soy sauce and yoghurt. During food processing and storage hydrocyanic acid, urea and ethanol act as precursors to the formation of ethyl carbamate. In stone fruit spirits, ethyl carbamate is formed when compounds in the stones are degraded to cyanate that reacts with the ethanol. Another source of ethyl carbamate is urea, resulting from the degradation of the amino acid arginine by yeasts during fermentation, which in turn reacts with ethanol (Lachenmeier 2005b; Schehl *et al.* 2007).

Although there is an extensive literature dating back to the 1940s on the genotoxicity and carcinogenicity of ethyl carbamate in industrial settings, public health concerns related to its detection in food and beverages were only raised in 1985, when relatively high levels were found in some alcoholic beverages by Canadian authorities (Dennis *et al.* 1989; Zimmerli and Schlatter 1991). In 1989, the California Department of Health Services (Salmon *et al.* 1991) undertook major reviews of the available carcinogenicity data. It is now generally accepted that ethyl carbamate is a genotoxic carcinogen in animals and probably can cause cancer in humans (International Agency for Research on Cancer 2010).

The European Food Safety Authority (2007), in reviewing ethyl carbamate in alcoholic beverages, found median levels of up to 5 µg/L for beer and wine, 21 µg/L for spirits other than fruit brandy, and 260 µg/L for fruit brandy. Exposure to ethyl carbamate was estimated to be close to 4 µg/person per day in general and a high of 33 µg/person per day when consuming fruit brandy as the main alcoholic drink. Based on the exposure estimates and animal cancer data, the European Food Safety Authority concluded that ethyl carbamate in alcoholic beverages indicates a health concern, particularly with respect to stone fruit brandies. For consumers of particular brands of spirits made from cyanogenic plants, like Brazilian cachaça from sugarcanes and Serbian šljivovica from Damson plums with higher than average levels of ethyl carbamate, the risk could be considerable.

The commercial spirit industry has mostly adopted available mitigation methods to limit the formation of ethyl carbamate. As an example, in 1988 wine and other alcoholic beverage manufacturers in the United States agreed to control the level of ethyl carbamate in wine and in drinks with higher alcohol content. However, cottage production of stone fruit brandies is a hobby for many people and the awareness of the mitigation methods might not have filtered through to the home brewing public and the small-scale producer. Pilot studies in Lithuania, Hungary and Poland, as well as follow-up studies in 16 European countries and Brazil pointed to several possible problems related to ethyl carbamate contamination in home produced fruit spirits (Lachenmeier *et al.* 2009a; Lachenmeier *et al.* 2007; Lachenmeier *et al.* 2009b; Lachenmeier *et al.* 2011; Lachenmeier *et al.* 2010). Past risk assessments have probably considerably underestimated ethyl carbamate exposure, especially from traditional fruit spirit producing countries, such as Hungary, Austria, Romania and Slovenia (Lachenmeier *et al.* 2005).

The downside of alcohol consumption

One common downside of alcohol consumption is an increased energy intake. Alcoholic beverages of all sorts have a high energy content with alcohol containing almost as much energy as fat – 27 kJ/g or 6 kcal/g for alcohol compared to 37 kJ/g or 9 kcal/g for fat. One standard drink contains 10 g of alcohol, equal to at least 270 kJ or 64 kcal, as alcoholic drinks also contain varying amounts of carbohydrates, which contributes to extra energy. A full strength can of beer (355–375 mL) provides about 550 kJ or 131 kcal, while a standard restaurant glass of wine of 150 mL provides about 440kJ or 105 kcal. Spirits contain an average of 40 per cent alcohol, which correspond to 270 kJ or 64 kcal for a standard serve of 30 mL (Furlong 2011). On a volume basis, spirits contain more energy than beer and wine. However, a typical serving of beer is several times the size of a serving of whisky. By that measure, 'a standard serving of beer' has more energy than 'a whisky', while 'a glass of wine' is in the middle.

The average alcohol consumption by adults is equivalent to around 10 per cent of the total daily energy intake in several developed countries. The role of alcohol energy in body weight control has been studied by using three different approaches: epidemiology (alcohol intake and body weight), psycho-physiologic investigations (alcohol and appetite regulation) and metabolic studies (effects of alcohol intake on energy expenditure and substrate oxidation). Epidemiologic evidence does not show a clear relation between daily alcohol energy intake and body weight. However, most studies report that people do not compensate for the alcohol energy by decreasing non-alcoholic food energy intake. Except in alcoholics, alcohol energy is usually added to total food energy intake. Therefore, moderate alcohol drinkers tend to have a higher energy intake than non-drinkers (Westerterp-Plantenga and Verwegen 1999). However, young adults who attempt to achieve a 'healthy lifestyle' have been shown to make trade-offs between the food and alcohol they consume, and the amounts of physical activity they undertake (Giles and Brennan 2014).

There are, of course, much more serious social and toxic risk effects of alcohol, if consumed in excess, than an increased body weight. The degree of risk of harmful use of alcohol varies with age, gender and other biological characteristics of the consumer. Harmful drinking is a major determinant for neuropsychiatric disorders, such as alcohol use disorders and epilepsy, and diseases such as cardiovascular diseases, cirrhosis of the liver and various cancers (Shield *et al.* 2013). Drinking of alcohol at risky levels can also have serious social and economic consequences for individuals other than the drinker and for the society as a whole (Sacks *et al.* 2013). Sudden cessation of long term, extensive alcohol consumption is likely to produce withdrawal symptoms, including severe anxiety, tremors, hallucinations and convulsions.

Risky levels of alcohol consumption contribute to a significant proportion of the societal disease burden. For example, alcohol consumption at socially and physically inhibiting levels can be attributed to unintentional and intentional injuries, including those due to road traffic accidents, violence and suicides (Rehm *et al.* 2003). Fatal injuries attributed to alcohol consumption tend to occur in relatively young age groups (Zador *et al.* 2000). It has been estimated that more than 300,000 young people between the age of 15 and 29 die from alcohol related causes per year. This corresponds to nine per cent of all deaths in this age group (World Health Organization 2011a). Alcohol consumption also poses a risk to the wellbeing and health of people around the drinker. An intoxicated person can harm others through violent behaviour, or negatively affect co-workers, relatives and friends as well as strangers.

Harmful use of alcohol is a global problem, at both the individual and the societal level, where the social and cultural norms are violated. Additionally, it can cause harm to the unborn generation, as excessive alcohol consumption by an expectant female may cause foetal alcohol syndrome and pre-term birth complications, which are detrimental to the health and development of neonates (May *et al.* 2014). Beyond the immediate physical and mental health risks, a child growing up in a family with heavy alcohol consumption increases the risk for the child to experience neglect and abuse in the environment that can influence them throughout their adult life.

Binge drinking – drinking five or more drinks on one occasion for males or four or more drinks on one occasion for females – can increase the risk of many harmful health conditions. These include self-inflicted traffic injuries, falls, drowning, burns and unintentional firearm injuries (Smith *et al.* 1999). Violence affects others in the perpetrator's immediate surroundings, including intimate partner violence and child maltreatment. About 35 per cent of victim reports stated that the offender was under the influence of alcohol at the time of the abuse (Greenfield 1998).

Heavy drinking can harm the liver. In the liver, enzymes first convert alcohol into acetaldehyde. During this step, a molecule called NADH (nicotinamide adenine dinucleotide) is produced. Acetaldehyde is further metabolised into acetic acid, water and then carbon dioxide that is discharged through the individual's breath (Lieber 1998). People who drink daily will have elevated levels of NADH, which can lead to the accumulation of fat in the liver, a condition called fatty liver. A liver clogged with fat is not only less efficient in performing its duties, but it can reduce oxygen and nutrient access for the liver cells. Left untreated, this causes the liver cells to die and form fibrous scar tissue leading to liver cirrhosis (Tsochatzis *et al.* 2014) a leading cause of death among excessive alcohol drinkers (Heron 2007).

Over time, excessive alcohol use can lead to the development of several chronic diseases. These include neurological problems, including dementia, stroke and neuropathy (Corrao *et al.* 2002, 2004). Sometimes psychiatric problems can be seen, including depression, anxiety and suicide attempts (Castaneda *et al.* 1996). Cardiovascular problems are common, including myocardial infarction, cardiomyopathy, atrial fibrillation and hypertension (Rehm *et al.* 2003), as well as diseases like pancreatitis and gastritis (Lesher and Lee 1989; Kelly *et al.* 1995). In general, the risk of cancer increases with increasing amounts of alcohol. Typically, cancers of the mouth, throat, esophagus, liver, colon and breast have been associated with excessive alcohol consumption (Baan *et al.* 2007).

The most serious effect is alcohol poisoning with high blood alcohol levels suppressing the central nervous system and causing loss of consciousness, low blood pressure and body temperature, coma, respiratory depression and death (Sanap and Chapman 2003).

Restrictions on alcohol consumption

Public perceptions of the influence of alcoholic beverages on health and social wellbeing are derived from the individual's social and cultural environment. Customs around drinking of alcoholic drinks range from total abstention, due to cultural and religious considerations or general concerns about alcohol's devastating societal consequences, to unrestricted drinking under self-imposed social control. Judging from consumption patterns, moderate levels of drinking are adopted by a majority, albeit a minority appears to be impervious to health advice, as displayed by regular binge drinking occasions. Similarly, scientific conclusions are diverse, covering findings of beneficial health effects and facilitation of social interactions at moderate consumption levels to a harmful health impact and social disarray at abuse levels. A special case is the alcohol dependency syndrome or alcoholism that is universally seen as destructive for affected individuals and their families.

The magnitude and pattern of alcohol consumption are influenced by a variety of factors at the individual as well as the societal level. Economic development, culture, availability of alcohol, and the level and effectiveness of alcohol policies are pertinent factors in explaining differences in vulnerability between societies, historical trends in alcohol consumption, and alcohol related harm (Babor *et al.* 2010). The near universal rules of discouraging solitary drinking and favouring the sociability, sharing, and reciprocity of communal drinking provides a basis for a highly effective informal social control of drinking, in terms of both consumption and behaviour. These self-imposed protocols are considered to have a far greater effect on levels of consumption and drinking behaviour than any controls imposed by legislators and policy makers (The Social Issues Research Centre 1998).

The most consistent and widespread self-imposed protocol influencing alcohol consumption is the different customs by males and females. There is an informal convention that in the majority of societies alcohol is considered more suitable for males than females, and thus at least some informal restrictions on female drinking are found in most cultures (Heath 1995). Drinks considered suitable for females are often weaker, sweeter and softer than the hard liquors favoured by males (Papagaroufali 1992). It might be that restrictions on females' drinking originated as a purely pragmatic means of protecting the health of offspring, or it could be that, because of physiological differences, females need less alcohol to experience the same effects as males. However, this informal control seems to have partly broken down, with young females increasingly seen to be adopting binge-drinking behaviours (Smith and Foxcroft 2009). It has been shown that young females who engage in binge drinking are more likely to hold positive beliefs that they have fun by drinking excessively and that reducing inhibitions are a pleasant outcome of drinking (Johnston and White 2004).

Another informal, but stricter, form of alcohol avoidance is the voluntary teetotalism movement embracing the practice of complete personal abstinence from alcoholic beverages. The teetotalism movement was first started in Preston, England, in the early nineteenth century (Gately 2008). Later in that century an organisation now known as the International Organisation of Good Templars, or IOGT International, began as one of a number of fraternal organisations for temperance or total abstinence with a structure modelled on Freemasonry. It admitted males and females equally, and it made no distinction regarding ethnic belonging of the members. IOGT International is now the largest worldwide community of non-governmental organisations with a mission independently to enlighten people around the world about a lifestyle free from alcohol and other drugs (Blocker *et al.* 2003). Some common reasons for choosing teetotalism are psychological, religious, health, medical, familial, philosophical and social, or sometimes it is simply a matter of taste and preference. Religion is the most common reason for abstention. Other reasons for abstention are health consciousness in general or a medical history making alcohol consumption problematic. Some people are advised not to drink because they are taking certain medications or due to pregnancy.

People's social and cultural environment can both inhibit and facilitate excessive drinking of alcohol, as some people, independent of home environment, can have a healthy relationship with alcohol, others might succumb to alcoholism. Alcoholism is a broad term for compulsive and uncontrolled consumption of alcoholic beverages, usually to the detriment of the drinker's health, personal relationships and social standing. The World Health Organization estimates that there are 140 million people suffering negative effects of drinking alcohol worldwide, including people who have developed alcohol-derived diseases (Adewale and Ifudu 2014). Attitudes and social stereotypes can create barriers to the detection and treatment of alcoholism, perhaps more so for females, because of socio-cultural traditions that they should drink in moderation or not at all (Blum *et al.* 1998). Hence, fear of stigmatisation may lead females to deny that they are suffering from alcoholism and to hide their drinking. This makes it less likely for family and friends to understand that they have become alcoholics and are in need of help. In contrast, reduced fear of stigma may lead males to display their drinking publicly or more readily, and to drink excessively in groups. The gendered differences might lead family and friends to be more likely to suspect that a male they know is an alcoholic, than a female. Alcoholics Anonymous (AA) is an example of an informal fellowship of males and females, who share their experience of alcoholism to develop strength and support each other to recover from debilitating alcoholism, as they have a common problem in trying to overcome the craving to drink. It is an informal society of more than two million recovering alcoholics throughout the world. Their primary purpose is for their members to stay sober and help other alcoholics to achieve sobriety (Kurtz 2013).

Despite informal societal efforts to limit the harmful effects of excessive drinking, there are still large groups in the society that are not following the direction of responsible consumption of alcohol. Many countries have imposed age limits for alcoholic beverage purchase, in order to limit alcohol abuse by young people who are still impressionable and may be led by their peers to embark on binge-drinking sessions. The introduction of further official alcohol restrictions poses a difficult balance for a tolerant society, where responsible drinking has been adopted by a majority of the population; but attempts at prohibition have been tried, with less success.

Although religious movements were among the first to limit or outright ban alcohol consumption, these were later followed by state-sanctioned prohibitions. Prohibition is the legal act of prohibiting the manufacture, storage, transportation and sale of alcoholic beverages. The earliest records of prohibition of alcohol date back to the Xia Dynasty, ca. 2070 BC–ca. 1600 BC, when alcohol was banned throughout the kingdom of China. It is said that Emperor Yu tried a tasteful alcoholic drink and felt that future rulers might overindulge in the beverage with a possible loss of power (Xu and Bao 1998). In 14 countries with a majority Muslim population and some parts of India, state-sanctioned bans of alcohol consumption were imposed for religious reasons and are currently in place. Equally, much of the impetus for the prohibition movement in the Nordic countries and North America in the early twentieth century came from moral convictions of pietistic Protestants. The first half of the twentieth century saw periods of prohibition of alcoholic beverages in several countries. After some years, prohibition became a failure in North America and elsewhere, as organised crime took control of the distribution of alcohol. Prohibition generally ended in the late 1920s or early 1930s in most of North America and Europe. Although prohibition was lifted, Nordic countries, with the exception of Denmark, continue to have strict controls on the sale of alcohol, with government monopolies in place for selling spirits, wine and stronger beers.

Socio-cultural traditions supported by governmental regulation are still strong impetuses to protect population health and reduce the social burden caused by the harmful effects of alcohol abuse in many countries, and it is one of the objectives of the World Health Organization's global strategy to ease worldwide alcohol consumption. The strategy includes evidence-based policies and interventions that can protect health and save lives if adopted, implemented and enforced. The strategy also contains a set of principles that should guide the development and implementation of policies; it sets priority areas for global action, recommends target areas for national action and gives a strong mandate to WHO to strengthen action at all levels (World Health Organization 2014c).

Conclusion

Alcohol consumption is well situated within the socio-cultural risk discourse developed by Douglas (1966) and by Douglas and Wildavsky (1982), where the culture, faith, social environment and physical environment, including the climate of the society, are all part of the developed customs and traditions in relation to alcoholic beverages. This has not changed dramatically since the earliest use of alcohol drinking, as it continues to have this social and cultural grounding, with alcohol consumption integrated into the core systems of myths and ritual practices within emergent cultures. Cultural traditions and rules both prescribe the use of alcohol for social, profane and religious ceremonial celebrations, but proscribe continuous or excessive inebriation. Drinking in the twenty-first century meets largely similar individual, collective and cultural customs to those of ancient times. Alcohol consumption at the low-risk levels practiced by females and males in most countries can actually be beneficial to health and, as a cultural facilitator, improve human interaction and social wellbeing. However, for a minority of the population, daily heavy drinking, occasional hazardous drinking or binge drinking can create significant individual risks, including public health and safety issues.

In contemporary societies where access to alcoholic beverages is largely unlimited, it can be freely bought, but it can also be produced in the home. With common health warnings about the risk of consuming excessive volumes of alcoholic beverages, people in many countries drink alcohol in moderation. Research acknowledges that for healthy people, moderate drinking is currently assessed as being safe. Nonetheless, anything in excess of moderate drinking can clearly be risky. Binge drinking can damage a person's health, increase the risk of accidents and injuries and act as an instigator of or exposure to physical assault. Years of heavy drinking can lead to liver disease, heart disease, cancer and pancreatitis. Excessive alcohol consumption is also a significant factor within family violence crimes; it causes problems at work, and with social relationships among friends.

Public perception of the influence of alcoholic beverages on health and social wellbeing demonstrates wide habitual variations, from total abstention to free for all drinking under self-imposed social control. Similarly, scientific conclusions are diverse; ranging from beneficial health effects and facilitation of social interactions at moderate consumption levels to a harmful health impact and social disarray at abuse levels. Judging from consumption patterns, moderate levels of drinking are adopted by a majority. However, a minority group appears to be impervious to health advice as evidenced by regular binge-drinking occasions. A special case is the alcohol dependency syndrome or alcoholism that is universally seen as destructive for affected individuals and their families.

There is still a strong impetus to protect population health and reduce the social burden caused by the harmful effects of alcohol abuse in many countries. WHO has initiated such protective global and national frameworks.

6   The risks and benefits of dietary supplements

Introduction

Humans' overall increased longevity is a manifestation of people's innate ability to understand the need to adapt to their social, cultural and physical environment. Throughout historical periods, people have adjusted their way of living and shown resilience against adversity to sustain their preferred way of living. The socio-cultural risk discourse as presented by Douglas (1966, 1985) and Douglas and Wildavsky (1982), stresses the significance of societal wellbeing and sustainability for the common good; hence, to eat well is situated within our social and cultural environment and our religious beliefs. In contemporary society, the philosophy of eating well is enforced almost daily: the importance of healthy foods, exercise and consuming adequate levels of essential nutrients in the right proportions. A critical component in maintaining good health and achieving a balanced diet is access to diverse food choices throughout the year. However, food choices are strongly influenced by socio-cultural traditions developed within society's social and physical living environment and especially by what food each season produces.

Humans are best suited to eat a varied diet to achieve a proper nutrient balance. This should include a combination of small portions of meat, fish and eggs, and larger portions of fruit and vegetables, some bread or other cereal products, and a mix of dairy products, if the last can be digested. A balanced diet containing all essential food groups will easily provide all the necessary macronutrients like protein, fat and carbohydrates, and equally all the essential micronutrients like vitamins and minerals, as well as protective flavonoids and antioxidants (Lichtenstein *et al.* 2006). Despite the availability of sufficient food alternatives to gain a healthy balance in most countries, large parts of the population believe that this is not sufficient to remain healthy.

There is an emerging perception among individuals who are already healthy that they might be at risk of malnutrition, even with the best of diets. The perceived risk of malnutrition and vitamin deficiencies have paved the way for commercialisation of a fear of insufficient nutrients through the promotion of extensive use of dietary supplements in the belief that at least the supplements will do no harm. This is particularly the case in the era of fad diets (as discussed in Chapter 7), where vitamins and other supplements are being used as diet enhancers. Many of those following restrictive dieting programmes have started to take supplements as a form of insurance, because they feel that essential nutrients may be missing from their diets, or to boost the immune system to strengthen resistance to disease.

According to Beck (1992) and Giddens (1990, 1991), the urge to take evasive action to avoid risks might be a reaction to the undesired side effects of technological and industrial progress in a risk-focused society. Every day we are made more aware of these risks, and consumers are compelled to attempt to negotiate and minimise risks as best they can. The twenty-first century is also an age of rising anxiety about what evidence to believe and whom to trust. Many of the risks we face today are initially invisible, with actual harm only evident many years later. The public is exposed to a wide variety of information in the media, with health science results translated, often sensationalised and further manipulated by commercial interests. In the risk society discourse, it is increasingly proposed that it is the responsibility of the individual to manage their own risks; hence, dietary supplements have become important resources for harm reduction in the public's mind (Nichter 2003). In this form of 'self-government', people are encouraged to manage their own lives through choice, take responsibility for their future and maximise their own potential (Rose and Miller 1992).

A United States survey explored the drivers for supplement use. People participating in the research felt that their lifestyles were under constant pressure in the modern risk society, and they felt a desire to take precautionary action in the form of various dietary supplements. Young people were found to take dietary supplements, especially vitamins, to counterbalance unhealthy lifestyle choices. They agreed that their unhealthy behaviours did have consequences and felt that they were responsible enough to attempt to compensate for them. Middle-aged and older people taking supplement were found to be more worried about an increasingly toxic environment and indicated that they took dietary supplements, especially antioxidants and 'blood purifiers', to rid themselves of perceived harmful residues from preservatives and pesticides in foods. Since toxins cannot be completely avoided, they attempt to reduce them before they accumulate to dangerous levels in the body (Nichter and Thompson 2006).

In the same survey, some of the people using dietary supplements perceived 'natural' herbal supplements as being safer and having fewer side effects than conventional medicines. They substituted pharmaceuticals with herbal medicines. The word 'natural' carries with it connotations of genuine, pure, unadulterated, especially when juxtaposed against conventional notions of pharmaceuticals as being chemically synthesised and potentially harmful. In this group, people using supplements merged a concern for the wellness of the individual body with the health of the environment and with their spiritual wellbeing (Nichter and Thompson 2006; cf. Douglas 1966, 1985; Douglas and Wildavsky 1982).

Disagreements between the view of science and socio-culturally based public perception have been particularly apparent when official studies have shown that a supplement was generally ineffective. Two-thirds of regular and occasional users said that they would continue to take the supplement and questioned whether the scientific assessments were accurate, except in cases where harmful substances were identified and removed from the market (Blendon *et al.* 2001). On the contrary, advice coming from friends, as well as friends' experiences, was the most important influence on the use of supplements (Douglas 1966, 1985; Douglas and Wildavsky 1982). Additionally, laypeople's involvement in the co-production and evaluation of knowledge served to diminish scientific authority (Nowotny 2000; Nowotny *et al.* 2001).

Another central influencer on public perception is supplement advertising that reflects and reinforces popular motivations for using supplements. Advertisements often emphasise the natural treatment of illness and suggest opportunities to maximise use of time and enhance performance, beauty and overall fitness. Advertisements targeting the elderly promise youth and vitality; males are offered virility and sex appeal through a variety of herbal supplements; females are presented endless opportunities for weight loss, beauty in the form of healthy hair, skin and nails, and relief from hormonal changes due to menstruation, pregnancy and menopause. Even athletes hoping to get a legal edge in their sport are offered products for enhanced endurance, body-building and a faster recovery time (Nichter and Thompson 2006).

The increasing use of dietary supplements is puzzling particularly because, when comparing contemporary with historical time, it is unambiguous that the nutritional value of the general food supply has improved considerably with enhancements in food production, storage and preparation. Hence, the assumption that the average diet is lacking in sufficient nutrients to maintain health is an anomaly of risk perception. In this case, the public's socially and culturally influenced perception of nutritional risk is diametrically opposed to expert opinion of nutritionists and dieticians. The latest scientific findings clearly demonstrate that many dietary supplements provide little gain and that some can even do more harm than good – facts that are often disregarded by the public (Guallar *et al.* 2013).

The history of dietary supplements

Dietary supplements have existed in many different forms and combinations, and have a long history of use. In general, they consist of concentrated sources of nutrients or other substances with a nutritional or physiological effect. The purpose with taking a supplement is to complement the normal diet (Yetley 2007). The supplements can be vitamins, minerals, herbs or other plants, and a range of other substances isolated from a natural source. They are taken in the form of a pill, capsule, tablet, powder or liquid. Supplements are supposed to complement the diet and are not considered a substitute for food. It is estimated that there are currently more than 50,000 different formulations of dietary supplements on the market. Worldwide in 2011, dietary supplements generated about US$85 billion in sales from all commercial outlets. The USA is the world's largest market and China has the fastest growing consumption of supplements. Growths of the consumer market in China and other emerging markets are partly driven by the rise of the middle class populations (Anon 2012).

The identification, isolation and purification of individual nutrients in the early twentieth century raised the possibility that optimal health outcomes could be realised through nutrient supplementation (Lichtenstein and Russell 2005). This was nothing new. Herbal remedies had been in use for much of human history to treat diet imbalances and related diseases. Here they had a role to fulfil in compensating for lack of well-balanced and nutritional food. Plainly, the use of medicinal plants is the most common form of traditional medication worldwide. Herbal remedies have also been used by modern medicine for a considerable time. Substantial parts of commercial pharmaceuticals currently on the market are derived from botanical sources (Schmidt *et al.* 2007). Examples include aspirin (from willow bark), quinine (from the quinine tree) and digoxin (from the foxglove plant). In contemporary society, herbal extracts have entered western cultures making up a large part of the growing worldwide dietary supplement market.

Herbal supplements, sometimes called botanicals, are the oldest form of dietary supplements. Written evidence of herbal remedies dates back over 5,000 years to the Sumerians, who created lists of beneficial plants. In ancient Egypt, herbs are mentioned in Egyptian medical papyri depicted in tomb illustrations. Seeds likely used to treat maladies have been found in the archaeological sites of Bronze Age China dating from the Shang Dynasty in the second millennium BC. Over a hundred of the 224 drugs mentioned in an early Chinese medical text were herbs (Hong 2004). The international trade in herbal supplements is now a considerable part of the global economy, and the demand is increasing in both developing and developed nations. There are currently more than one thousand companies producing medicinal plant products (Newmaster *et al.* 2013).

Other common dietary supplements, apart from herbal supplements, include preparations comprising individual or a combination of vitamins and minerals. The human body needs vitamins in order to function properly and maintain good health, but only in minute amounts. For example, this knowledge was not available to sailors in the past, who often died in large numbers from scurvy during lengthy voyages. During the eighteenth century, scurvy killed more British sailors than enemy action. It was not until 1747 that James Lind, a Scottish military surgeon, scientifically proved in the first-ever clinical trial that scurvy could be treated and prevented by supplementing the diet with citrus fruit (Greenstone 2009). Nonetheless, it took almost another 200 years before the active compound protecting against scurvy could be isolated and identified, by Albert Szent-Györgyi and Charles Glen King, in 1932. The compound was named ascorbic acid or vitamin C (Svirbely and

Szent-Györgyi 1932). Humans are one of the few organisms that cannot form their own vitamin C, and thus need to rely on a continual supply of the vitamin; however, humans need very small amounts of it. Any diet containing fresh fruit and vegetables will suffice.

The discovery of the benefit of vitamin C was the beginning of a vitamin obsession. The development was largely driven by a singlehanded determination of one person, dual Nobel Price winner Linus Pauling. In 1970, Pauling published the book, *Vitamin C and the Common Cold*, urging the public to take 3,000 milligrams of vitamin C every day, which is about 50 times the recommended daily allowance (Pauling 1970). Pauling believed that the common cold would soon be a historical footnote. Despite study after study showing that Pauling's assertions could not be clinically supported (Heimer *et al.* 2009), he went even further, proposing a range of mechanisms in which high doses of vitamin C could be effective in delaying death by cancer (Cameron *et al.* 1979). Subsequent studies have consistently shown that vitamin C does not treat cancer or limit cancer risks (Lee *et al.* 2003). However, the perception that the common cold could simply be treated by taking vitamin C has been difficult to disband, and sales of not only vitamin C but also of other vitamins, have taken off and have since remained high.

Following the introduction of vitamin C supplements there are now many types of combination preparations on the market. Manufacturers adjust production according to the varying demands for the range and amount of vitamins, minerals and other ingredients by consumers. Among the most common are basic, once-daily products containing all or most vitamins and minerals deemed essential, with the majority in amounts that are close to intake recommendations. Special purpose supplements promoting better performance or superior energy, weight control or improved immunity usually contain herbal and other ingredients, such as echinacea and glucosamine, in addition to vitamins and minerals.

Consumption of multivitamin and multi-mineral supplements increased from 30 per cent of the US adult population in 1994 to almost 40 per cent in 2004, while overall use of dietary supplements over the same period increased from 42 to 53 per cent (Gahche *et al.* 2011). The US supplement industry reached US$30 billion in annual sales in 2011, including US$12 billion for vitamin and mineral supplements (Anon 2012). Figures show a steady increase in multivitamin supplement use, but a decline in the use of individual vitamin supplements. Similar trends have been observed in the United Kingdom and in other European countries. This is despite the findings that current intakes of vitamins from food across a range of different European countries are adequate, except for vitamin D (Mensink *et al.* 2013). Researchers have found that, in most cases, supplements made very little difference to the proportion of individuals below recommended vitamin intake levels. This might be due to the common finding that those who take supplements are not those with low micronutrient intakes from food. The trend is rather that individuals who use dietary supplements generally report higher dietary nutrient intakes from their food supply and overall healthier diets. This has been demonstrated in studies of dietary data (Rock 2007), although self-reporting does not necessarily completely reflect the actual intake of food and supplements.

The range of herbal supplements

Herbal supplements are sold in many different forms. It could be as fresh or dried products, liquid or solid extracts, tablets, capsules, powders or in tea bags. For example, fresh ginger root can be used as a spice and is often found in the produce section in food stores. Ginger as a herbal supplement can be sold dried and packed in tea bags, capsules or tablets, but ginger is also available in a liquid form as a drink. A particular group of chemicals or a single chemical may be isolated from a botanical and sold as a dietary supplement, usually in tablet or capsule form.

Ginkgo is one of the most commonly used herbal supplements and is considered relatively safe. St John's wort has been used for centuries, and it is suggested that it can be used to treat mildly depressed patients with an aversion to prescription medication. Ginseng is today mostly used as a stimulant and is common in energy drinks. The list of herbal remedies is exceedingly long. Table 6.1 lists potential health benefits and possible harm linked to some of the more common herbal supplement ingredients.

There are now at least 29,000 different formulations of herbal products available on the market (Marwick 2002). Public expectations of benefits associated with taking herbal supplements are widespread, while the risks are noted less commonly. Research indicates that there is evidence of risks linked to side effects of taking supplements. The side effects range from minor to severe and in some cases can even cause death. Nonetheless, it is a common belief that products labelled 'natural' are always safe and beneficial, but this is not necessarily true.

Table 6.1 Potential health benefits and possible harm from taking some common herbal supplements (Nichter and Thompson 2006; National Health Service 2011)

Herb	Potential Benefits	Possible Harm
Gingko	Memory improvement	Relatively safe, possible bleedings
St John's Wort	Mental illness treatment	Medicine interaction
Ginseng	Stimulant and energy booster	Cardiovascular disturbance
Echinacea	Immune system boost	Allergy, liver damage
Saw Palmetto	Prostatic hyperplasia	Headache, gastrointestinal effects
Kava	Treat anxiety and insomnia	Serious liver damage
Valerian Root	Calming effects	Restlessness, heart palpitations
Black Cohosh	Premenstrual pain, menopause	Rash, gastrointestinal effects
Comfrey	Pain in muscles and joints	Liver damage and death
Ephedra	Enhance athletic performance	Heart attack, stroke and death

Inconsistencies between labelling information and content of herbal supplements

Herbal supplements, in contrast to pharmaceuticals, are rarely clinically tested, hence the implied classification of 'natural' herbal supplements as being safe is rarely backed by appropriate research findings. Herbs, such as comfrey and ephedra, can cause serious harm and some herbal supplements can interact with prescription or over-the-counter medicines. There is also the situation that herbal supplements may not provide any proven health benefits over and above the effect of a placebo, but might at least be safe to use as long as they are true to the provided labelling. However, testing has shown that herbal supplements on sale for public consumption can contain vastly different ingredients or concentration of ingredients to what is stated on the label.

Researchers in Canada tested 44 bottles of popular supplements sold by 12 companies (Newmaster *et al.* 2013). They used a deoxyribonucleic acid (DNA) barcoding test to detail the genetic fingerprint of the ingredients and to discover if what was stated on the label corresponded with the actual content of the supplement. A DNA test is the most accurate scientific measurement for mapping comprehensively what ingredients the drug, herbal tablet or powder contains. The researchers found that in the supplements tested the labels listed popular herbs, which were often diluted or entirely replaced by cheap fillers, like soybean, wheat and weeds. A bottle labelled as St John's wort contained nothing but powdered rice. They also found that numerous supplements contained completely different herbs from those named on the labels. For instance, the study found that one product advertised as the North American black cohosh, a popular remedy for hot flashes and other menopause symptoms, contained the related Asian baneberry plant, which can be toxic to humans. This confirmed previous research that has shown that 25 per cent of black cohosh preparations instead contained three Asian Actaea species (Baker *et al.* 2012).

Herbal supplements adulterated with ingredients not listed on the label could pose serious health risks to consumers. For example, they identified black walnut contamination in a gingko product and contamination of many products with Santa Maria feverfew. This latter plant can trigger respiratory and skin reactions in people. One of the bottles tested even contained Alexandrian senna, a powerful laxative made from an Egyptian yellow shrub (Newmaster *et al.* 2013).

Product substitution occurred in 30 of 44 (68.2 per cent) of the products tested and only 2 of the 12 (16.7 per cent) companies had products without any substitution, contamination or fillers. Consumers would assume that if the local pharmacy or health food store carry a particular herbal supplement, it should have been tested as not being harmful to human health, but research has demonstrated that this is not always the case, as labelling often did not even reflect the herbal content. Some of the contaminants can have significant medical effects detrimental to human health.

Adulteration problems may be inadvertent. Cross-contamination can occur in fields where different plants are grown side by side and picked at the same time or in factories where the herbs are packaged. Rice, starch and other compounds are sometimes added during processing to keep powdered herbs from clumping, just as rice is added to saltshakers.

The testing of herbal supplements indicates that product adulteration and deliberate ingredient substitution occur, as species of a lower market value were substituted for those of a higher value. This practice not only constitutes product fraud but, according to the World Health Organization (2002), the adulteration of herbal products can be a threat to consumer safety.

Scientists and consumer advocates indicate that the research provides evidence that some sections of the herbal supplement industry do not follow honest practices. However, the industry representatives argue that the problems are not widespread (Newmaster *et al.* 2013).

The discovery of discrepancies and incorrect labelling with herbal supplements is further strengthened by data collected by the Drug-Induced Liver Injury Network in the USA (Navarro *et al.* 2014). The National Institutes of Health established a network with the aim of tracking patients who suffer liver damage from certain drugs and alternative medicines. The network includes doctors at eight major hospitals throughout the USA. The network investigated 845 patients with severe drug-induced liver damage, who were treated at hospitals in the network between 2004 and 2012. It focused only on cases where the investigators ruled out other causes and could identify a drug or a supplement with a high degree of certainty.

The findings suggest that dietary supplements accounted for nearly 20 per cent of drug-related liver injuries that turned up in hospitals, up from seven per cent a decade earlier (Hayashi *et al.* 2015). While many patients recovered, once they stopped taking the supplements and received treatment, a few required liver transplants or died because of liver failure. Uninformed young people were not the only consumers at risk, as many were middle-aged females who turned to dietary supplements that promise to burn fat or speed up weight loss.

One product that patients reported they frequently had used was green tea extract. This extract contains catechins, a group of potent antioxidants that are supposed to increase metabolism. The extracts are frequently marketed as fat burners, and catechins are commonly added to weight loss products and energy boosters. Most green tea pills are highly concentrated, containing several times the amount of catechins found in a single cup of green tea. In high doses, catechins can be toxic to the liver and a small percentage of people appear to be particularly susceptible.

It has been estimated that only 30 per cent of dietary supplement companies follow basic quality control standards that would help prevent adulteration of their products, and only in 15 per cent of clinical trials had the specific ingredients in the herbal supplement been quantified (Wolsko *et al.* 2005). Of roughly 1,000 plants, clinical trials had been published only for 156 plants supporting specific pharmacological activities and therapeutic applications. While for about half of the plants there was some support for therapeutic use, there was strong evidence that five plants were so toxic or allergenic that their use ought to be discouraged or forbidden (Cravotto *et al.* 2010). Supplement contamination and incorrect labelling can cause dangerous health issues as the risks can be high, but this message appears not to have filtered down to consumer behaviour, as the public seems not to be perturbed by the negative findings in their personal risk/benefit assessment, when choosing to consume herbal supplements.

The scope of vitamins and minerals included in dietary supplements

Vitamins are vital nutrients that cannot be synthesized by the body; they are required in limited amounts to sustain life and must be obtained through the diet. A human being needs 13 vitamins to maintain health – vitamins A, C, D, E, K and the eight B vitamins – thiamine, riboflavin, niacin, pantothenic acid, biotin, pyridoxine, folate and cobalamin (World Health Organization 2004a). Contrary to the definition, the body can actually make vitamins D and K. Table 6.2 shows a brief description of the different vitamins and their significance for the human body.

Vitamin A deficiency is rare except in some developing countries (Roncone 2006). The eight B vitamins often coexist in the same foods. Deficiency of vitamin B9 (folate) in early embryonic development has been linked to neural tube defects. Thus, females planning to become pregnant are usually encouraged to increase vitamin B9 intake (Pitkin 2007; Lamers 2011). Vitamin B12 (cobalamin) deficiency is a legitimate concern for vegans since it is scarcely available from plant products (Watanabe *et al.* 2014). Vitamin C deficiency is rare but people who get little or no vitamin C for many weeks can get scurvy (Combs 2008; McKenna and Dawson 1993). Large doses of vitamin C supplements may cause a range of symptoms, such as abdominal bloating and cramps, diarrhoea, heartburn and headache (Jacob and Sotoudeh 2002). In children, vitamin D deficiency causes rickets, while in adults it can

Table 6.2 Potential health benefits of vitamins and possible harm from taking vitamin supplements (Institute of Medicine 1997, 1998, 2000, 2001)

Compound	Potential Benefits	Possible Harm
A vitamin	Vision, immunity, reproduction	Nausea, headache, blurred vision
B vitamins	Cell metabolism	No current reports of harm
C vitamin	Antioxidant, immunity, collagen	Diarrhoea, cramps, insomnia
D vitamin	Bone health, cell communication	Nausea, constipation, weakness
E vitamin	Antioxidant, gene expression	No current reports of harm
K vitamin	Blood coagulation, bone health	No current reports of harm

lead to osteomalacia (Holick 2004). Forthright vitamin E deficiency is rare (Takahashi *et al.* 1990; Calzada *et al.* 1997) as is vitamin K deficiency.

Minerals are necessary to build strong bones and teeth, control body fluids inside and outside cells, and turn food into energy. Essential minerals include calcium, copper, iodine, iron, magnesium, phosphorus, selenium and zinc, although there are also many other types of minerals that serve as important parts of a healthy diet (World Health Organization 2004a). Table 6.3 shows a brief description of the different minerals and their significance for the human body.

A lack of calcium can lead to rickets in children or osteoporosis and osteomalacia in later life (Guyton and Hall 2001; Tuck and Datta 2007; Campbell *et al.* 1994). Symptoms of copper deficiency include defects in connective tissue, anaemia and possibly specific aspects of central nervous system dysfunction (Harris 1997). Iodine deficiency can cause mental retardation, hypothyroidism, goitre, cretinism and varying degrees of other growth and developmental abnormalities (Wolff 1969). A lack of iron can lead to anaemia with impaired physical work performance (Willis *et al.* 1988). Early signs of magnesium deficiency include loss of appetite, nausea, vomiting, fatigue and weakness (Rude 2010). Phosphorus is so ubiquitous in various foods that near total starvation is required to produce dietary phosphorus deficiency. There are indications that selenium deficiency seldom causes overt illness. However, it might lead to biochemical changes that predispose to illness associated with other stresses (Institute of Medicine 2000). Because of the ubiquity of zinc

Table 6.3 Potential health benefits of minerals and possible harm from taking mineral supplements (Institute of Medicine 1997, 2000, 2001)

Mineral	Potential Benefits	Possible Harm
Calcium	Bone health, blood vessel and muscle function, cell signalling	Hypercalcaemia, heart arrhythmia, soft tissue calcification
Copper	Blood cell formation, infant growth	Stomach pain, diarrhoea, and damage to liver and kidneys
Iodine	Thyroid hormone formation, protein synthesis	Hypothyroidism, goitre, mental retardation, growth abnormalities
Iron	Component of proteins, including enzymes and haemoglobin	Constipation, nausea, vomiting and stomach pain
Magnesium	Regulation of a diverse range of biochemical reactions	Diarrhoea, nausea and abdominal cramping
Phosphorus	Buffers pH, energy metabolism, catalytic protein activation	Calcification of the kidneys, increased porosity of the skeleton
Selenium	Defence against oxidative stress, regulation of redox status	Selenosis with hair and nail brittleness and loss
Zinc	Cell and enzyme generation, wound healing	Suppression of immune response, anaemia and bone weakening

and its involvement in so many core areas of metabolism, features of zinc deficiency are frequently quite basic and nonspecific, including growth retardation, alopecia, diarrhoea, delayed sexual maturation and impotence, eye and skin lesions, and impaired appetite (Institute of Medicine 2001).

The inability of vitamin and mineral supplements to prevent chronic diseases

From the above descriptions of the beneficial effects of vitamins and minerals, it is obvious that these compounds are all necessary for the body to maintain good health. This has been known for a reasonably long time, with possibly the best example being the complete cure of scurvy with vitamin C, as mentioned previously. Scurvy is a terrible disease that troubled humans long back through recorded history, but is now a condition rarely seen. Many other vitamins and micronutrients are required for good health. Antioxidants, like selenium, and vitamins A, C and E, fight free radicals that can damage DNA, cell membranes and the lining of arteries. Deficiencies can cause all sort of diseases, some of them very serious. Several studies have shown that people who eat more fruits and vegetables that contain high levels of antioxidants have a lower incidence of cancer and heart disease and they live longer. Consequently, if people eat numerous portions of fruits and vegetables they ought to be healthier and, as a parallel, if these natural products can be substituted by supplemental antioxidants, this could easily also be expected to lead to healthier people. This is the main basis for the massive growth of the supplements industry selling multivitamins and high-dose mineral supplements in a bewildering variety, but it is grounded on unsubstantiated logic.

Remarkably, studies involving tens of thousands of people have shown that high doses of vitamins and mineral supplements, rather than being helpful, lack beneficial effects or can sometimes even be harmful to health. The likely reason for this is that humans are adapted to getting nutrients from whole foods. Most nutrients require enzymes, synergistic co-factors and organic mineral-activators to be properly absorbed. While these are naturally present in food, they are often not included in synthetic vitamin preparations (Shayne 2000).

An evaluation of 38,772 mature females found that several commonly used dietary vitamin and mineral supplements, including multivitamins, vitamins B6 and folic acid, as well as minerals like iron, magnesium, zinc and copper, were associated with a higher risk of total mortality. Supplemental iron was of particular concern, since it is dose dependent and strongly associated with increased total mortality risk. Only calcium was associated with a decreased mortality risk, but without a clear dose response relationship (Mursu *et al.* 2011).

Equally, a study of 35,533 males found that the risk of prostate cancer increased for the males taking vitamin E, selenium or both. Although the increased risk was small, it was clear that neither of these supplements were helpful against prostate cancer (Klein *et al.* 2011).

One study systematically reviewed published research on the efficacy of vitamin supplements for primary prevention in community dwellings occupied by adults with no nutritional deficiencies. This population group is the typical supplement customers (Fortmann *et al.* 2013). After reviewing 27 trials of single, paired or multivitamin supplements randomly assigned to more than 400,000 participants, the authors concluded that there was no clear evidence of a beneficial effect of supplements on overall cause mortality, cardiovascular disease or cancer.

Another study evaluated the efficacy of a daily multivitamin to prevent cognitive decline among 5,947 elderly males (Grodstein *et al.* 2013). After 12 years of follow-up, there were no differences between the multivitamin and placebo groups in overall cognitive performance or verbal memory. They concluded that the use of a multivitamin supplement in a well-nourished elderly population did not prevent cognitive decline. This conclusion was further supported by a review of some other studies that evaluated supplementation with multivitamins, B vitamins, vitamins E, C and omega-3 fatty acids, in persons with mild cognitive impairment or mild to moderate dementia. None of the supplements improved cognitive function (Lin *et al.* 2013).

Other trials have assessed the role of vitamin and mineral supplements in primary or secondary prevention of chronic disease and have consistently found no beneficial effects or even possible harm. Several clinical trials have shown that beta-carotene, vitamin E, and possibly high doses of vitamin A supplements increase mortality and that other antioxidants, folic acid and B vitamins, and multivitamin supplements have no clear benefit (Miller *et al.* 2005; Huang *et al.* 2006; Miller *et al.* 2010; Bjelakovic *et al.* 2013; Fortmann *et al.* 2013).

The evidence from recent trials and practice, combined with biological considerations, suggests that any effect, either beneficial or harmful, is probably small. The reality is that for the general population with no clear evidence of micronutrient deficiencies, most supplements do not prevent chronic disease or death. The supplements do not give people eating a balanced diet and without health issues any benefits; hence, supplements do not improve the health of already healthy people and they should be avoided, as some might even be harmful (Gahche *et al.* 2011). The research demonstrates that supplements are only needed where there is a demonstrable micronutrient deficiency with targeted recommendations for nutrient supplements to certain segments of the population, like fast growing children, pregnant females, those suffering from general malnutrition or alcohol abuse, or the frail elderly in a nursing home setting (Caulfield *et al.* 2006; Feinman and Lieber 1998; Kulnick and Elmadfa 2008).

Conclusion

People's religious beliefs and social and cultural environment influence their attitudes toward food and their idea of what constitutes healthy living

(Douglas 1966, 1985; Douglas and Wildavsky 1982). It becomes a daily habit to follow guidelines in eating healthy foods, to exercise and to consume adequate levels of essential nutrients in the right proportions. Still a large section of the population believes that their diet is insufficient to sustain health. Based on scientific results that are now emerging, it is important that the public risk perception of diet insufficiency in a balanced diet be challenged. Although herbal supplements have a role to play as an alternative to modern medicine in treating mild disturbances to health and well-being, their use should be supported by scientific evidence and the purity of the ingredients assured.

The situation is slightly different for nutrient supplements. The most promising data in the area of nutrition and positive health outcomes relate to dietary patterns, not nutrient supplements. This suggests that other factors in food or the relative presence of some foods and the absence of other foods are more important than the level of individual nutrients consumed. In most cases, eating plenty of fruit and vegetables as part of a balanced diet will provide all micronutrients and vitamins needed for a healthy person. The focus should be directed toward buying nutritious foods, rather than dietary supplements. Hence, nutrients ought to come from food, not supplements, whenever possible.

However, the perceived need to take dietary supplements has been ingrained in the public's mind through intensive and numerous marketing campaigns claiming health benefits. In a society increasingly dominated by business-focused advertising, public counter messages easily get lost unless well targeted. The current body of research into dietary supplements undoubtedly demonstrates this situation. It is essential that the public's risk perception of diet insufficiency be altered and communicated, but it also requires questioning of the commercial interests behind promotion of supplements. The socio-cultural risk discourse highlights how commercial advertising has become entrenched in contemporary society, challenging socio-culturally based healthy eating traditions, and explains why official recommendations and public perceptions of risks need to be part of the debate.

7 A socio-cultural risk perspective on distorted diets

Introduction

Research shows that the fundamentals of habitual food consumption and the representative lifetime diet of an individual are grounded in early life (Resnicow *et al.* 1998), and food choices established in childhood or adolescence may significantly spread into adulthood (Mikkila *et al.* 2004). Many facets of daily life, such as fashion choices, body image, the brand of car or dietary habits embraced, provide distinguishing characteristics about the upbringing of the individual. However, these characteristics are also strongly influenced by pressure from a shifting social and cultural environment. The perception of body image and dieting are often a result of socio-cultural pressure. Dieting is the practice of deliberately attempting to change habitual consumption patterns in the short term to achieve or to maintain what is perceived as an ideal weight. Reducing food intake might involve unintentional risk taking, as the advice presented in the popular mass media often focuses on a generalised healthy individual. The dieting advice in the popular press might also give the reader a false impression that the dieting advice is medically sound, hence without risks, but many of the diets in the popular mass media are not scientifically tested or based on medical advice.

Undeniably, choices made about eating habits have come under intense scrutiny. Food consumption can be seen as a strong indicator of prosperity, education level, social class and feelings about the self (Celimli-Inaltong 2014). The societal focus on nutritional habits has increased, almost proportionally to the growth in overweight and obese individuals, but also in response to a surge in health consciousness. Food consumption and body image are conceptually influenced by societal practices and traditions, and within the community setting of the socio-cultural risk discourse a preferred body image is identified with a prescribed food intake to sustain a person's healthy living (Douglas 1966, 1985; Douglas and Wildavsky 1982).

Unfortunately, the ideal body image dictated by contemporary mass media is virtually impossible for people to achieve without excessive dieting, extreme exercise regimes or both (Cusumano and Thompson 1997).

The simple principle espoused publicly for maintaining an ideal weight is to balance the intake of food and beverages with the preferred lifestyle on an enduring basis; a food consumption that satisfies energy and nutrient needs to maintain a healthy body and to support everyday activities. However, official health promotion activities targeting the obesity explosion have largely been unsuccessful in counteracting a prevailing cult of excessive slimness and rather have reinforced a 'medicalised' notion of the problem of excess weight, thereby legitimising intermittent risky dieting practices (Germov and Williams 1996). As a result of an increased promotion of healthy living and warnings of possible health issues with being overweight or obese, a plurality of populist diets has come on the market with little regard to their long-term effects. The rise of these countless populist diet strategies are tantalising a receptive public. Deliberate imbalances between food intake and output through restrictive or skewed diets are thus common and have caused community concerns over many decades, especially in societies where the norm to be thin is promoted. Poor diet quality is a worldwide risk factor and a major cause of mortality and disability (Lim *et al.* 2012).

Body image and what is considered a healthy lifestyle is analysed in this chapter from the socio-cultural risk discourse perspective, but restrictive diets also fall within the risk society discourse (Beck 1992), as some of them contribute to nutritional imbalances and an increase in disordered eating posing serious risks to individual health. Distorted diets are not only about restricting overall food consumption or creating a skewed diet by limiting food intake only to specific food groups. They are also about substituting food with herbal supplements and pharmaceuticals and thus a medicalising of body sustenance. Popular diet recommendations range from the healthy to the unhealthy, but also to the risky and the fatal.

Chapter 3 dealt with risks associated with excessive energy intake through energy-dense food and beverage consumption as factors among a multitude of causes to overweight and obesity. This chapter will look at the other side of the issue, by exploring the risks posed by skewed dietary patterns that can lead to malnutrition, due to inadequacy of either energy or micronutrients. Common malnutrition among underprivileged populations is mainly due to inadequate food supply, poor nutritional quality of accessible food items or limited food choices within the available budget, while in privileged populations it is mainly due to poor dietary habits or excessive dieting amidst an abundant food supply. More specifically, the chapter focuses on the risk to public health posed by poor dietary habits and dieting among mainly privileged populations or population groups within a country, where the people have the financial recourses to source and secure a balanced and healthy food diet.

Skewed dietary practices

At the individual level, food consumption and inclination to diet depends on the individual's age, gender, level of education and socio-economic status, but it also relates to the societal level, as food availability, convenience and quality characteristics are linked to the overall national income of the society. The choice of food is closely associated with habits, social and cultural traditions and taste preferences, but also influenced by social class perception.

In examining the food habits of over 5,000 US adults in 2001–2002 it was found that more than half of the individuals had tried to control their weight in the previous 12 months, mainly through dieting, but also through increased exercise (Weiss *et al.* 2006). The focus on dietary habits is not a new phenomenon. The phrase 'you are what you eat' can be traced to early Christianity where the body and blood of Jesus were represented by bread and wine (Gilman 2008), but is now more of a token statement indicating a strong association between physical wellbeing and eating (Celimli-Inaltong 2014).

Choice of food and the preferred taste of food are interconnected with social, cultural and religious traditions. Food preferences are 'embedded within a social and cultural milieu involving habits, norms, rituals and taboos' (Pietrykowski 2004:312). Food preferences and taste are developed during the individual's early years within their social and cultural family environment, but are also influenced by socially and historically embedded phenomena. These multitudes of influences create the individual's identity, but also reflect perception of societal social class status (Bourdieu 1984). Where the societal structure gives the framework for social identity, the agency personalises the individual's identity and, through daily practices, the person will identify with the character she or he is as consumer (Celimli-Inaltong 2014).

In the past, females were more likely to be linked with gluttony than any form of food abstention or dieting. If a female was gluttonous, it was often branded as the most terrible of sins; she was shameful and scandalous (Okholm 2014). It was something females were warned against and encouraged to feel guilty about, much as females in contemporary Western culture are. Females are made to feel guilty if not aspiring to a thin ideal. It is unmistakeable that social, cultural and religious traditions and social norms influenced the eating habits of medieval females, much as popular culture and societal archetypes affect female consumption in today's society (Chadbourn 2014). The focus is still mainly on females, with the gendered health discourse based on a combination of traditional health issues revealing how patterned ways of communicating about health contribute to the façade of being 'natural' and customary differences between females and males (Payne 2014).

The gendered health discourse is conveyed primarily through the media, and it shapes how people think about identifying and treating health issues, as well as how females and males interpret their bodies' meaning and worth (Brenton 2014). A survey that followed 1,902 young adults over ten years from 1998–1999 to 2008–2009 found that dieting and unhealthy weight control behaviours were prevalent, especially for females (Neumark-Sztainer *et al.* 2012). Close to 38 per cent in 1998–1999 and 44 per cent in 2008–2009 of the females, but only about 10 per cent and 19 per cent of males, respectively, reported intermittent dieting or persistent use of unhealthy weight control behaviours. Adolescent females, in particular, were highly aware of their appearance and invested significant cognitive and emotional resources into their preferred physical body image. Several studies demonstrate that, in this developmental period, young females are overly concerned with weight and shape, and they are prone to adopt unhealthy eating habits to gain a preferred appearance (Nanu *et al.* 2014). This strategy results in body perception and behaviour negatively influencing the psychological wellbeing of females more than males during adolescence (Vogt Yuan 2010). Research has indicated that 35 to 60 per cent of females are chronic dieters (Polivy and Herman 2007), with a heightened risk to health, in that dieters are eight times more likely to develop eating disorders than non-dieters (Patton *et al.* 1990).

This presents a conundrum. There is constant pressure from the mass media for individuals to adopt new slimming regimes, which conflicts with the pressure from the food industry to direct food consumption to more profitable, energy-dense food products (Vogel and Mol 2014). In the middle are public health experts, who are advocating for a balanced diet and better access to healthy food. The mixed messages emphasise the conflict between official dietary recommendations based on science and the power of relentless advertising and promotion that influence public perception.

Official dietary advice

Dietary advice is not new. The English undertaker William Banting was one of the first who developed an enduring diet that was not extreme. In 1863, he wrote a booklet called *Letter on Corpulence, Addressed to the Public*, which contained the specific plan for the 'Banting Diet' he had successfully followed. Banting's own diet was four meals per day, consisting of meat, greens, fruits and dry wine. The emphasis was on avoiding sugar, saccharine, starch, beer, milk and butter. Banting's regimen became popular for many years, and it has become a model for modern diets (Groves 2003).

The initial publishing of diet advice has since grown exponentially, with a multitude of new diet recommendations published each year by government authorities and public health organisations. Publications in the public health domain cover a diverse range of balanced diets with a focus on health and healthy living. Examples of healthy diets include the 'Mediterranean Diet', the 'Dietary Approaches to Stop Hypertension Diet' (DASH), the 'Therapeutic Lifestyle Changes Diet' (TLC), and the 'Mayo Clinic Diet'. These enduring diets are all relatively easy to follow, nutritious and safe, as well as suitable for diabetics and heart disease risk groups.

Public health authorities should have an important role to play in influencing dietary patterns and healthy living as a strategy to limit increases in societal health costs. However, from a socio-cultural risk perspective, governments and official authorities have limited avenues to regulate or influence individual dietary choices and to successfully counter dieting misinformation. As a less legalistic approach, public health authorities in many countries issue diet recommendations in an attempt to influence population consumption habits. Eighty-one countries across the globe have developed and implemented dietary guidelines. Although their impact on consumption and nutritional outcomes has not been widely studied, there is some evidence to indicate that they have improved awareness of proper nutrition (Hawkes 2013). However, the influence of more general food knowledge campaigns on actual consumer behaviour appears to be limited. For example, ten public information campaigns presented throughout Europe point to an increased awareness and knowledge about nutrition, but the campaigns are presumed to have had little impact on actual behaviour and nutritional outcomes (Capacci *et al.* 2012). Nonetheless, formalised education strategies do have an impact on general food knowledge and nutrition specific details; hence, targeted education is proving to be more effective than general information at impacting individual food habits (Webb and Block 2004; World Bank 2007; Headey 2011). Unfortunately, home economics, where basic dietary information is included in the teaching, has declined as part of the curriculum across the world (Lichtenstein and Ludwig 2010).

The reluctance to follow official healthy eating recommendations might be because benefits of changing the diet are not seen as outweighing the barriers for behavioural change (Ma *et al.* 2002). Except for health professionals, who have the knowledge about the vital role that nutrition plays in supporting a healthy body, most people prioritise other aspects of food over its importance to health. Eating habits are very difficult to influence on an enduring basis, as they augment complex patterns of feelings, values and traditions established already in the early childhood years and remaining at a subconscious level throughout people's life. Abstract knowledge imparted by official agencies is rarely sufficient in itself to motivate a change in eating habits. A favourable response would be more likely if the new knowledge were presented within the framework of the individual's milieu, along with social, cultural and religious considerations (Stanfield and Hui 2010), but this is rarely the case.

The basis for nutritional information

Eating is usually driven by hunger or appetite, where hunger is a physiological mechanism controlled by the central nervous system, while appetite is a desire for food related to past experiences in response to stimuli such as smell, taste and appearance. Hunger can lead to consumption of many foods outside the cultural frame of reference in order to survive, while appetite can give rise to an uncontrolled eating behaviour that can lead to excessive weight gain (Stanfield and Hui 2010).

To manage dietary risks, it is vital for governments as well as individuals to have access to accurate nutrition information. Since the 1960s, nutrition science has been dominated by two conflicting interpretations. One dominating view reasons that people do have access to information about how to select healthy food and to maintain a healthy weight, although with the shortcoming that people do not always implement the knowledge that they have available. Despite the assumption of availability of basic knowledge about healthy eating, variable diet advice has skyrocketed, with over 600,000 articles published in the scientific literature over a 50-year period, along with thousands of diet books (Taubes 2014). The publications purport to convey significant information in relation to weight control and diseases related to food.

The protocol of science requires an initial hypothesis and the process of testing whether the proposal is proved or disproved. In nutrition science, the hypotheses cover assumptions about what foods or dietary patterns help or hinder the pursuit of a healthy life and longevity. The hypotheses are ultimately about what happens to people over decades, thus meaningful trials are very expensive and extremely difficult to execute. Thousands of people would need to be enrolled in trials, and they would need to change their eating habits for years or decades to amass enough heart attacks, cancers and deaths to establish whether the dietary intervention was beneficial or detrimental. This would be extremely costly and logistically challenging, but without such trials, the ultimate proof of the effects of dietary interventions will not be known (Taubes 2014). The lack of evidence contributes to the current diversity of opinion on the subject of healthy diets, which can rarely be refuted by existing facts. Innovative ideas proliferate and new crash or fad diets are popping up almost daily.

Novelty dieting programmes promoted in popular mass media often have weight loss as their specific focus, and not a holistic healthy food emphasis. Most do actually lead to quick and sometimes dramatic weight loss, but only for the weight to creep back up again at the end of the dieting period. Countless fashion diets are based on dubious research or no research at all, prescribing hazardous eating practices that can be detrimental to health. Clinicians and dieticians regularly stress that these diets with a single focus can pose significant health risks and might be of minimal long-term benefit to overall wellbeing (Bacon and Aphramor 2011). A danger with fashion diets is their particularly short-term weight loss focus that involves drastic changes to normal eating habits, when small changes over a longer timeframe would be more beneficial.

Regrettably, constant diet changes, or yo-yo dieting, can lead to physical illness and depression, especially if the weight oscillates up and down following the latest diet pattern (Skaznik-Wikiel and Polotsky 2014). Such fluctuations may cause malnutrition and increase the risk of heart disease and other health problems (Daee *et al.* 2002). Yo-yo dieting has been defined as the process of going on and off diets repeatedly, which results in weight loss, but is unlikely to result in a sustained weight decrease. The exact prevalence of yo-yo dieting is not known, but there is evidence that it is a common and widespread phenomenon (Qazi and Keval 2013). Qazi and Keval (2013) highlight factors that trigger frequent dieting episodes among females, such as socio-cultural pressure to lose weight, physical appearance and mental perception of the 'right' body image. Long-term risks to health and wellbeing might not be on the minds of the users, as they are more likely to focus on short-term gains rather than on possible future negative implications of the diet. In a study of 869 Australian female high school students aged 14, 15 and 16 years, the prevalence of unbalanced eating, unhealthy dieting and distorted body image were 33, 57 and 12 per cent, respectively. Over one-third had used at least one extreme dieting method – crash dieting, fasting, slimming tablets, diuretics, laxatives and/or cigarettes – in the past month. Motivating factors for disordered eating and unhealthy dieting behaviours were, for example, peer pressure, media glorification and the perception that extreme dieting strategies were harmless (Grigg *et al.* 1996).

With all the focus on weight in our society, encouraged by a multibillion-dollar weight loss industry, it is not surprising that millions of people fall prey to fashion diets and bogus weight loss products. Conflicting claims, testimonials and hype by so-called 'experts' can confuse even the most informed consumer about what to eat.

Idiosyncratic body image perception is an additional contributing aspect of this issue. People might think they are overweight when they are not, as body image is very subjective. Sullivan and Brown (2013), in their study of perception of healthy weight in the United Kingdom, found that 32 per cent of females and 15 per cent of males of normal weight, thought that they were overweight. More than 40 per cent of females who were underweight thought that their weight was about right, and 29 per cent of females of normal weight were dieting to lose weight. Body image is based more on perception than on scientific facts; social and cultural capital, agency, social identity, social media and current social networks are all factors that influence an individual's body image. Personal perception of weight does not necessarily reflect the scientific definition, but has more to do with how people perceive themselves when looking in the mirror. Poor body image can be linked to low self-esteem, deprived social identity and individual interpretation of the ideal body. Western society's thin body image contributes to dieting, overexercising and eating disorders, such as anorexia nervosa, bulimia and binge-eating disorders. The push to be thin can influence a person's overall wellbeing and mental health status by contributing to depression and anxiety (Mask *et al.* 2014).

Faith and ethically based diets

The mass media's influence on eating habits is but one factor in a complex matrix. Dietary choice is additionally affected by a variety of other factors, including religion, culture, tradition and ethical beliefs that are relatively impervious to the influence of mass media. In every culture, food is a crucial determinant of self-constitution, as demonstrated by anthropologists and sociologists, and dietary choices are means of expressing adherence to a social and cultural group (Douglas 1992; Douglas and Wildavsky 1982). Some religions, such as the Hindu, Islamic and Jewish faiths, prescribe special diets, and for many individuals dietary practices reflect religious persuasion (Sabaté 2004; Douglas 1969).

Ethical attitudes towards animals, and vegetarianism in particular, tends to be a marker of whiteness and middle class status, as well as gendered politics (Adams 1995). Taylor (2010:72) and Foucault (1983:229) indicated that food in ancient Greece was once the focus of a complex set of restrictions. It inspired a greater discursive interest than sexual activity, thus a marked contrast to the modern West, in which sexual activity rather than food became the privileged site of moral restriction, scientific inquiry and individuating reflexivity. Eating is moral, as far as people feel bound to common dietary rules and feelings of guilt for their transgressions. Eating is disciplinary as far as we are instilled with specific eating habits or are inherently constituted to eat in certain ways that are highly difficult to get away from because they have become our habitual means of relating to our bodies, emotions and selves (Taylor 2010).

Since early civilisation, there has been an inexorable interlinking of food and religion, as humans strive to interconnect nourishment of the body with the sustenance of the soul (Blix 2001). Most religions have dietary norms or instructions, which might be observed more or less closely. Different denominations within the same religion may have slightly different food recommendations. The rationale behind the prescribed dietary practices might be based on religious text and tradition. However, some religious customs and laws can be traced to early concerns about health and safety in consuming food and beverages. In the past, preservation techniques for food were limited. Therefore, religious leaders, who traditionally were the most educated in the society, developed rules about the safe consumption of food and beverages as part of religious laws that remain in most religions today, despite advancement in food preservation. Douglas (1969) describes the rationale behind not eating pork, as it would give off a strong smell and be difficult to preserve for an extended period in warm climates, thus making it an unhealthy food to consume.

In addition, attentions to specific eating practices, such as avoiding overeating, not drinking alcoholic beverages or consuming oral stimulants, and vegetarian diets, are recommended in various religious practices. The practice of fasting or severely restricting intake of food and drink during certain periods became prevalent, and it continues to be practiced by different faiths. Although food is an important part of religious observance for different faiths, the precise role of food in cultural practices and religious beliefs is complex and varies considerably among individuals and communities.

For example, vegetarianism is the practice of abstaining from the consumption of red meat, poultry, fish and seafood and the flesh of any other animal. It often includes avoiding by-products of animal slaughter. Vegetarianism is adopted for different reasons. In many societies, including some religious denominations, controversy and debate have arisen over the ethics of eating animals. The main ethical objection to eating meat relates to the killing of animals as being unacceptable and morally unjustifiable. Ethical vegetarians may also object to the agricultural practices underlying the production of meat, or cite concerns about animal welfare, animal rights, environmental ethics and religious issues (Pluhar 2010). Other reasons for vegetarianism include health, political, environmental, cultural, aesthetic or economic motives.

There are several varieties of the vegetarian diet. An ovo-vegetarian diet includes eggs but no dairy products, a lacto-vegetarian diet includes dairy products but no eggs and an ovo-lacto-vegetarian diet includes both eggs and dairy products. A pesco-vegetarian diet includes consumption of fish and seafood and it is a type of semi-vegetarian diet. Adding seafood to an otherwise vegetarian diet can make it easier to meet nutrient needs, while still maintaining a mainly plant-based diet (Tuso *et al.* 2013; Barr and Chapman 2002).

A vegan, or strict vegetarian, diet excludes all animal products, hence avoiding eating eggs, dairy, beeswax and honey, as the production of these foods causes animal suffering and possibly premature death. A group of vegans also avoid animal products, such as leather for clothing and goose fat for shoe polish. Various packaged or processed foods, including cakes, cookies, candies, chocolate and marshmallows, often contain animal ingredients, and they may be of special concern (Senghore 2013).

Raw veganism is a diet that combines the concepts of veganism and raw foodism. It excludes all food and products of animal origin, as well as food cooked at a temperature above 48°C (118°F). A raw vegan diet includes raw vegetables and fruits, nuts and nut pastes, grain and legume sprouts, seeds, plant oils, sea vegetables, herbs and fresh juices. There are many different versions of the diet, including fruitarianism, juicearianism and sproutarianism. In terms of health, some raw vegans believe that cooking foods destroys the complex balance of micronutrients, while others strive for physical, spiritual and mental health (Tuso *et al.* 2013; Senghore 2013). Such types of diets prove how far people are prepared to go in support of beliefs and cultural traditions.

The weight-loss conundrum

On the other side of the spectrum are intermittent diet patterns. Short-term weight loss, rather than ethical or religious devotion, usually with no concern for long-term weight maintenance, is the driving force behind some idiosyncratic diets and eating patterns, often called 'fad' or 'crash' diets, which usually enjoy temporary popularity. Fad or crash diets are general terms that describe diet plans that involve making extreme and rapid changes to food consumption, often favoured by individuals wanting to lose weight fast. Such diets have been around for centuries, and although some of them sound senseless now, history proves that eager dieters have always looked for desperate measures. The anorexic and bulimic poet Lord Byron popularised the 'Vinegar Diet' in the 1820s. It involved cleansing the body by drinking plenty of vinegar and water daily inducing vomiting and diarrhoea (Baron 1997; Foxcroft 2012). During the second half of the nineteenth century, a 'Starvation Diet' was all the rage within the middle class and aristocracy of Western Europe. The diet was used to live up to the popular notion of frailty and the associated spiritual purity and femininity (Bennet and Gurin 1982). The 'Fletcher Diet', invented in 1903, involved chewing each morsel of food 32 times and spitting out the remains. The idea was that the body would absorb the nutrients it needed without the person gaining any weight (Christen and Christen 1997).

One of the most dangerous diets seems to be the 'Cigarette Diet' promoted in 1925 by cigarette companies. They boasted that cigarette smoking had appetite-suppressing qualities and should precede any meal. In the short term, nicotine increases energy expenditure and can reduce appetite, which may explain why smokers tend to have lower body weight than non-smokers and why smoking cessation is frequently followed by weight gain (Chiolero *et al.* 2008). The 'Inuit Meat-and-Fat Diet' was an early version of the Atkins diet. It was introduced in 1928 to mimic the dietary habits of the Inuit people living off caribou, raw fish and whale blubber, and consuming very few fruits or vegetables (Searles 2002). Slimming soaps involved products like 'Fatoff', 'Fat-O-NO' and 'La-Mar Reducing Soap' among others. In the early 1930s, they were claimed to have magical fat blasting ingredients when used while bathing, despite using similar ingredients to ordinary hand soap. Slimming soaps are still advertised for sale (SUTLA 2014). Some people adopted the 'Tapeworm Diet' when it was introduced in 1954. The diet proposed swallowing tapeworm eggs with the aim to reduce the amount of calories that became absorbed by the body, hence to eat without gaining weight. The Tapeworm Diet made a new appearance on the Tyra Banks show in the USA in late 2009, not to promote the diet but to dissuade people from trying it by showing samples of some flat long tapeworms (Banks 2009).

Knowledge about nutrition and understanding of healthy eating have increased, but the increase has not necessarily changed our behaviour. It is documented that many of the above diets cause nutrient deficiencies from starvation, lung cancer from smoking, seizures, meningitis or even dementia from ingesting tapeworm eggs. Nonetheless, it has not stopped the introduction of a new range of extreme weight loss diets ready to be adopted by unsuspected customers unaware of possible risks. As with previous diets, contemporary diets often focus on short-term results of losing a few kilograms. Unfortunately, the weight will come back on again as quickly as it was lost if lifestyle changes are not adopted simultaneously. An analysis of diet studies covering a 25-year period found that it was possible for participants to lose an average of 5 to 10 per cent of their weight (Perri and Fuller 1995). Although it was also shown in another study of crash dieters during a four to five year follow up period that a majority regained the lost weight and reached at least the same weight as before undertaking the diet programme (Hensrud *et al.* 1994).

Diets, especially 'fashionable' or 'crash' diets, are geared to reduce dramatically the number of calories consumed. The diets are based on unrealistic conditions, as few people can maintain a strict diet over a longer period. It becomes too restrictive in food choices, it is socially difficult to sustain and the commitment will easily dissipate over an extended period. Additionally, crash diets can make the user feel unwell and unable to function properly because the diet is nutritionally unbalanced. An unbalanced diet can lead to poor concentration and low energy already after a short period. There is evidence from large-scale observational studies that weight cycling or yo-yo dieting is linked to increased mortality (Blair *et al.* 1993).

Some diets recommend cutting out certain food groups, such as meat, fish, wheat or dairy products. However, cutting out certain food groups altogether could remove important nutrients and vitamins from the diet that the body needs to function properly. For example, the Atkins diet is very low in carbohydrates as it limits consumption of pasta, bread and rice, which are basic energy sources (Atkins 2004). These types of diets may produce weight loss, but they are often high in protein and fat that can in turn induce illness. In addition, low carbohydrate diets can cause side effects, such as bad breath, headaches and constipation. Low carbohydrate diets often include foods high in saturated fat, such as butter, cheese and meat. Although currently debated, there is still a prevailing view that too much saturated fat in the diet can raise cholesterol levels and increase the risk of heart disease and stroke (Mustad *et al.* 1997; Hunter *et al.* 2010).

Furthermore, some crash diets are based on eating a single food or meal, such as cabbage soup or raw foods. Others make farfetched claims, for example, that you should cut out certain foods from your diet based on your blood type. Intermittent fasting, which includes the increasingly popular 5:2 diet, is a pattern of eating normally for five days a week, and fast on the other two days. Proponents of the 5:2 diet propose that it can help you live longer and protect you against diseases (Harrison 2013).

Often, there is little or no scientific evidence to back up dieting claims and it can be difficult to keep to such diets over extended periods. If followed over long periods, these diets, if unbalanced, can be a risk to good health. They may create weight loss in the short term, but a better strategy is to make lifestyle changes and lose weight gradually through a well balanced diet and regular exercise.

Socio-cultural perspectives on the adherence to diet advice

The gap between the scientific view of risk and the perception of risk by ordinary people is basically ignored by governments and experts when issuing advice. The experts' ignorance of sociological frameworks and the fundamentals of the socio-cultural risk discourse that fashion people's everyday life has resulted in expert guidance being given without a social and cultural context, thus missing the core construct that people's traditional eating patterns are generationally derived and difficult to alter with abstract information. Eating habits are enforced by social interaction within social status groups and networks (Delormier *et al.* 2009).

Hitherto, nutrition interventions have used models that aim to modify people's psycho-social characteristics, such as influencing knowledge, self-efficacy and attitudes (Contento 2007), and in its most current approach, 'food, bodies and eating are disembodied and disengaged from the social contexts in which people live their lives' (Warin *et al.* 2007:98). Sociological and social anthropological studies of food are grounded on a divergent perspective, with focus on food cultures, social and religious traditions and the collective character of eating patterns among like-minded population groups (Douglas 1984; Murcott 1988). In contrast to behavioural policies, the sociological discipline analyses eating arrangements within the social group or social network, and it aims to explain patterns in relation to their socio-cultural environment (Murcott 1995). The sociological framework recognises that the collective features of a society and its norms fundamentally influence whole populations as well as individual's unique behaviour (Rose 1992).

Attempting to foster dietary change requires continual efforts to sustain alternative behaviours as well as an understanding of population dynamics. Eating patterns characteristic for distinctive populations are implicitly embedded in configurations of social practices and relations, and are shaped specifically by their social agents (Delormier *et al.* 2009). Social practices are skilful procedures, methods or techniques that are appropriately performed by social agents. Individuals, while encouraged to act in ways that are practical and appropriate, do not just react to social structural constraints, but interact via their agency, in a range of socially structured situations (Giddens 1984). Important structures include interpretive schemes that allow people to communicate and share understandings during social interactions (Kechidi 2005). Referring to 'healthy' or 'junk' food portrays individual items on a health continuum related to discourses about food and health in society, with social structures through interpretive schemes shaping food choice practices. Accordingly, research with adolescents has shown that eating practices are deeply embedded in the contexts of home and school as well as in relationships with parents and peers (Backett-Milburn *et al.* 2006; Wills *et al.* 2005). However, significant differences between the eating habits of females and males have been documented, and in seeking to improve nutritional status, it is essential to clarify why such differences occur. Research shows that females demonstrate a more in-depth understanding of nutrition and seek nutrition counselling more frequently than males do (Arganini *et al.* 2012). As an example, fewer males than females knew the current recommendations for fruit and vegetable intake, and fewer males were aware of the links between fruit and vegetable consumption and disease prevention. These findings indicate that males' poorer nutrition knowledge explains a significant part of their lower intake of fruit and vegetables (Baker and Wardle 2003).

Apart from fruit and vegetables, females eat more cereals, milk, dairy products and whole grain products, while red meat, particularly pork, sausages, eggs, alcohol and high sucrose foods are more prominent in the diet of males. The reasons for the different eating behaviours and the different attitudes towards nutrition can be found in psychological and socio-cultural factors. A number of researchers have noted that meat products are commonly associated in everyday life with such qualities as strength, power and virility, and that the consumption of red meat tends for this reason to function as a symbol of masculinity (Twigg 1984; Adams 1987, 2010; Fiddes 1991). In contrast, vegetables are viewed as females' food, making them undesirable to males (Adams 1987). Overall, males' attitude towards nutrition is more straightforward and pleasure-oriented, and less focused on weight than the attitudes of females. Females might have a more indecisive approach and demonstrate less satisfaction with their weight than males (Kiefer *et al.* 2005). Additionally, gendered differences in food choices appear to be attributed partly to females' weight control focus, hence be related to their stronger beliefs in healthy eating (Wardle *et al.* 2004).

Furthermore, results suggest that barriers to healthy eating in males include cynicism about government health messages and a rejection of healthy food on the grounds of poor taste and an inability to satisfy their personal food desires. These reactions can be seen to relate to masculine ideals such as rationality, autonomy and strength (Gough and Connor 2006). In surveying newspaper articles in relation to males and their diet, Gough (2007) found a persistent adherence to hegemonic masculinities predicated on health defeating diets, special occasion cooking of hearty meals and a general distancing from the feminised realm of dieting. Dieting is thus more prevalent in females, whereas males control their weight with exercise and implement diets only for health reasons (Kiefer *et al.* 2005). However, a number of dietary surveys confirm a connection between the nutritional status of both females and males who have higher levels of education or higher incomes (Prättälä *et al.* 1992; Sweeting *et al.* 1994; Osler *et al.* 1990); hence, eating habits are also influenced by education and socio-economic standing. While well-balanced and healthy diets are associated with greater affluence, energy-dense diets poor in nutrients, are preferentially consumed by people associated with lower socio-economic status and of more limited economic means (Darmon and Drewnowski 2008).

In view of the disease burden associated with suboptimum dietary patterns, there is a need to better elucidate whole population trends, to create relevant policy alternatives to populist dietary advice, and to encourage food industry developments that contribute to global improvements to the overall diet quality (Imamura *et al.* 2015).

Conclusion

Individual dietary patterns are typically established in early life with the choice of food closely associated with enduring habits grounded in the social and cultural milieu of the individual. Dieting is the practise of deliberately attempting temporarily to change the habitual consumption pattern for short-term gain, most commonly to achieve or maintain what is perceived as an ideal weight. It is often a result of socio-cultural pressure. Dieting might involve deliberate risk taking by people who are too trusting of popular mass media dieting advice and constantly willing to try novel diet recommendations that are inundating the public domain. Such diet recommendations range from the healthy or simply unhealthy to the risky and fatal.

Novelty diet programs promoted in popular mass media often have weight loss as their specific focus, rather than a holistic healthy food emphasis. Most do actually lead to quick and sometimes dramatic weight loss, but only for the weight to creep back up again at the end of the diet period. Countless fashion diets are based on dubious research or no research at all, prescribing hazardous eating practices that can be detrimental to health. However, long-term risks to health and wellbeing are unlikely to be of concern for the person feeling the need to lose weight.

Poor body image can be linked to low self-esteem, ambivalent social identity, and distorted individual interpretation of the ideal body. Western society's 'thin body image' contributes to dieting, overexercising and an environment conducive to eating disorders. To not live up to this ideal body image can influence a person's overall wellbeing and mental health and contribute to depression and anxiety. With all the focus on weight in Western societies, encouraged by a multibillion-dollar weight loss industry, it is not surprising that millions of people fall prey to fashion diets and bogus weight loss products. Conflicting claims, testimonials and hype by so-called 'experts' can confuse even the most informed consumer.

Rather than adopting short-term dieting fads, small enduring changes to the habitual dietary pattern are more likely to be successful in reaching a healthy body weight. It should be noted that to be thin is not the same as being healthy, and to be slightly overweight is not synonymous to being unhealthy. Official authorities have so far largely failed in influencing habitual food consumption towards sustaining a healthy body weight, as evidenced by continued increases in the worldwide obesity rate.

Governments and experts, when issuing dietary advice, ignore the gap between the scientific view of risk and the perception of risk by people. Food and health advice need a social and cultural context to be made relevant to the targeted population group. Without this socio-cultural framework, advice will not achieve the aim of creating a more health conscious population. People are habitual eaters, habits are developed over generations and attempts to change population consumption patterns with abstract information will fail.

Thus, a health discourse that ignores the social and cultural environment around food and society's diverse ethnic cultures will not change people's eating habits. In view of the disease burden associated with suboptimum dietary patterns, the focus should be on better elucidating diverse population needs for healthy food consumption advice, to create relevant policy alternatives to populist dietary promotions, and to encourage the food industry to contribute to improvements to overall diet quality.

Part III

The risk society perspective of modern industrialisation

Beck's (1992) risk society discourse focuses on modern industrialisation and the risks posed by new procedures and products released for public consumption before being scientifically tested in clinical trials over a longer period. Globalisation of food production has created world markets, and the traditional nation states' power and control have diminished due to the domination of multinational food corporations (Urry 2014b:ix). Multinational food production has widened the distance between production and consumption and made it more difficult for the individual consumer, as well as experts, to keep track of products from their origin through processing interventions to the consumption stage.

Scientific experts might propose that a product is safe to consume, but people's perception of how safe a product is does not necessarily correspond with the scientists' findings, as risks can take a long time to be recognised. Furthermore, continuous innovation and development in farming methods and enhanced technology and production systems, but also improved scientific accuracy, provide continuous challenges. The time pressure for a product to be declared safe from a scientific perspective does not imply that it will be considered safe also in the future when the scientific methodology has improved and the product has been tested on a larger population. Hence, a product that initially is considered safe but might be considered hazardous when further research results become available. Re-analysing the product with new testing methods can give very different results for its impact on people's health and the environment than the initial findings.

The time delay between the launch of the product and conclusive safety results might take years or decades, thus making it difficult for people to trust producers, experts and scientists, as it gives people the impression that shifting science and expert opinions cannot be trusted.

The development of genetically modified food (GM) (see Chapter 8) is one example where consumers have questioned the long-term safety of food, but also its influence on other food crops and weeds growing close to the GM field. The fear of the unknown, and the difficulty faced by producers, scientists and experts in guaranteeing the absence of any negative health effects from food products, have raised questions about future implications of genetically altered food. Currently, some governments and consumer groups are still questioning the science, and the demands for detailed labelling of products are still a contested issue between producers and consumers.

However, it is not only the production of food that causes risks to people's health in modern industrial food production, as during the whole process, from growing to consumption, a product can be a risk to public health through pathogens slipping through deficient quality systems (see Chapter 9). This is an issue with opposite opinions to the GM challenge, in that it is often ignored by the public but highlighted by experts.

The issues around the origins of food and weaknesses in the whole production chain have reignited the question of organic food as an alternative to industrial production of food, and reraised the question of whether people would be safer and healthier if they were mainly eating organic food (see Chapter 10). The myths that a growing population cannot be fed without commercial industrialised food have been questioned in the twenty-first century. Can the risks with industrial production of food be more or less eliminated by going back to traditional small-scale production and using organic methods of production?

In the following chapters, food production, processing and consumption are analysed from the risk society perspective of modern industrialisation.

8 The genetically modified food credibility gap

Introduction

Genetically modified (GM) foods are products of advanced manufacturing processes of late modernity driven by a perception that conventional food production cannot feed the world's growing population. This perception has created a demand for new plants that are genetically modified to grow faster, be less labour intensive, be time and cost efficient, be able to tolerate long transports, keep their freshness, and have the ability to withstand diseases. New products have been allowed to be released into the human and animal food chain without following usual scientific practice that requires extensive and multiple testing of food and environmental safety over an extended period. Genetically modified foods are good examples of what Beck (1992) refers to as creating new risk uncertainties and fundamental disagreements over knowledge, values and how to proceed, where new technology and products, especially consumption products, have not been exposed to rigorous testing over a sufficient time period. This includes testing of environmental impacts and possible cross contamination. The introduction of GM foods have led to intractable controversies in which old strategies for negotiating conflict have failed as the disagreements are too fundamental for a consensus to be found (Pellizzoni, 2003).

The controversy revolves around the wisdom of humans manipulating natural organisms. Genetically modified foods are products derived from organisms whose genetic material (deoxyribonucleic acid [DNA]) has been deliberately altered by human intervention through the forced introduction of genes from a non-related organism, in a way that does not usually occur naturally. Such technology is also called genetic engineering or transgenics. Scientists first discovered that DNA could be transferred between dissimilar organisms in 1946. Genetic engineering has since been applied experimentally and commercially to produce a large range of genetically modified organisms (GMOs). The first GM plant was produced in 1983, through the creation of an antibiotic resistant tobacco plant, proving that genes could be inserted and subsequently inherited by the progeny (Horsch *et al.* 1984).

Although many scientists are supportive of the use of genetic engineering, the technology is not universally endorsed. The potential threat to public health and the environment posed by GM technologies is a hotly contested topic between scientists and the public, as well as between scientists. Genetically modified foods are considered an unacceptable risk in parts of both the developing and developed world. Recently, in the developing world, even during the famine in Zambia in 2002, President Levy Mwanawasa refused GM maize offered by the USA as food aid because it could endanger the health of the starving people in his country (Breithaupt 2003). In the developed world, bans on GM products spread through the European Union (EU) member states, which lead to a trade war with the USA. The latter is a country where the GM technology is widely used and accepted. The US government filed a lawsuit in 2003 through the World Trade Organization (WTO), claiming that the failure of the EU to lift its moratorium on the import and approval of GM crops and food products was in breach of WTO rules (Moore 2003).

The use of GM technology is a difficult conundrum to resolve. Proponents claim that using the technology is a necessity if we want to be able to feed the world's growing population in the future (Raven 2014). Detractors claim that short-term gains are soon to be reversed by eroding biodiversity of traditional cultivars and the evolution of herbicide resistant 'superweeds', which can jeopardise future agricultural sustainability (Mortensen *et al.* 2012).

Public opposition to GM foods

Much of the opposition to genetic engineering of food is focused on the practice of inserting a genetic code from one organism into another unrelated organism, which is seen as manipulating nature, initially with the sole purpose of benefitting agribusinesses. What could have been a public relations triumph for biotechnology, with a promise to provide the world with more nutritious and less expensive food using fewer resources, has become a serious fight driven by dislike of corporate power, especially multinational company control, and lack of transparency. This has created fears of uncontrolled environmental and health effects (Beck 1992, 1999; Douglas 1992; Douglas and Wildavsky 1982). The introduction of GM food products is a typical example of the risk society discourse highlighting discrepancies between science and public perception, but also the limited knowledge of the product's long-term influence on the eco-system.

Consumers in many countries are voicing serious concerns about the substantial risks that are involved in eating GM food and the harm it can cause, while many scientists believe that the GM food presented on the market for human consumption poses no greater risk to human health than conventional food. This is probably the most powerful dichotomy between public perception of risk and the scientific view that exists in the food area. Of particular public concern is the claim that GM food causes cancer and allergies, but also the capacity of GM crops to contaminate non-GM counterparts. The battle over genetic engineering of food crops is being waged on multiple fronts, by farmers, legislators, activists and scientists around the world, all trying to separate fear from fact. Fears over the safety of GMOs have given rise to a vitriolic public debate, consumer boycotts and a political battle that is difficult to resolve (Howarth 2012).

However, there are many other issues to consider when evaluating the use of genetic modification besides health concerns. Key areas related to GMOs that need further attention include the effect of GM crops on the environment, the impact of such crops for farmers and their financial returns, the effect on pesticide resistance of weeds, and the power of multinational corporations to control breeding material through intellectual property rights. Environmental concerns have recently been raised also at government levels. Although herbicide-tolerant crops have enabled farmers to substitute more toxic and persistent herbicides with glyphosate, overreliance on glyphosate and a reduction in the diversity of weed management practices have contributed to the evolution of glyphosate resistance in some weed species (Fernandez-Cornejo *et al.* 2014).

Genetic modified technology explained

The transmission of DNA is a process in which an organism incorporates genetic material from another organism without being the offspring of that organism, such as between prokaryotes, organisms like bacteria whose cells lack a defined nucleus, and eukaryotes, organisms whose cells contain a defined nucleus like plants and animals, or between unrelated eukaryotic species. This is called horizontal gene transfer. It is distinguished from the transmission of genetic material from parents to offspring during reproduction, which is known as vertical gene transfer. It should be clear that horizontal gene transfer has been part of the natural evolution of eukaryotic genomes, but mainly between organisms that are either intimately associated or through occasional cell to cell contacts in mutualistic or parasitic relationships (Bock 2010). Nearly every food crop grown today has been genetically altered many times through a breeding process that uses natural genetic variety, spontaneous mutations and cross breeding of related varieties to create and select the desired traits. Selective breeding has been used for thousands of years to improve plant traits, and it began with the domestication of wild plants into uniform and predictable agricultural cultivars. High yielding varieties have been particularly important for progress in agriculture. However, these procedures are time consuming and it may take ten or more years to transfer a trait from a donor species into a crop cultivar via conventional strategies (Khan and Liu 2009). Genetic engineering is very different to selective breeding in that it transfers genes coding for desired traits between completely unrelated organisms by direct manipulation of the genes. Thus, it is a shortcut the scientists have devised to speed up the work of selective breeding of plants and to introduce attributes that would not be possible with traditional techniques.

Genetically engineered plants are generated in a laboratory by altering their genetic makeup and are initially tested in the laboratory for desired qualities before undergoing field trials and possible commercialisation. Genetic modification can involve either the insertion or deletion of genes to create a genetically modified organism. When genes are inserted, they usually come from a different species, which is a form of horizontal gene transfer. The techniques used might involve attaching the genes to a virus that penetrate the recipient cell. Additional methods include the physical insertion of extra DNA into the nucleus of the intended host with a very small syringe, using electroporation by introducing DNA from one organism into the cell of another by use of an electric pulse, or with very small particles fired from a particle gun; the biolistic method. Some methods exploit natural forms of gene transfer, such as the ability of Agrobacterium tumefaciens to transfer genetic material to plants, or the ability of lentiviruses to transfer genes to animal cells. Most GM plants have been generated by the biolistic method or by Agrobacterium tumefaciens mediated transformation (Khan and Liu 2009).

Organisms that have been genetically modified in the past include microorganisms, such as bacteria and yeasts, insects, plants, fish and mammals. GMOs are widely used in medical research; they are the source of GM foods and are also used to produce goods other than food. Currently available GM foods stem mostly from plants, but in the future foods derived from GM microorganisms or GM animals might be introduced to the market (Smith *et al.* 2010; Uzogara 2000). Most existing first generation GM crops have been developed to improve yield, through the introduction of resistance to plant diseases or increased tolerance to herbicides (Chen and Lin 2013). In the future, second generation genetic modification could be aimed at altering the nutrient content of food, reducing its allergenic potential or improving the efficiency of food production systems (Ruiz-Lopez *et al.* 2014; Jabed *et al.* 2012; Key *et al.* 2008).

Genetically manipulated food is already very much part of modern industry production although there are strongly critical opponents. Beck and Holzer (Beck 1992, 1999; Beck and Holzer 2007) refer to risks of prematurely using new technologies that are not fully understood until long after their introduction. One view is that when the risks of GM foods are understood the damage might already be done and responsibility for the GM products obscured. There are lingering questions in relation to the full impact of certain GM organisms on the balance of the overall environment and possible direct or indirect effects on public health. Green activists propose that GM crops are a potential hazard, arguing that their genes could spread to related plants through cross-pollination. A commonly cited event involved the spread of GM maize pollen to native wild maize varieties in Mexico, the ancestral home of maize. Mexico imposed a moratorium on the planting of transgenic maize in 1998 in order to protect genetic diversity of their landrace varieties. Despite the moratorium, early in the new century, research found that 1 per cent of

Mexican landrace and wild maize varieties carried genes that had jumped from GM varieties. Hence, cross-pollination can seriously threaten the nature of traditionally grown crops, which have implications for the local people's social and cultural food supply of biologically diverse plants – a diversity that is a precious global resource (Soleri and Cleveland 2006).

Genetically engineered traits

So far, new traits introduced through genetic engineering have mainly targeted benefits to farmers and industries with few benefits flowing directly to consumers. A primary focus has been cash crops in high demand by farmers such as soybean, corn (maize), canola (rapeseed) and cotton, with cottonseed oil as a food oil. Agricultural traits include improved disease and stress resistance, herbicide resistance and pest resistance, while industrial traits include production of biofuel or drugs and products with an ability to absorb toxins for use in bioremediation of pollution. Only scant attention has been given to consumer's food preference for enhanced quality like improved shelf life and nutritional composition.

Herbicide resistance is the most prevalent genetically engineered trait introduced so far. Crops have been commercialised that are resistant to the herbicides glyphosate or glufosinate. As weeds have grown resistant to glyphosate, companies have started to develop crops engineered to become resistant to multiple herbicides to allow farmers to use a mixed group of two, three or four different chemicals (Batista and Oliveira 2009).

Genes encoding for insecticidal proteins from Bacillus thuringiensis (Bt) have been inserted into tobacco, corn, rice and many other crops (Sanahuja *et al.* 2011). Papaya, potatoes and squash have been engineered to resist viral pathogens such as the cucumber mosaic virus, which, despite its name, infects a wide variety of plants (Abrol and Schankar 2012).

Tolerance to non-biological stresses like drought, frost, soil salinity and nitrogen starvation have been attempted through genetic engineering and, if successful, could increase yield when plants are grown under harsh environmental conditions (Zurbriggen *et al.* 2010). Genetically modified fish have been developed with traits that drive an over-production of growth hormone for use in the aquaculture industry to increase the speed of development and potentially reduce fishing pressure on wild stocks. GM salmon can mature in half the time it takes non-GM salmon and achieve twice the size (Smith *et al.* 2010).

Improved shelf life was actually the first GM trait to be allowed on the market for human consumption, by adding an antisense or reverse orientation gene to a tomato. The ripening process was slowed to prevent softening and rotting, while allowing the tomato to retain its natural flavour and colour. In 1994, the Food and Drug Administration approved the transgenic Flavr Savr tomato for marketing in the USA. However, the tomato was so delicate that it was difficult to transport, and it was withdrawn from the market (Bruening and Lyons 2000). Another attempt to improve shelf life involves an apple that has been genetically modified to resist browning. A gene in the fruit has been modified so that the apple produces less polyphenol oxidase, a chemical involved in the browning reaction (Haroldsen *et al.* 2012).

Improvements to the nutritional profile of oils have been achieved by genetically engineering soybeans to facilitate processing and provide healthier oils. Other examples include a GM cassava with lower levels of toxic cyanogen glycosides (Sayre *et al.* 2011) and golden rice with increased levels of vitamin A as a possible way of preventing vitamin A deficiency, which is common in some developing countries. *Camelina sativa*, a member of the mustard family, has been modified in research laboratories to produce plants that accumulate high levels of oils of similar composition to beneficial fish oils (Ruiz-Lopez *et al.* 2014). Additionally, pigs have been genetically engineered to produce omega-3 fatty acids through the expression of a roundworm gene (Kang 2005). Chinese and Argentinian scientists genetically engineered dairy cows with human genes to produce milk with the same composition as human breast milk (Yang *et al.* 2011). Researchers from New Zealand also developed a genetically engineered cow that produced allergen free milk (Jabed *et al.* 2012). All but the soybeans have so far been confined to research laboratories, except some field trials for the golden rice.

Goats have been genetically engineered to produce milk with spider web silk proteins in their milk for industrial purposes (Römer and Scheibel 2008). Oilseeds can be modified to produce fatty acids for detergents and GM algae can produce biofuels. Maize seeds have been genetically modified to convert its own starch to sugar to speed the process of making ethanol for biofuel (Johnson *et al.* 2008). While the current focus is on using plants for biofuels, such as ethanol and biodiesel, plants are a potential source of a much wider range of useful chemicals and biomaterials. Several companies and laboratories are working on engineering plants that can be used to make bioplastics, but such developments are still at a relatively early stage (van Beilen and Poirier 2008; Furtado *et al.* 2014).

Poplar and other plantation trees have been genetically engineered to be insect resistant or to contain less lignin, a complex polymer that form an integral part of the secondary cell walls of plants. With less lignin, it is easier to digest the pulp during pulping and bleaching for paper production. However, compromising the structural integrity of the plant might require increased use of pesticides because of a lessened disease resistance (Hall 2007).

Medical applications include pharmaceuticals produced from plants, with a GM product already approved for Gaucher's disease, a genetic disease in which fatty substances – sphingolipids – accumulate in cells and certain organs (Fox 2012). Bananas have been developed that produce human vaccines against infectious diseases such as hepatitis B (Kumar *et al.* 2005). Tobacco plants have been developed that can produce therapeutic antibodies. Although improving global health through molecular 'pharming' has been discussed for at least two decades, little progress has actually been made (Ma *et al.* 2013).

Genetically modified plants have also been used for bioremediation of contaminated soils. It is widely viewed as the ecologically responsible alternative to the environmentally destructive physical remediation methods currently practiced (Abhilash *et al.* 2009). Various GM plants expressing bacterial genes can be used to enhance degradation and remediation of herbicides, explosives and persistent organic pollutants, such as polychlorinated biphenyls (PCBs). PCBs are artificially constructed chemicals that are used in products like electrical equipment, surface coatings, inks, adhesives, flame retardants and paints. Exposure to PCBs can cause cancers of the digestive system, liver, skin and lymphatic system. PCBs have also been linked to reduced fertility in females, lower mobile-sperm count in males, and negative neurological health effects (European Food Safety Authority 2012). They may be released into the environment when waste containing PCBs is incinerated or stored in landfills. The use and production of PCBs is now banned worldwide, but because of their persistence, they are difficult to remove from the environment. Specific GM plants could potentially detoxify contaminated environments. There have also been attempts to remove heavy metals, such as mercury and lead, from soils through bioremediation. However, since only the chemical configuration, but not the elements as such, can be altered, the focus has been on hyper-accumulation above ground and removal of the soil surface (Meagher 2000). Although there have been many encouraging results in the past decade, there have also been numerous inconclusive and unsuccessful attempts at phytoremediation in the field (Gerhardt *et al.* 2009).

Planting of genetically modified organisms

Since the first commercial planting of a GM crop, farmers have embraced GM technology in a range of countries. Between 1996 and 2012, the total surface area of land cultivated with GM crops increased from 1.7 million hectares to 170 million hectares, incorporating 10 per cent of the croplands of the world. In 2012, GM crops were planted in 28 countries of which eight were developed countries, and 20 developing countries (James 2012).

As of 2013, approximately 90 per cent of corn, 93 per cent of soybeans and 90 per cent of cotton produced in the United States were GM varieties. Other GM crops commercially grown in the United States are herbicide-tolerant canola, sugar beets and alfalfa, as well as virus resistant papaya and squash (Fernandez-Cornejo *et al.* 2014). Estimates suggest that as much as 80 per cent of the US processed food may contain ingredients from a GM crop, such as corn starch, high-fructose corn syrup, corn oil, canola oil, soybean oil, soy flour, soy lecithin and cottonseed oil (Hallman *et al.* 2003). Despite this percentage found in processed food, there are only a few genetically engineered plant foods directly available on the US market including papaya, squash and sweet corn.

Canada is one of the world's largest producers of GM canola, with an adoption rate of 94 per cent of the total canola crop being herbicide tolerant. Canada also grows GM maize, soybean and sugar beet. It is one of very few countries to grow triple stacked maize; that is a crop variety with three modified genes, one gene for European corn borer control, a second for rootworm control and a third for herbicide tolerance (James 2010).

Europe has relatively few genetically engineered crops, with the exception of Spain where 24 per cent of maize or corn grown was genetically engineered in 2010. This equalled 80 per cent of the Bt maize MON 810 grown in Europe with smaller amounts in five other countries: Portugal, Poland, the Czech Republic, Slovakia and Romania. In 2012, Poland discontinued planting Bt maize because of regulation inconsistencies in the interpretation of the law on planting approval between the EU and Poland. Sweden, Germany and the Czech Republic briefly grew the Amflora potato before it was withdrawn from the market (James 2010; James 2012). The European Union had a de facto ban on the approval of new GM crops from 1999 until 2004.

Genetically modified cotton, canola and carnations are grown in Australia. A notable 98.5 per cent of all the cotton grown in Australia in 2010 was transgenic, of which over 91 per cent featured the stacked genes for insect resistance and herbicide tolerance (James 2010). In 2011, GM plants were grown in all states except South Australia and Tasmania, which have extended their moratoriums until 2019.

In New Zealand, no GM food is grown and no medicines containing live genetically modified organisms have been approved for use. However, medicines manufactured using GMOs that do not contain live organisms have been approved for sale and imported foods with GM components are sold in New Zealand (MPI 2012).

There has been a rapid growth in the area of GM crops sown in developing countries. The five lead developing countries are India and China in Asia, Brazil and Argentina in Latin America, and South Africa in Africa. In 2012, developing countries grew a majority, 52 per cent, of the total GM harvest for the first time. Brazil and Argentina are the second and third largest producers of GM food behind the USA, followed by India and China. Brazil is growing GM soybean, maize and cotton, and had the largest increase in GM crop area with a year on year increase of 21 per cent. India currently only grows GM cotton, while China produces GM varieties of cotton, poplar, petunia, tomato, papaya and sweet pepper. The use of GM crops in India has been controversial. Although Indian regulators cleared a GM eggplant for commercialisation in 2009, a moratorium had to be imposed on its release after opposition by some scientists, farmers and environmental groups (Anon 2010). South Africa was, in 2012, the major commercial grower of GM crops in Africa, with smaller amounts grown in Burkina Faso (maize), Egypt (cotton) and Sudan (cotton) (James 2012).

Genetically modified food controversies

To assess the safety of GM food products official authorities generally gauge whether or not the food is substantially equivalent to non-genetically engineered counterparts that are already deemed fit for human consumption. Although such appraisals should at least provide some public assurance, there are still widespread popular perceptions that eating GM food can be harmful to health (Martinez-Poveda *et al.* 2009; Bawa and Anilakumar 2013). Based primarily on such concerns, but also on wider trepidations about the risk to the environment, anti-GMO activists have lobbied for restrictions on growing modified crops and on selling such food. Additionally, they demand labelling of GM food when sold to the consumer. Various scientific research projects have provided partial support for concerns emphasised by anti-GMO activists related to negative environmental aspects attributed to GMOs (Waltz 2009).

Because of the pervasive public unease about risks associated with biotechnology, there is an urge for more public information about the risks themselves, and a desire for a choice of non-GM varieties to be able to avoid the possibility of being exposed to genetically engineered food products. There is also the general impression of a fast moving social and technological society in which people feel powerless to influence the production, distribution and correct labelling of GM food. These issues give rise to an extensive anxiety, which augment the further need for assurances of a safe food supply (Hunt 2004; Beck 1992).

When assessing attitudes to natural and GM foods in a representative sample of adults from France, Germany, Italy, Switzerland, the UK and the USA, there were surprising degrees of similarities across the six countries in seeing 'natural' as very positive. On the contrary, there were widespread opposition in all countries towards genetic engineering of food, as it was thought of as the opposite to natural food. However, the strength of the attitudes varied, with the highest negative attitudes to GM food in continental Europe and the lowest in the USA (Rozin *et al.* 2012). Similarly, a survey of US consumers found that 34 per cent were very or extremely concerned about GM food (Deloitte 2010), while almost twice as many, or close to 60 per cent, European consumers thought that GM food could pose a threat to their health and that of future generations (Eurobarometer 2010). It had previously been shown that risk perceptions exerted a greater effect than perceptions of the benefit on public attitudes towards agro-biotechnology. UK consumers were more susceptible to negative attitudes towards GM food than US consumers (Moon and Balasubramanian 2004).

Concerns over GM crops typically stem from both health and environmental issues. Slightly more than half of the Europeans, but only 13 per cent of Americans, felt that GM crop production could be detrimental to the environment (Eurobarometer 2010; Kopicki 2013). Furthermore, the issue of GM derived feed used in animal production was claimed to be of major concern to about half of the sample of Canadian consumers (Komirenko *et al.* 2010). The Food Standards Australia New Zealand (FSANZ) 2007 survey in Australia, where GM labelling is mandatory, found that 27 per cent of consumers looked at the label to see if it contained GM material when purchasing a grocery product for the first time. Overall, there were less serious concerns about GM food in the USA compared to Europe, but a 2013 poll by *The New York Times* still indicated that three quarters of Americans showed some trepidation and 93 per cent wanted GM labelling (Kopicki 2013).

In contrast to public perception, there is fundamental scientific consensus that current food products on the market derived from genetically engineered crops pose no greater risk to human health than conventional foods (Nicolia *et al.* 2014). No reports of ill effects have been documented in the human population from GM food, although causality might be difficult to substantiate (Key *et al.* 2008), and it might take a long time before the effects occur (cf. Beck 1992). Foods derived from GMOs are rarely tested on humans before commercial release, since it is difficult to design meaningful and longitudinal clinical studies to test them. Scientists instead examine the genetic modification, its protein products, and any intended changes that those proteins make to the food, which does not necessarily guarantee that it is safe for human consumption.

One of the well-known risks of genetically modifying a plant or animal that is later used as food is the introduction of an allergen. Testing for allergens is part of the research and development of GMOs intended for animal and human consumption, and passing those tests is part of the regulatory requirements prescribed by food authorities before the food can be marketed (Batista and Oliviera 2009). The opposite can also be true, in that genetic engineering can be used to remove allergens from food, and this can potentially reduce the risk of food allergies. A hypoallergenic strain of soybean was shown to lack the major allergen that is found in the GM unaltered beans and a similar approach has been tried in ryegrass. These findings demonstrate that the production of hypoallergenic grass is a possibility (Herman *et al.* 2003; Bhalla *et al.* 1999).

Checks are implemented to see whether the food derived from a GMO is 'substantially equivalent' to its non-GMO derived counterpart. This examination is supposed to provide a way to detect any negative non-intended consequences of the genetically engineered food. If the newly incorporated protein is not similar to that of other proteins found in food or if anomalies arise in the substantial equivalence comparison, further testing is required (Kuiper *et al.* 2001). However, the application of the substantial equivalence concept has been criticised as potentially flawed, and there are concerns that some current safety tests could allow harmful substances to enter the human food chain. It has even been suggested that all GM foods should go through extensive biological, toxicological and immunological testing and that the concept of substantial equivalence should be abandoned (Levidow *et al.* 2007).

Consensus among scientists and regulators points to a continuing need for improved testing technologies and protocols to better identify and manage risk. In particular, the variety and complexity of genetically engineered traits and modes of action expected in the near future, as well as improved knowledge of genetic factors that can affect composition, raise questions about the need for expanded requirements for future safety testing. In 2012, the European Food Safety Authority Panel on Genetically Modified Organisms stressed that 'novel hazards' could be associated with transgenic crops that would not be present in conventional crossbreeding (European Food Safety

Authority 2012). However, there is no universal consensus on methods to be used since it is very difficult to test a food compared to an individual chemical.

There is less consensus among scientists about potential harmful environmental effects from the release of transgenic organisms. Advocacy groups including Greenpeace, the World Wildlife Fund, Organic Consumers Association and the Center for Science in the Public Interest have long raised concerns that such potential risks have not yet been adequately investigated (Levidow *et al.* 2007). Genetically modified crops are planted in fields much like regular crops. There they interact directly with organisms that feed on the crops and indirectly with other organisms in the food chain. Pollen from GM plants is distributed in the environment as for any other crop. This distribution has led to concerns about the effects of genetically engineered crops on other species and about gene flow to other plants, to animals and bacteria. Genes from a GMO may pass to another organism just like an endogenous gene. The process is known as outcrossing and can occur in any new open-pollinated crop variety, with newly introduced traits potentially crossing into neighbouring plants of the same or closely related species. There are concerns that the spread of genes from modified organisms to unmodified relatives could produce species of weeds resistant to herbicides. These new genes could contaminate nearby non-GM crops or organic crops, and disrupt the whole ecosystem (Prakash *et al.* 2011).

One concern raised is the possibility of a horizontal gene transfer from plants used as feed to animals, which would subsequently enter the human food chain, or directly from plants used as food to humans. However, the risk of horizontal gene transfer between plants and animals has been shown to be very low and equivalent to gene transfer from conventional foods that have always been part of human consumption and human diets. Any risks associated with the consumption of genetic material will remain, but it is minimal since breakdown of DNA during food processing and passage through the gastrointestinal tract reduces the likelihood that intact genes capable of encoding foreign proteins will be transferred to the gut microflora or human cells (Jonas *et al.* 2001). Of particular concern is the antibiotic resistance gene commonly used as a genetic marker in transgenic crops that could be transferred to harmful bacteria, creating superbugs that are resistant to multiple antibiotics, but also this risk is currently considered to be low (van den Eede *et al.* 2004).

There is a view that GM crops provide benefits to the environment through a reduction in the use of pesticides. This has not been substantiated; on the contrary, it has been shown that the spread of glyphosate resistant weeds has brought about substantial increases in the number and volume of herbicides that are required to prevent destruction of the crops. Herbicide resistant crop technology has led to a 239 million kg increase in herbicide use in the United States between 1996 and 2011, while Bt crops have reduced insecticide applications by 56 million kg. Overall, pesticide use increased by an estimated 183 million kg, or about 7 per cent. Weeds that are more resistant continue to emerge, and some farmers are finding it necessary to return to the practice of yearly ploughing as part of their strategy for weed control (Benbrook 2012).

A major use of GM crops is in insect control. Regulatory agencies assess the potential for transgenic plants to affect non-target organisms before approving their commercial release. Still, there are concerns that these toxins could target predatory and other beneficial or harmless insects as well as the targeted pest. Another problem with such crops is resistance that evolves naturally after an insect population has been subjected to intense selection pressure in the form of repeated use of a single insecticide. The pink bollworm has been found to be resistant to the first generation Bacillus thuringiensis (Bt) cotton in parts of Gujarat, India. Bollworm resistance to first generation Bt cotton has also been identified in Australia, China, Spain and the United States. A primary pest targeted by Bt maize in the United States is the western corn rootworm and it has now been found to have developed resistance against the Bt toxin. Armyworms resistant to Bt maize were first discovered in Puerto Rico. The European corn borer, one of the primary insects Bt is meant to target, has also been shown to be capable of developing resistance to the Bt protein (Gassmann *et al.* 2011; Wan *et al.* 2012; Tabashnik *et al.* 2013).

Additionally, there are fears that the genetic diversity of crops might decrease as GM varieties limit the number of cultivars being used or that they might indirectly affect the diversity of other organisms (Jenkins 2013). A further factor is that traditional food crops are discarded for financial reasons and multinational agribusinesses are buying up land to grow crops, not for the local but for the global market, hence creating food shortages for the local population (Shiva 2000; Isenhour 2014).

The escape of GMOs into neighbouring crops is of concern to farmers whose crops are exported to countries that have not approved harvests from modified crops. In 2000, Aventis StarLink corn, which had been approved only as animal feed due to concerns about possible allergic reactions in humans, was found contaminating corn products in US supermarkets and restaurants. This corn became the subject of a widely publicised recall, which started when Taco Bell branded taco shells sold in supermarkets were found to contain the GM corn. Consequently, sales of StarLink seeds were discontinued (Lemaux 2008). In another example, American exports of rice to Europe were interrupted in 2006 when the US crop was contaminated with rice containing the LibertyLink modification, which had not been approved for release (Berry 2011). In May 2013, glyphosate-resistant GM wheat that was not yet approved for release was discovered on a farm in Oregon, growing as a weed or 'volunteer plant' in a field that had been planted with winter wheat. The discovery threatened US wheat exports (Reuters 2013). These examples highlight the threats the risk society discourse are concerned about and it demonstrates as highly likely that the modern industry, despite strict regulation of how GM food should be produced and distributed, are compromised in reality, as emphasised by for example, Beck (1992, 1999), Beck and Holzer (2007) and Hunt (2004).

Regulating genetically modified organisms

The centrality of food in society, culture and everyday life has created an environment for potentially highly emotive engagements, and agri-biotechnology has attracted fierce debates over perceived new risks in the second modernity – globally centred risks – as different from the first modernity – nation state centred risks (Beck 1992; Urry 2014b:xi). Such perceived new risks are construed as qualitatively different from natural disasters, in that they are manufactured, emerge out of technological advances of second modernity and have novel impacts (Beck 1992, 1999; Giddens 1998). Threats to life-sustaining quality of air, food and water are mostly invisible and their long-term effects are largely unknown. These potentially unlimited spatial and temporal conditions are outside ordinary people's influence, which makes them powerless to take evasive action (Beck 1997b). Commonly, governments are seen as complicit in facilitating progress, yet unable to manage the risks or control the consequences, because possible novel impacts exceed the limits of existing evidence and scientific knowledge (Beck 2003; Giddens 1998).

The presumption that genetic engineering would become a strategic technology for the twenty-first century, much as nuclear power and information technology were in the twentieth century, has been challenged by press and public reactions (Bauer 2005). The European press, in particular, questioned the prudence of technocratic processes that facilitate an expansion in the availability of GM food, while the evidence of harm and safety remained inconclusive. The most deeply contested issue centred on the status of scientific knowledge, evidence and methodology, as well as on claims about expert partiality, ignorance and the suppression of evidence that was inconvenient for the policy agenda. Food retailers in several countries joined in the argument by shifting company policy on GM food based on a business rationale linked to the newspaper coverage, a consumer boycott and the financial unfeasibility of retaining products that did not sell (Austin and Lo 1999).

As a reaction to the negative press, governments have attempted to assess and manage through legislation potential risks associated with the use of genetic engineering technology, the development and release of GMOs, and the conditions for sale of GM food to consumers. However, the fierce resistance to GM food in parts of the world led to differing government responses, with some of the most marked differences occurring between the USA and Europe.

In the United States, a policy framework and governing regulatory activities were developed to ensure safety for the public, but also to guarantee the continuing development of the biotechnology industry without overly burdensome requirements. The policy is focused on the final product of the genetic engineering process, rather than on the process itself. It stipulates that there is no reason to bar the technology in the absence of proven scientific risks since genetic engineering is part of a continuum of agricultural innovations with the same kind of risks as those seen for traditionally produced food. Therefore, existing regulatory oversight is considered sufficient to safeguard the public (Marsden 2003).

The European Union approach is very different, as it is primarily based on the precautionary principle, with a focus on genetic engineering as a new technology that may have unintended hazardous consequences. The legislation is one of the more stringent in the world, with all food containing a GMO considered to be a new product. Each new product is subject to an extensive, science-based assessment by the European Food Safety Authority (EFSA). Exceptions are crops not intended for food use, which are generally not reviewed by authorities responsible for food safety. The EFSA opinions are presented to the European Commission, who then drafts a proposal for granting or refusing the authorisation of the GM product, which in turn is decided on by member states. The criteria for authorisation cover safety, freedom of choice, labelling and traceability. The EU differentiates between approval for cultivation within the EU and approval for import and processing. While only a few GMOs have been approved for cultivation in the EU, a number of GMOs have been approved for import and processing. The cultivation of GMOs has triggered a heated debate about coexistence of GM and non-GM crops within member states (Davison 2010).

Canada has an extensive science-based regulatory framework used in the approval process of agricultural products produced through biotechnology. Plants or products modified through genetic engineering are referred to in the Canadian legislation as plants with novel traits or novel foods. The Canadian Food Inspection Agency, Health Canada and Environment Canada are the three agencies responsible for approval of products derived from biotechnology. The three agencies work together to monitor development of plants with novel traits, novel foods and all plants or products with new characteristics not previously used in agriculture and food production. Canadian law requires that manufacturers and importers submit detailed scientific data for safety assessment, including information on how the GM food crop was developed, its composition and nutritional data of the novel food compared to the original non-modified food, to make it possible to assess potential new toxin formations and the potential for causing an allergic reaction (Evans and Lupescu 2012).

All GM foods intended for sale in Australia and New Zealand must undergo a safety evaluation by Food Standards Australia New Zealand (FSANZ). FSANZ must approve any food produced from GM crops, or produced using genetically engineered enzymes, before it can be marketed in Australia or New Zealand. The GM food regulation has two provisions – mandatory pre-market approval, including a food safety assessment, and mandatory labelling requirements. Each new genetic modification is assessed individually for its potential impact on the safety of the food by comparing the GM food with a similar, commonly eaten conventional food from a molecular, toxicological, nutritional and compositional point of view. The Office of the Gene Technology Regulator in Australia and the

Environmental Protection Authority in New Zealand oversee the development and environmental release of any GM organisms and issue licenses for their use (Crothers 2011).

Other countries seem to be polarised around the attitudes to regulations in the USA or the European Union depending on their relationships with the respective trading block. Thus, Latin American countries tend to be more supportive of GM crops, while African countries tend to take the more restrictive approach adopted by the European Union. However, there are also international attempts to harmonise the legislative approach for the worldwide growing and marketing of GM crops. In 1982, the Organization for Economic Co-operation and Development (OECD) released an initial report into the potential hazards of releasing GMOs into the environment, as the first transgenic plants were being developed (Bull *et al.* 1982). Subsequently, the OECD joined forces with the World Health Organization (WHO) and the United Nations' Food and Agricultural Organization (FAO) to develop strategies for assessing the safety of genetically engineered crops and food. The OECD's Group of National Experts on Safety in Biotechnology issued two consensus reports for field testing of GM crops and principles for evaluating the safety of GM food, respectively (Organization for Economic Co-operation and Development 1992, 1993). Finally, the Codex Alimentarius Commission (CAC) of the FAO/WHO at its 26th session in 2003 adopted overarching principles for risk analysis and food safety assessment for foods derived from genetically engineered plants and microorganisms (Codex Alimentarius Commission 2003).

The use of the substantial equivalence concept is common as a starting point for the safety assessment of GM foods by most national and international agencies. As noted above, it relates to a comparison between the food derived from modern biotechnology and its conventional counterpart, focusing on determination of similarities and differences. Rather than trying to identify every risk associated with a particular food, the intention is to identify new or altered hazards relative to the conventional counterpart. If a new or altered hazard, nutritional anomaly or other safety concerns are identified, the associated risk should be characterised to determine its relevance to human health. The comparative method recognises the fact that existing foods often contain toxic components or anti-nutrients as well, but are still able to be consumed safely, since in practice there are some tolerable chemical risks taken with food. However, if the product has no natural equivalent, or shows significant differences from the unmodified food, further safety testing will be required (Codex Alimentarius Commission 2003).

There is a preference by consumers in many countries for specific labelling of foods with GM ingredients. The labelling requirements are driven by the right of the consumer to know what they purchase, and governments in several countries have introduced laws prescribing labelling of GM ingredients. In 2014, 64 countries required labelling of all gene-modified foods. The European Union, Russia, Australia, New Zealand, Brazil, Japan, China, as well as many other countries, with India the latest to be added in 2013, have all made GMO labelling compulsory, while other jurisdictions make such labelling voluntary or have plans to introduce labelling. GMO labelling is not required in the United States, although there have been numerous efforts to pass labelling laws in individual states (Center for Food Safety 2013).

A 2007 study on the effect of labelling laws found that once labelling went into effect, few products containing GM ingredients remained on the shelves. Businesses stopped carrying products with ingredients that had been genetically modified. The study also found that costs were higher in food exporting than in food importing countries. Food exporters like the United States, Argentina and Canada have adopted voluntary labelling approaches, while importers have generally adopted mandatory labelling (Gruère and Rao 2007).

There are several arguments put forward in favour of and against mandatory labelling of GM foods. The most obvious is that consumers should have a right to know what is in their food, especially concerning products for which health and environmental concerns have been raised. Opponents claim that labelling implies a warning about health effects, whereas no significant differences between conventional foods and modified foods have been detected. They also claim that labelling imposes a cost on all consumers, not just the concerned public. Segregation, identity preservation and systematic testing are costly activities, albeit essential to secure food safety.

The future of GM crops

Currently the most widely planted genetically engineered crops, including maize, soybean and cotton, are mainly used for animal feed and cooking oils, as well as for biofuel production and other non-food applications. Genetically engineered varieties of rice, wheat and potatoes are not yet commonly grown, since opposition to such staple foods has discouraged commercialisation attempts. So far, genetically engineered crops used directly as food include virus resistant papaya and squash, and recently Bt sweet corn. The question is whether it will be commercially possible to introduce a new generation of GM foods and not face fierce opposition to it.

With the global population expected to reach 9.7 billion by 2050 according to the United Nations, Department of Economic and Social Affairs, Population Division (2015), food demand is expected to almost double driven by the larger number of people and a growing middle class in developing countries. Although agricultural productivity has improved radically over the last 50 years, it is predicted that further improvements will be much more difficult. In particular, the rapid increase in rice and wheat yields that helped feed the world for decades are showing signs of dwindling. Climate change is also expected to have a detrimental impact, bringing higher temperatures and, in many regions, wetter conditions that can spread disease and insects into new areas. Drought, damaging storms and very hot days can be anticipated to influence crop yields adversely. Among these stresses, drought is the most serious problem for global agriculture, affecting approximately 40 per cent of the world's land area. Even worse, climate change is predicted to lead to extreme temperatures and more severe and prolonged drought in some parts of the world, which will have a dramatic impact on crop growth and productivity (Trenberth *et al.* 2014).

One advantage of genetic engineering is its potential to rapidly assist crops to adapt to environmental changes. While creating a new crop variety through conventional breeding takes more than a decade, genetic engineering can achieve the same change in less than six months. However, the downside of speeding up the process is the subsequent potential for increasing the risk that the food can have negative health effects if sufficient time is not allowed in order to perform scientific clinical trials to verify its safety (Beck 1992). Preparation of such regulatory packages can cost as much as US$35 million per transgenic event and take more than five years to complete (Lusser *et al.* 2012). Although genetic engineering allows plant growers to make changes that are more precise and that draw from a far greater variety of genes from the plants' wild relatives or from different types of organisms, developing crops that are better able to withstand climate change, this is not an easy task. Due to the multiple genetic changes needed and the quantitative nature of stress tolerance in plants, efforts to improve crop performance have been elusive and may require basic changes to the plant's physiology (Zhang *et al.* 2014).

Looking further into the future, there are likely advances in molecular biology that will allow endogenous genes to be deleted, modified or moved with far greater precision. In particular, new genome engineering tools 'Talens' and 'Crispr' allow geneticists to change chromosomes to exactly where they want them, and not randomly as is the case with current genetic engineering tools. Talens use special proteins fused with nucleases that cleave the DNA at a precisely the place required. The broken chromosome allows new genes to be inserted or other types of modifications to be made. Crispr, an even newer version of the technology, uses RNA (ribonucleic acid), which helps transfer the DNA code to other cell components, to zero in on the targeted genes. With both Talens and Crispr, molecular biologists can modify even a few nucleotides or insert and delete a gene exactly where they want on the chromosome, making the change far more predictable and effective. Gene editing combined with gene drive technologies, where nature takes care of driving a modified gene through a species population, could provide rapid change. Public perception and the performance of the engineered crop varieties will determine the extent to which these powerful technologies contribute towards securing the world's food supply (Voytas and Gao 2014).

It is too early to tell if crops modified without foreign genes will change the public debate over GMOs. These foods will still not be seen as 'natural', an important aspect in the public perception of risk. Wheat, accounting for 21 per cent of the calories consumed globally, would be an early candidate for the use of Talens and Crispr, since it is particularly sensitive to rising temperatures and is grown in many regions, such as Australia, that are prone to severe droughts. However, interfering with a grain that makes bread daily for countless millions around the world would be particularly offensive to many opponents of GM foods. Additionally, wheat is a commodity grain sold on the world markets; hence, approval of GM wheat in a leading exporting country would likely have repercussions for food markets everywhere. This risk society paradigm faces many challenges still to be resolved, as to assess if the wheat grain is safe can take more than a decade, and if it is shown not to be safe the damage done could be irreversible.

Lingering doubts

Natural food has a special image of being the best source of nourishment and being good for people's health; however, the fear of not being able to feed a growing population has created an industrialised scale of food production far removed from past traditions. Due to a perceived urgency, new products have been created by genetic modification of plants to make them more resist-ant against diseases, create higher yields and make them more adaptable to climate change. This might seem to be a worthy course. The problem is the gap between the scientific development and consumer trust and confidence in the new products. This is due to the inability of authorities and scientists to assure the public that the new products are not detrimental in any way and have no negative implications for public health or for the environment over the long term.

Consequently, GM food and the industrialisation of food products have become highly contentious issues. Beck started the discussion with the pub-lication of *Risk Society* (1992) and others have followed, accentuating the risks posed by novel products of modern industrialisation. Cross contami-nation of crops and neglect of strict regulatory requirements have already demonstrated that GM trial crops can contaminate the human food chain, despite not yet been approved for commercial release. These revelations have not enhanced consumers' confidence in the security of novel products.

Genetically modified and industrialised food production stripped or obscured of its natural origin are eminent examples of the issues the risk soci-ety discourse highlights, where there is a disregard for the need of trustworthy information that can impart sufficient knowledge for consumers to make an informed decision about what to eat.

Food production has become a mystery perceived as a secret 'black box' (Beck 2007; Latour 1999), and judged as a danger to people's health in a gen-eral sense that embraces definition of health as a state of complete physical, mental and social wellbeing and not merely the absence of disease or infirm-ity. Lingering public issues encompasses a broader societal sense of 'public health' incorporating land sovereignty, social justice and access to uncompro-mised food also for future generations, rarely considered in the evaluation of current risks by scientists and authorities.

Conclusion

In this chapter, different implications have been highlighted of novel products from genetic engineering of plants. To recap, genetic engineering is the transmission of DNA from one organism to another unrelated organism. Genetically engineered organisms are the source of GM foods. Currently available GM foods stem mostly from plants that have been developed to improve yield through the introduction of resistance to plant diseases or increased tolerance to herbicides. In the future, second generation genetic modifications could be aimed at altering the nutrient content of food, reducing its allergenic potential or improving environmental tolerance of food production systems. Proponents claim that using the technology is necessary if we want to be able to feed the world's growing population in the future, while detractors claim that short-term gains will soon be reversed by eroding biodiversity of traditional cultivars and the evolution of herbicide resistant 'superweeds' that can jeopardise agricultural sustainability.

The knowledge gaps between consumers and scientists are telling, as what could have been a good public relations strategy for biotechnology – to promise to provide the world with more nutritious and less expensive food using fewer resources – has been compromised. It has rather become a serious fight driven by dislike of corporate power and fears of uncontrolled environmental and health effects. GM food is an excellent example of what the risk society emphasises: the separation between science and public perception. The confrontation over genetic engineering of food crops is being waged on multiple fronts by farmers, legislators, activists and scientists around the world, all trying to separate fear from fact. Fears over the safety of GMOs are not slowing down: the public debate, consumer boycotts and political battles are still raging and seem to be difficult to resolve in the near future.

Looking further into the future, there might be advances in molecular biology that could allow existing genes to be deleted or modified with great precision. However, it is too early to tell if crops modified without foreign genes will change the public debate over GMOs. GMOs can hardly be seen as 'natural', which is an important aspect in the public perception of risk. The risk society paradigm provides an important approach through which to analyse issues around modern industrialisation and novel consumer products and the prospects of providing uncompromised food also for future generations. Genetically modified food is only one expression of several risk issues facing a modern industrialisation society in producing products for human consumption.

9 Risk perception of foodborne pathogens

Introduction

The risk society discourse focuses on modern industrialisation that has created vast geographical, social and cultural divides between consumers and producers. Multinational companies source food products and seek processing locations worldwide, and the products are distributed to customer markets globally. This makes it nearly impossible to trace the original product sources of complex food safety hazards and to take the appropriate action to avoid contamination (Beck 1992, 1999). There is a pervasive impression that risks in the global food distribution chain have become more difficult to expose, be acknowledged by the producer and redressed when something goes wrong; and this worries people.

A risk can be deceptive, and what actually constitutes a real risk can be difficult to assess, as it might be hidden and not obvious not only to the layperson, but to experts as well. This is specifically the case regarding foodborne pathogens. They cannot be seen or easily identified by direct observation and the harmful effects often show up well after consumption of the contaminated food. Foodborne pathogens are human-disease-causing microbial agents transmitted through food. Many consumers are concerned about the risks caused by diverse sources of contamination of food throughout the different production stages. This concern is well founded, as there are over 200 known microbial, chemical or physical agents occasionally found in food, which can cause acute illness when ingested (Acheson 1999). This chapter will focus on foodborne pathogens and the public's response to these threats to public health, as triggers of numerous illnesses.

The public's trepidations are based on anxieties, not only about the food's health impact, but also about the influence of contaminants in general on sustainable agriculture, ecology and food culture (Holm and Kildevang 1996). Public perception of possible harm from the diverse range of agents often differs considerably from expert opinion of the risks posed by the contaminants and their potential health consequences. The public frequently expresses more concern about anticipated illnesses caused by the combined sources of ingested chemical and physical agents, notwithstanding that these present less of a risk compared to the risk of harm posed by foodborne pathogens – a situation that the public is not always aware of as the source of their illness.

Risks that preoccupy most people are those primarily associated with something that can be seen with your own eyes, like a physical agent, which potentially can be avoided or managed. For example, a fly in the soup can be observed and can be removed. It might not be a health risk per se, but many people would find it nauseating and would not eat the soup. However, in contrast to physical risks that are visible, microbial and chemical risks that very much encircle us are invisible to the naked eye and thus more esoteric in the public's mind, causing fear, but not necessarily deliberate avoidance. Although consumers are commonly more familiar with, or knowledgeable about, microbial food risks compared to chemical risks (Fife-Schaw and Rowe 1996), the magnitude of dread is often greater for chemical than microbial contaminants. This risk anomaly can be explained by the fact that chemical agents are often seen as unnatural in the public's eye and thus feared more than what is seen as naturally occurring food dangers, like microbial contaminants. Consumers might feel a lack of personal control over the exposure to chemical contaminants, but believe they have control over microbial risks, especially during food preparation (Kher *et al.* 2013).

Similarly, research suggests that people are more likely to worry about risks caused by external factors, which they feel they have no power over, while being much less concerned about personal factors or factors linked to their own behaviour or lifestyle. People will present behavioural patterns and make choices that might contradict or be irrational, illogical or at least inconsistent with expert opinions and scientific knowledge about risks (Hilgartner 1990). Numerous investigations have demonstrated that the public is more concerned about food risks that the scientific community considers less likely to cause harm, for example, chemicals used in farm production and preservatives used in food processing. These risks are compared to risks that are scientifically assessed to be more likely to occur, such as microbiological hazards that can be exacerbated by inappropriate consumer food handling and cause severe food poisoning (Macfarlane 2002; Slovic *et al.* 1980; Wandel 1994).

In general, consumers tend systematically to overestimate some risks relative to the technical probability of harm occurring, whereas other risks are largely ignored. There is habitually a weak correlation between the perceived risk associated with a specific food safety concern and its actual probability of causing harm. Consumers place much importance on factors that may not contribute to technical risk estimates, while underestimating other factors, which potentially represent a substantial threat to human health (Miles and Frewer 2001). Accordingly, consumers exposed to a risk tend to focus on the severity of possible consequences rather than the probability of occurrence. This divergence of perspective is at the root of the disparity between technical and social definitions of risk, and it is the reason technical assessment of risk has proved an inadequate basis for the management of social risk, including food safety issues (Yeung and Morris 2001b; Beck 1992).

For example, there was a public outcry when variant Creutzfeldt-Jakob disease (vCJD) in humans was linked to consumption of beef from cattle affected by Bovine Spongiform Encephalopathy or Mad Cow disease (Dealer and Lacey 1990; McCluskey and Swinnen 2011). The Creutzfeldt-Jakob complex of diseases are all fatal human conditions, and 224 individuals were diagnosed worldwide specifically with vCJD during a 15-year period up to 2011 (World Health Organization 2012). This is in contrast to the findings that more than 70 per cent of chicken meat sold in supermarkets in the United Kingdom was contaminated by *Campylobacter* organisms (United Kingdom Food Standards Agency 2014). These organisms caused nine million individuals to become ill, albeit a relatively mild illness, at an estimated cost of €2.4 (US$2.97) billion each year in the European Union alone (European Food Safety Authority 2011a). The public saw it as less alarming. The latter disease is an ongoing real societal issue, whilst the former has proven to be of a transitional nature and much less of a problem than initially thought. The example demonstrates the discrepancy between risk perceptions driven more by the expected severity of the disease than the likelihood of illness as reflected in the actual number of people suffering from foodborne pathogens.

Although the public is increasingly concerned about food-related risks, the rise in food poisoning cases suggests that the public still makes decisions on food consumption, storage and preparation that are less than ideal from a health and safety perspective. Consumer studies concerning food safety knowledge and practices have shown that consumers are aware of and are thinking about food safety, but there are also many gaps in food safety knowledge and practices that may result in foodborne illness (Jevšnik *et al.* 2008; Patil *et al.* 2004).

The gap between lay and expert opinions about risks has been attributed to the existence of a 'perception filter' causing a disconnection between reality and scientific evidence and consumer perception of this reality. Consumer perceptions are based on human subjectivity, which ultimately determines purchasing and consumption decisions (Verbeke *et al.* 2007). Epidemiologic surveillance summaries of foodborne diseases indicate that consumer behaviours such as ingestion of raw or under-cooked foods and poor hygienic practices are important contributors to outbreaks of foodborne diseases (Patil *et al.* 2004). The perception by people, young and mature, that they know how to handle food safely is widespread, but self-reported food-handling procedures do not support this confidence (Unusan 2007).

Disease prevalence from foodborne pathogens

Microorganisms surround us, and the aggregate of microorganisms we as humans carry around in our gastrointestinal tract weigh up to two kilograms. They outnumber our human cells by a factor of ten to one (Sekirov *et al.* 2010). Most of these microorganisms appear to be beneficial and assist in maintaining processes necessary for a healthy body, but some of the microorganisms we carry around can become harmful under certain circumstances. Other detrimental microorganisms reside in the external environment ready for an attack through food if the circumstances are favourable. The increased complexity and length of food chains through globalisation of food markets and global food distribution have created increased opportunities for contamination by pathogens (Miles *et al.* 1999; World Health Organization 2007; Beck 1992).

It has been estimated that foodborne pathogens are responsible for millions of cases of infectious gastrointestinal diseases each year. These types of diseases cost billions of dollars in medical care and lost productivity, yet they are highly preventable with the correct production and handling of food. Foodborne illness is the result of consumption of food contaminated by pathogenic, or disease-causing, bacteria or viruses. There are around 30 pathogens known to cause foodborne illness (Thomas *et al.* 2013). Common foodborne pathogens include the *Salmonella* species, *Campylobacter jejuni*, Enterohaemorrhagic *Escherichia coli*, *Listeria monocytogenes*, *Clostridium perfringens*, norovirus and hepatitis A virus. New variations of foodborne diseases are likely to emerge in the future, as transfer of antibiotic resistance between microorganisms and evolution of virulence factors caused by changes in agricultural and food manufacturing practices occur, and as changes to the human defence status arise. Additionally, changes to the immune system due to declining acquired immunity and increasing proportions of immune-compromised individuals are likely to intensify (Newell *et al.* 2010).

Symptoms of a foodborne illness vary depending on the cause. The incubation period ranges from hours to days, depending on the microorganism involved, the contamination level and how much of the food was consumed. The longer incubation periods make it more difficult to identify the source of the illness, as after an extended period of several days it can be difficult to attribute the symptoms to the correct food item and separate it from other communicable diseases or food intolerances. Symptoms of foodborne disease can range from mild and self-limiting vomiting and diarrhoea, sometimes associated with fever and aches, to severe neurological conditions. Severe neurological conditions are rare, but can create long-term health problems and even death (Thomas *et al.* 2013).

The total burden of foodborne disease is unknown, as cases are not always reported. However, according to an estimate by the World Health Organization (WHO), it is assumed that globally there are nearly 1.7 billion cases of which 1.8 million people die each year from diarrhoeal diseases, mainly attributed to contaminated food and drinking water (Newell *et al.* 2010; World Health Organization 2013a). More refined research by the Centers for Disease Control and Prevention (CDC) has shown that one in six people in the USA are estimated to get ill due to foodborne diseases each year, or 17 per cent of the population. A calculation undertaken in 2011 in the United States estimated that 47.8 million illnesses, 127,839 hospitalisations and 3,037 deaths had occurred as a result of foodborne disease. The calculation is based on combining estimates of major known pathogens and unspecified agents, and the overall annual estimate of the total burden of foodborne illness that year (Morris 2011). The cost to society has been estimated at US$77.7 billion based on a replication of the CDC data, which was added to a more detailed cost of illness model including economic estimates for medical costs, productivity losses and illness related mortality. The refined cost of illness model provides a more inclusive pain, suffering and functional disability measure, which was based on a monetised quality adjusted life year estimate (Scharff 2012).

A comparable situation was highlighted in a European survey. It showed that an estimated 16 per cent of Netherlands' population were affected by illness caused by foodborne pathogens each year (de Wit *et al.* 2001). The Public Health Agency of Canada estimates that each year approximately one in eight Canadians, or four million people, get sick due to domestically acquired foodborne diseases (Thomas *et al.* 2013). In Australia, there are an estimated 5.4 million cases of foodborne illnesses each year – one in four Australians becoming ill due to ingesting contaminated food. This causes 18,000 hospitalisations and 120 deaths (Hall *et al.* 2005).

In light of the high incidence of disease caused by foodborne pathogens relative to other agents, it is striking that the public does not rank these food related risks at their corresponding level of seriousness. In 2010, a survey was undertaken with a sample of approximately 27,000 individuals, 15 years of age and over, representing the population in the 27 European Union member states. When prompted to rank possible issues associated with food, the number one concern was chemical residues from pesticides in fruit, vegetables and cereals. This was followed by concerns about antibiotics or hormones in meat, cloning of animals for food production, and pollutants such as mercury in fish and dioxins in pork. Concerns about bacterial contamination of food came in as number five, despite being a major cause of food related illness (Eurobarometer 2010).

In another project, ten focus group discussions were held in five countries: Poland, Ireland, the Netherlands, France and Brazil. Again, consumers expressed higher concerns about chemical, as compared with microbial, contaminants. Chemical contaminants were more strongly associated with the potential for severe consequences, long term effects and lack of personal control and thus ranked higher (Kher *et al.* 2013), while disease caused by foodborne pathogens were seen as of short duration and of little discomfort.

A recent survey by the University of Florida showed that consumers ranked food safety in general near the top of their list of concerns, with 85 per cent of respondents calling it extremely or highly important, trailing only the economy and health care. However, again the survey found that more participants named chemical hazards like growth hormones, additives and preservatives as health risks rather than bacteria, despite the fact that it is the bacteria that cause major foodborne diseases (Rumble and Leal 2013).

These findings support the view that the consumer perception of risks in relation to food are more likely to be in the reverse order to the food safety ranking of risk, as identified by experts (Slovic 2000; Verbeke *et al.* 2007).

There have been numerous attempts to educate consumers on how to avoid getting sick from foodborne pathogens. Proposed precautionary methods include avoiding cross contamination, proper heating of raw food, vulnerable populations to avoid specified foods, cold storage of leftover food and thorough hand washing. The limited success is reflected in outbreaks of campylobacteriosis (cross contamination), salmonellosis (inappropriate heating), listeriosis (vulnerable populations – young, elderly and people with low immune resistance), clostridium perfringens toxicosis (inappropriate cold storage), and norovirus illness (lack of hand washing). In the following, we will discuss these five groups of pathogenic microorganisms.

Cross contamination by Campylobacter

Campylobacteriosis is a leading cause of human gastroenteritis in the developed world and has been estimated to cost the society around US$4 billion annually in the USA alone (Wilson *et al.* 2008). As the name of the disease implies, *Campylobacter* species are literally curved rods, which is reflected in the Greek meaning of the name and the way they look. *Campylobacter jejuni* is the dominating species causing 90 per cent of human campylobacteriosis, with most of the rest caused by *Campylobacter coli*, both ubiquitous in nature and found in the gut of farm animals where they thrive at temperatures between 37 to 42°C causing very few ill effects for the animals.

Most people who become ill with campylobacteriosis get diarrhoea, cramping, abdominal pain and fever within two to five days after exposure to the organism. Foodborne illness caused by campylobacter can be severely debilitating, but it is rarely life threatening. The diarrhoea may be bloody and can be accompanied by nausea and vomiting. The illness typically lasts about one week. On rare occasions there are long term consequences of this infection, called sequelae, beginning several weeks after the diarrheal illness. People can develop arthritis; others develop a rare disease called the Guillain-Barré syndrome. The Guillain-Barré syndrome affects the nerves of the body and it leads to paralysis, which requires intensive medical care. It is estimated that approximately one in every 1,000 reported campylobacteriosis cases leads to the Guillain-Barré syndrome (Humphrey *et al.* 2007).

Chicken meat is the most common source of campylobacteriosis globally. It only takes less than 500 campylobacter organisms to cause illness. Even one drop of juice from raw chicken meat can carry enough bacteria to infect a person (Friedman *et al.* 2000). The most common way of being infected is to cut raw poultry meat on a cutting board, and then use the unwashed cutting board or utensils to prepare vegetables or other raw or lightly cooked foods. The campylobacters from the raw meat thus gets onto the other foods through cross-contamination. Identification of suspected exposure routes have linked naturally contaminated raw foods like chicken with important food handling malpractices, contaminated contact surfaces and ready to eat foods. In a model domestic kitchen, 29 per cent of food preparation sessions showed that bacteria was transmitted to other foods such as salads, cleaning materials and food contact surfaces (Redmond *et al.* 2004).

The risk of such cross-contamination has been known for a long time, but public reaction is not concurrent with existing cross-contamination dangers. A Danish study of food handling behaviour showed that young males, after leaving home, had the riskiest kitchen practices with little knowledge of cross-contamination potentials (Rosenquist *et al.* 2003). Similarly, only 34 per cent of young female college students staying in dorm accommodations in the north of Jordan were considered to have an adequate understanding of food safety practices. Their circumstance related more to the difficulties with cooking conditions and food sources of foodborne pathogens, than knowledge about possible food cross-contamination (Osaili *et al.* 2011).

Governments in some countries have attempted to limit the spread of campylobacteriosis. New Zealand, which has been badly affected, introduced in 2006 a number of voluntary and regulatory interventions to reduce campylobacter contamination of poultry. Two years later, the rate of the disease had more than halved (Sears *et al.* 2011). Performance standards established by the US Department of Agriculture in 2011 have so far been less successful since campylobacteriosis continued to increase with the incidence in 2013 being 13 per cent higher than the average incidence over the period between 2006 and 2008 (Crim *et al.* 2014). Within the EU clear directions and binding procedures are still inadequate (European Food Safety Authority 2011a). Although in Denmark 'campylobacter free' chicken meat can be marketed at a premium price, providing that it comes from flocks that meet required monitoring standards (Krause *et al.* 2006). The campylobacter risk management programme, which was introduced by the UK Food Standards Agency, aims to more than halving the number of the most contaminated birds (United Kingdom Food Standards Agency 2013).

However, it is a shared responsibility in the overall risk society to limit the incidence of campylobacteriosis. Governments can set a maximum limit for acceptable safe contamination levels. The industry can change their systems in producing, transporting and processing campylobacter free chicken. Nevertheless, until the contamination of poultry carcases can be reduced, consumers must take responsibility for limiting their own risk of being affected by the disease by adhering to safe preparation practices.

Salmonella surviving inappropriate heating

Salmonellosis is another common and widely distributed foodborne disease that is caused by a group of bacteria called *Salmonella*. Foodborne outbreaks of salmonellosis are routinely observed and frequently reported. This demonstrates that vulnerable people only need a very low dose for them to fall ill (Newell *et al.* 2010). Salmonella species are hardy and can survive several weeks in a dry environment and several months in water. It is estimated that tens of millions of human cases of salmonellosis occur worldwide every year and that the disease contributes to more than hundred thousand deaths worldwide (World Health Organization 2013b). EFSA has estimated that the overall economic burden of human salmonellosis could be as high as €3 (US$3.7) billion a year in the European Union (European Food Safety Authority 2014a). In the USA, it has been estimated that there are over one million cases of salmonellosis each year with Salmonella being the leading cause of the 2,612 deaths from foodborne illness recorded annually (Scallan *et al.* 2011).

Over 2,500 different *Salmonella* strains, called 'serotypes' or 'serovars', have been identified to date. *Salmonella* Enteritidis and *Salmonella* Typhimurium are the two most important serotypes of salmonellosis transmitted from animals to humans in most parts of the world (World Health Organization 2013b). Symptoms of infection include diarrhoea, fever and abdominal cramps 12 hours to three days after infection. The illness usually lasts four to seven days, and most people recover without treatment. Vulnerable people including the elderly, infants and those with impaired immune systems are more likely to have a severe illness. The rate of diagnosed infections in children under the age of five is higher than the rate for all other people (Lampel *et al.* 2012). A small number of people develop Reiter's syndrome with pain in their joints, irritation of the eyes and painful urination. This is called reactive arthritis. It can last for months or years and can lead to chronic arthritis, which is difficult to treat (Dworkin *et al.* 2001).

Salmonella bacteria are commonly found in domestic and wild animals. The bacteria are prevalent in animals such as poultry, pigs, cattle and in pets, including cats and dogs, birds and reptiles, such as turtles. Salmonella can pass through the entire food chain from animal feed, primary production, and all the way to households or food service establishments and institutions. Salmonellosis in humans is generally contracted through the consumption of inappropriately heated food of animal origin, such as eggs, meat, poultry and milk, although other foods, including green vegetables contaminated by manure, have been implicated in its transmission (Blaser and Newman 1982; Crum Cianflone 2008).

From a risk society point of view, action to reduce the incidence of salmonellosis must involve the whole food chain, from agricultural production, to processing, manufacturing and preparation of foods in both commercial establishments and in the home. In 2003, governments across the European Union implemented an enhanced salmonella control programme with targets set for poultry flocks, for example, laying hens, broilers and turkeys, and also for pigs. The outcome from this programme was that human cases of salmonellosis were almost halved over the following five years, 2004–2009. The programme demonstrated that it is possible to reduce the disease incidence (European Food safety Authority 2014a).

Listeriosis affecting vulnerable populations

Although the number of people affected is relatively small, listeriosis is a leading cause of death amid foodborne illnesses. In particular, the disease poses a risk to vulnerable members of the population with a fatality rate as high as 30 per cent among people at risk. *Listeria monocytogenes*, the responsible organism, is hardy, salt tolerant, can survive and even grow at refrigeration temperatures, albeit slowly, unlike many other pathogens. In susceptible individuals, fewer than 1,000 total organisms may cause the disease. It is notable for its persistence in food manufacturing environments where it can survive in drains and on door seals. It is ubiquitous in the environment and can be found in moist environments, soil and decaying vegetation (Lampel *et al.* 2012).

There are two forms of listeriosis. The non-invasive gastroenteritis form has a relatively short incubation period, from a few hours to two or three days. Symptoms range from mild to intense nausea, vomiting, aches, fever and, sometimes, diarrhoea. It usually does not require any medical treatment. The severe, invasive form of the illness can have a very long incubation period, estimated to vary from three days to three months. It is a more deadly form as the infection can spread through the bloodstream to the nervous system. This can lead to meningitis (Lampel *et al.* 2012). Pregnant females may experience mild, flulike symptoms; but more seriously, it may lead to premature birth or miscarriage. It can also cause meningitis in newborn children (Ramaswamy *et al.* 2007). People with weak immune systems are also more vulnerable, such as people affected by AIDS or other chronic diseases, people who are taking immune suppressing arthritis drugs or undergoing cancer chemotherapy. The elderly are especially vulnerable to this pathogen, as their immune systems are often weakened due to their increased age (Muñoz *et al.* 2012).

Several food groups have been associated with *Listeria monocytogenes*. Examples include dairy products and soft serve ice cream, raw vegetables and meat products. Ready to eat products like soft cheeses, fermented raw meat sausages, hot dogs and deli meats, raw and smoked fish and other seafood are frequently associated with listeriosis (Lianou and Sofos 2007).

Pregnant females in particular should be aware of the risk of listeriosis. It is recommended that females avoid pate and soft cheeses during pregnancy. However, research and anecdotal evidence suggests that pregnant females still underestimate the risk of ready to eat foods, such as cold meats and pre-packed salads. In 2006, researchers from Wollongong University, Australia surveyed 586 females attending antenatal clinics. They found that while 81 per cent of the females identified soft cheeses as a high-risk food, only 68 per cent identified deli meats, and 50 per cent identified coleslaw as food to avoid during pregnancy. More than 57 per cent had an incomplete knowledge of foods with high listeriosis risk, and approximately 25 per cent continued the consumption of these foods, which have been associated with a relatively high frequency of cases of listeriosis (Bondarianzadeh *et al.* 2007).

Inappropriate cold storage facilitates *Clostridium perfringens* growth

Clostridium perfringens is an anaerobic, spore-forming microorganism that produces enterotoxin. It is believed to be the second leading bacterial cause of foodborne illness in many countries, second only to salmonellosis. In the USA, it is estimated to cause one million illnesses each year. Although vegetative cells of *Clostridium perfringens* are destroyed at temperatures over 60°C, its very tough spores can survive normal cooking temperatures (70°+C) and even boiling. They later germinate and grow to high numbers if the food is not chilled properly. Once the contaminated food is consumed, and reaches the intestines, the bacteria start to produce enterotoxin. Outbreaks caused by *Clostridium perfringens* occur regularly, they are often affecting a large number of people, and they can cause substantial morbidity. Meat and poultry have been implicated in 92 per cent of outbreaks with an identified single food source (Grass *et al.* 2013).

Foodborne illness caused by *Clostridium perfringens* can take two forms. The gastroenteritis form is very common, with a usually mild cramp and watery diarrhoea that start within eight to 16 hours. For most people, symptoms disappear by themselves within 24 hours, although the symptoms can be more severe and last up to a week or two in very young people and the elderly. The other illness, popularly called 'pigbel' or, to use the scientific term, enteritis necroticans, involves production of ulcerative β-toxin and is more severe and often fatal, but it is a rare illness. Symptoms include pain and gassy bloating in the abdomen, diarrhoea, possibly bloody, and vomiting (Lampel *et al.* 2012).

Beef, poultry, gravies and dried or pre-cooked foods are common sources of *Clostridium perfringens* infections, although the organism is also found on vegetable products, including spices and herbs, and in raw and processed foods. *Clostridium perfringens* infection often occurs when foods are prepared in large quantities and kept warm for a long time before serving. Hence, outbreaks often happen in institutional settings, such as hospitals, school cafeterias, prisons and nursing homes or at events with catered food where large quantities of food are prepared several hours before consumption and then left at room temperature before serving.

Government authorities have issued food-handling recommendations in order to limit the risk of getting *Clostridium perfringens* food poisoning. Recommendations state that meat dishes should be served hot or be refrigerated until they are served, large cuts of meat should be thoroughly cooked, and for rapid cooling of large dishes like stews, they should be divided into several smaller, shallower containers before refrigeration (United States Food Safety and Inspection Service 2010).

Inept hand washing can spread norovirus

Norovirus is a leading trigger for gastrointestinal illnesses affecting people of all ages and is estimated to cause almost one fifth of all acute gastroenteritis cases worldwide and up to 200,000 deaths in developing countries each year, mostly in infants and the elderly (Ahmed *et al*. 2014; Patel *et al*. 2008). Common names for the illness are viral gastroenteritis, acute nonbacterial gastroenteritis, stomach flu and winter vomiting disease. The virus is an environmentally hardy organism that not only can be transmitted by food and water, but also can easily be transmitted through person-to-person contact, through airborne virus particles, and through contact with environmental surfaces. Norovirus is quite resistant to disinfectants and detergents (Barker *et al*. 2004) and highly stable in the environment where it can survive for long periods outside a human host, depending on surface and temperature conditions. One study showed the virus surviving for more than a week on several surfaces used for food preparation (D'Souza *et al*. 2006), while in water it can survive several months. This was demonstrated with the detection of the norovirus in shellfish, eight to ten weeks after the contamination (Greening and Wolf 2010).

Foodborne norovirus illnesses have been linked to consumption of ready-made foods contaminated by food handlers, environmental contamination of produce or molluscs harvested from contaminated water. Salad ingredients, fruit and oysters are the foods most often implicated in norovirus outbreaks. However, any premade food that is handled by staff carrying an infectious illness can be contaminated. In most cases, contamination has been associated with improper sanitation controls, including inept hand washing. Illness have also been related to consumption of contaminated water, including municipal water, well water, stream water, commercial ice, lake water and swimming pool or recreational surface water exposure, as well as floodwater (Lampel *et al*. 2012).

The infectious dose of norovirus is very low: it might only involve less than twenty viral particles in a worst case scenario, while affected people excrete very high levels of virus particles that can contaminate food and the environment (Lopman *et al*. 2004). Symptoms usually start within one or two days of eating the contaminated food, but may start in as few as 12 hours. The first symptom is often intensive vomiting along with watery diarrhoea that is not bloody and severe cramps. It has been described as being accompanied by intense pain and nausea so powerful that even when the stomach is empty people affected feel the urge to continue to vomit. Norovirus illness is self-limiting, but can be very debilitating because of the high rate of vomiting. Most people get better in a day or two. Dehydration is the most common complication, especially among the very young, the elderly and patients with underlying medical conditions (Parashar *et al*. 2001; Glass *et al*. 2009).

The rapid spread of the infection is particularly evident in areas where large populations are enclosed within a confined environment, such as in institutions, college campuses, schools, military settings, hotels, restaurants, recreational camps, hospitals, nursing homes, day care facilities and cruise ships, and emergency accommodation after natural disasters, such as hurricanes and earthquakes (Lampel *et al*. 2012).

The spread of norovirus infections can be exemplified by the case where a woman vomited on the floor of a restaurant with 126 people dining at six tables. Staff quickly cleaned up the area and people continued eating. Three days later 52 people had reported a range of symptoms, from fever and nausea to vomiting and diarrhoea. There was a direct correlation between the risks of infection of people at other tables and their distance to the sick woman (Marks *et al.* 2000).

Norovirus continues to pose a significant burden on cruise ships, causing an average of 27 confirmed outbreaks annually over a five-year period (Wikswo *et al.* 2011). Amid such outbreaks, the question is what passengers can do to avoid an infection. The research is currently limited in exploring actual pre-ventative practices during an outbreak, as no vaccine exists that can protect against norovirus infection, and simply applying some antibacterial gel before eating at the buffet is not enough. Norovirus spreads easily to things people touch, and other people can pick up the virus that way. In general, frequent hand washing with soap and warm water and being careful in not touch-ing suspect surfaces can minimise the risk of catching a norovirus infection in any setting. Unfortunately, hand washing practices are often left wanting. In a Canadian study at Ontario University, students' compliance with hand hygiene recommendations were assessed at the height of a suspected norovi-rus outbreak at the university residence. The data based on observed prac-tices were compared to post outbreak self-reporting surveys administered to students to canvass their beliefs and perceptions about hand hygiene. Despite knowledge of hand hygiene protocols, less than one in five of the students were observed to comply with prescribed hand hygiene recommendations. However, four in five of the students indicated that they practiced correct hand hygiene all the time during the outbreak (Surgeoner *et al.* 2009).

Avoidable lifestyle hazard

It is clear that foodborne illnesses are a common problem in most countries of the world with prevailing sanitary conditions influencing the relative fre-quency and severity of the diseases. Numerous scientific studies have been published covering the threat posed by foodborne pathogens, but still both industries and consumers often neglect food-handling advice that could reduce contamination risks (Gravani 2009). Not following simple hygiene pro-cedures can have wide-ranging consequences for the individual and be costly for the industry. It can be devastating for individual consumers, who become affected by debilitating diseases that cripple them from living a normal life – diseases that can last for years and cause premature death. Risk avoidance is frequently not taken as seriously as it should be, thus risking diseases among unassuming populations. Industry might need to manage massive food recalls and pay extensive compensation to injured customers.

In the area of food risks, optimistic biases are much greater for lifestyle risks, such as food poisoning contracted in the home or illness experienced because of inappropriate dietary choices, than for industry technologies applied in the food production. At the same time, people often perceive that they know more about risks associated with different lifestyle dangers, and that they are in greater control of personal exposure to these lifestyle hazards, than might be the case (Frewer *et al*. 1994). Fact-based as well as perceived knowledge influence personal behaviour; hence, based on a high perceived knowledge and control, people will assume that they know enough about potential risks associated with home prepared food to deal with it effectively (Frewer *et al*. 1994). Nonetheless, in a study about the risk of food poisoning following domestic food preparation, Griffith *et al*. (1998) found that 95 per cent of consumers engaged in less than ideal hygiene practices, due to lack of knowledge or failure to implement known food safety procedures.

The disinclination of consumers to process information and make rational decisions is due to multiple reasons. For example, the information might fail to target particular needs or correspond with timely interests of consumers, thus it may be irrelevant or inadequate at the time of buying or cooking the food (Verbeke 2005). In some cases, it may even be perfectly rational for consumers to remain imperfectly informed about food safety issues even when information is free, as the available information might also contradict cultural, social and religious traditions. When opportunity costs of information processing become too high compared to expected benefits people's motivation to change behaviour will be constrained (McCluskey and Swinnen 2004).

In response to growing consumer uncertainty about food safety, and the perceived decline in consumer trust, regulatory bodies have increasingly stressed the importance of transparency in policy decision-making processes, as well as developing mechanisms in order to understand the concerns, attitudes and values of the public (Frewer *et al*. 2005). However, most consumers primarily receive information about food and food manufacturing through the popular press and television (Marks *et al*. 2003). Extensive media coverage of an event can contribute to a heightened perception of risk and amplify its consequences. Food scares are prime examples and are typically accompanied by a flood of media coverage that can lead to a temporary decline in demand for the product in question. The level of panic might greatly exceed what science would argue is appropriate, given the real risks (McCluskey and Swinnen 2011).

Food risk perceptions vary considerably within the social domain, with gender and education level consistent predictors. Other predictors include the nature of the perceived threat, trust in regulatory authorities, available information sources, and health and environmental concerns (Ellis and Tucker 2009). Both social and individual factors can intensify or diminish perceptions of risk (Flynn *et al*. 1998), with risk perception influenced by familiarity and dread. Food safety scares prompt a high level of immediate alarm, but if familiarity is high, the anxiety can taper off fairly quickly (Slovic 2000), while unfamiliarity with new food technology advances increases the persistence of dread (McCluskey and Swinnen 2011).

Although the mass media's effects on public perception are complex, their impact can be significant. This is particularly the case for negative information, as there is much criticism that mass media coverage is too negative. However, negative reporting catches people's interest, more so than positive stories, as the negative stories are often given a greater place, reported more prominently, which perhaps enhances the trust in negative or risky stories. This might be the situation when health risks are indicated, with credibility increasing with the severity of the risk (Siegrist and Cvetkovich 2001). Microbial food safety scares have a significant impact in terms of consumer behaviour, economics and politics. The power of the media to influence an ignorant public has important implications for government risk communication, education and management. Since initial beliefs affect not only overall risk perceptions, but also the way in which consumers process new information, it is important to enhance consumer understanding of microbial risks through education and by providing consumer relevant information (McCluskey and Swinnen 2011).

Conclusion

From a risk society perspective, microorganisms might be invisible, but they can affect many more people than is usually the case with risks that we 'see' or can avoid by reading the product label to gain knowledge about the food source, production and potential chemical contamination. However, ubiquitous microorganisms surround us all in the environment, in food and on and in our bodies. Many of them are helpful and even essential to life, as the vast number of microorganisms in the gut assist with food digestion. Nonetheless, there is also a range of pathogenic microorganisms that can cause mild to severe illness or even death.

To minimise contamination and growth of pathogenic microbes in food, joint engagements are required between government, industry and consumers. Governments have to set up and implement food safety regulatory systems that are robust with regular surveillance activities. Market forces provide strong incentives for industry to take great care in preventing food safety lapses as these can result in loss of brand reputation, create costly recalls and lower sales. However, since it is impossible to avoid any contamination in food production completely, consumers have to be vigilant.

Even when governments and industry perform their food safety functions according to guidelines, consumers can create new risks if they fail to practice good food safety in food storage, handling, preparation and cooking of food. Simple measures such as hand washing, separating cooked from uncooked food and refrigerating food not consumed within a short timeframe are simple strategies that will minimise food poisoning risks.

Unfortunately, consumers generally underestimate the likelihood of microbial food safety incidents to occur because of household practices and therefore frequently fail to adopt appropriate risk management strategies. Improving consumers' risk perceptions and, in turn, their food safety awareness is an enormous challenge, but it is essential to reduce microbial food safety risks.

10 Organic food – reinventing traditional food production?

Introduction

The risk society discourse criticises the global food industry for creating an environment of mistrust and a lack of information in contemporary food production, as it raises questions in the public's mind about long-term effects of the use of novel technologies like genetic engineering or a plethora of chemical compounds. This is particularly pertinent since harmful consequences of the food consumed today might take decades to materialise in exposed people, animals or the environment. It is understandable, then, that a movement has emerged to explore and to reinvent traditional food production and manufacturing, to turn the back to global food and to embrace local food production.

Fruits and vegetables were traditionally grown organically. Animals were allowed to venture outside into the sun for grazing, and tomatoes, apples and oranges had uneven shapes, but they tasted as we imagine tomatoes, apples and oranges should taste. Organic food was the food our ancestors produced and consumed for most of human agriculture, all the way to the baby boomers' parents, with many baby boomers themselves growing up on organic food.

The commercialisation and large-scale production of food have since replaced organic methods by introducing continuously refined and more efficient techniques, with the aim of increasing yields and improving shelf life. This development has been driven by urbanisation and the need to feed a growing population who do not have the means to grow their own food. Additionally, urban sprawl has forced food production to move well outside urban areas. It has increased transportation, and as food production became globalised, there was a need to develop food crops that could withstand long transportation and repeated reloading.

A public reaction to what has been characterised by some as bland and chemical-infused commercial food has seen a revitalisation of traditional organic production methods. The lack of public information available about how modern food production systems work, and the amount of chemicals used to boost throughput, further frightened parts of the community.

Different human life-cycle stages, and especially when having children to care for, can spark reflective shopping practices and incite a move to favour 'traditional' food, particularly among food conscious and ethically minded consumers. Mass media reporting shocking news about conventional food products and product health scares often supports this confrontation: 'news capable of creating a "cognitive dissonance" among consumers' (Hjelmar 2011:336).

There is an emotional side linked to the growing and purchasing of organically produced food, but there is also a public risk perception that modern industrialised food production uses practices and inputs damaging to the environment and yields food that can be harmful to public health. Further, demand for organic food is partially driven by consumers' perceptions that organic food is more nutritious than current industrialised food (Barański *et al.* 2014). Scientific opinion is duplicitous when comparing the environmental and health impacts of organic and industrial food production systems, not taking either side, and is almost silent on the importance of emotional facets of risk.

Although a focus on healthy living among middle and upper class population groups encouraged a return to traditional organic food production methods, its application has not been that simple, as the whole commercial production system needed to be adjusted and chemical residues in the soil removed. Additionally, organic produce is more labour intensive to grow and some products might have a shorter shelf life. These changes make the products more expensive and out of reach for a large section of the population. The high cost can thus create potential health inequalities as, if organic food is a healthier alternative, it will divide people not only according to social class, but also on health and possibly life expectancy.

This chapter discusses the history of organic food and its emergence as an alternative food source – for those who would like to use it and can afford it – exploring issues of health and safety, and the impact of social class on access to this alternative food.

The reintroduction of traditional food

The renewed attention among a widening public to healthy eating and food quality has increased the market for organic food. Purchasing of organically produced food can be seen as a reaction to perceived food safety risks, nutritional deficiencies associated with conventional food production systems, and a desire among parts of the public to improve their health, but also to secure, protect and care for the environment and to improve animal husbandry (Harper and Makatouni 2002). The risk society paradigm focuses on the difficulty the public encounters in accessing accurate information and knowledge to be able to identify responsible individuals and their level of control over products produced and the potential long-term effects of product ingredients on people's health and the environment (Beck 1992).

The recognition of organic food as superior by parts of the public has increased rapidly. Since 1990, the world market for organic food has grown from a small niche market to reach a market value of US$64 billion in 2012, a calculation based on information available from 164 countries (Willer and Lernoud 2014). This had increased by US$4 billion compared to 2010, but is only marginally different from 2011, mainly due to fluctuations in exchange rates and a revision of North American data, according to information from the Research Institute of Organic Agriculture and the International Federation of Organic Agriculture Movements (Willer and Lernoud 2014). The leading market is the United States, with an annual turnover of US$28.1 billion. In the European Union, US$25.9 billion was spent on organic food. Germany leads with US$8.7 billion, and is followed by France with US$5.0 billion. The countries with the highest annual average per capita spending were Switzerland with US$234 and Denmark with US$197. In 2012, approximately 44 per cent of the world retail market for organic products was in the United States. It was followed by Germany with 14 per cent and France with 8 per cent. Canada, the United Kingdom and Italy all had a retail market for organic products of 4 per cent, followed by Switzerland with 3 per cent. Other countries made up 19 per cent of the retail market for organic products (Willer *et al.* 2014).

In 2008, more than two-thirds of US consumers bought organic products, and more than one-quarter bought organic food at least weekly (Forman and Silverstein 2012). The fresh produce category makes up the main part of the organic food and drink sales. Fruits and vegetables such as apples, oranges, carrots and potatoes are typical first purchases for consumers buying organic products. Their newly harvested nature appeals to consumers seeking healthy and nutritious foods. Dairy products and beverages are the next most important organic product categories. Consumers often enter the organic market by first purchasing organic produce such as fruits and vegetables, and subsequently widen their purchases to include other organic products (Dettmann and Dimitri 2010). Consumers choose organic food in the belief that the organic products are more nutritious, have fewer additives and contaminants, and are grown more sustainably and often closer to the consumer market (Shepherd *et al.* 2005).

The increased consumer demands, together with the concerns of farmers about land degradation, have been the main drivers for the growth in organically managed farmland. The increase has been at the level of a compounding rate of close to 9 per cent per annum over the ten years between 2001 and 2011 (Paull 2011b). As of 2012, more than 1.9 million farmers in 164 countries reported growing organic food and worldwide almost 38 million hectares of agricultural land were farmed according to organic principles. It represents approximately 0.9 per cent of the total world farmland. About one-third of the world's organic agricultural land and more than 80 per cent of organic farmers are small-scale operations in developing countries and emerging markets (Willer and Lernoud 2014). The high percentage reflects that in many developing countries industrialisation of food production has not yet reached them.

The retail market for organic food in industrialised economies has been growing by about 20 per cent annually. A major driver of market growth in all geographic regions has been the increasing adoption and acceptance of organic food by mainstream retailers. It is possible to buy organic food in large supermarkets. There was a temporary decline in the growth rate of organic food at the time of the global financial crisis (GFC) that started in 2008. After several years of double-digit growth, the overall organic market expanded by 5 per cent in 2009, with a varying response in different markets. The statistics from 2012 demonstrate that the overall global market for organic food and drink has overcome the GFC downturn with growth recovering to pre-crisis levels (Willer *et al.* 2014).

There has been criticism that organic agriculture could not feed the current or future world population, should it become the dominant food production system. On the contrary, in a 2010 United Nations study de Schutter (2010) concluded that organic and other sustainable farming methods that come under the umbrella of 'agroecology' would be sufficient to produce enough food to feed the future world. Two years earlier, an examination of farming in 24 African countries concluded that organic or near-organic farming demonstrated yield increases of more than 100 per cent (United Nations 2008). In further support of organic farming methods, a report compiled by 400 international experts stressed that the way the world grows food needs to change radically to meet future demand (International Assessment of Agricultural Science and Technology for Development 2009). It called on governments to focus more attention on small-scale farmers and sustainable practices, rather than assuming that large-scale factory farming enterprises and their focus on short-term efficiencies would be the only solution to feed the world.

The history of organic farming

Organic farming was the predominant cultivation method practiced for thousands of years as the original type of agriculture. This is still the case in many developing countries. Concurrent advances in biology and engineering at the beginning of the twentieth century swiftly and profoundly altered prevailing farming systems and began to spread over the world. Development of the combustion engine led to the introduction of tractors and other mechanised farm machinery. This allowed farmers to manage larger fields and agriculture to become more specialised to maximise use of the machinery. The chemical industries developed synthetic fertilisers, and an increasing range of pesticides for weed and insect control were introduced. Research in plant breeding led to the commercialisation of hybrid seeds requiring more input support. The fast adoption of herbicides, fertilisers and new machinery created less demand for manual labour and work assistance from animals. The era of large-scale agriculture was born. However, these new agricultural techniques, while beneficial in the short term, can have serious longer-term side effects, such as soil compaction, erosion and declines in overall soil fertility, along with health concerns about toxic chemicals entering the food supply (Stinner 2007).

In reaction to agriculture's growing reliance on synthetic fertilisers and pesticides, traditional farming systems were gradually rejuvenated. Already in the late 1800s and early 1900s soil biology scientists began to develop theories about how new advancements in biological science could be used in agriculture as a way to remedy side effects of large scale agriculture, while still maintaining higher production. In central Europe Rudolf Steiner's *Lectures on Agriculture*, presented in 1924, created the concept of biodynamic agriculture, an early version of what is now called organic agriculture (Steiner 1929). The system was based on Steiner's philosophy of anthroposophy rather than on a solid grasp of agricultural science (Paull 2011a). In the late 1930s and early 1940s, Sir Albert Howard and his wife Gabrielle Howard developed a more scientific model of organic agriculture inspired by traditional farming methods in India. A supporter of the movement, Lord Northbourne, coined the concept 'organic farming' and wrote the book *Look to the Land* explaining his ideas (1940). Northbourne considered the farm as an organism, emphasising the need to take a holistic and ecologically balanced approach to farming. He claimed that for this to be attained the farm itself must have a biological completeness, since every branch of work is interlocked with all others. He pointed to vegetables converted through animal digestion into manure that in turn supported the growth of new vegetables in a cycle of great complexity and highly sensitive to any disturbance of its proper balance.

Organic farming, in response to sustainability of land quality, came to rely on techniques such as crop rotation, green manure, compost and biological pest control. Organic farming was supposed to use natural fertilisers and pesticides, and to exclude or strictly limit the use of synthetic fertilisers, pesticides, plant growth regulators, livestock hormones and antibiotics, food additives, genetically modified organisms, human sewage sludge and nanomaterial.

In the 1970s, global organisations concerned with pollution and environmental degradation began to focus on organic farming. One outcome was the formation of the International Federation of Organic Agriculture Movements (IFOAM) in France in 1972. The aim of IFOAM was to dedicate itself to the spread and exchange of information grounded on the principles and practices of organic agriculture across national and linguistic boundaries.

However, it lacked a common language with which to communicate the espoused benefits to customers of the products and ensure trust in adherence to the principles of organic farming. Thus, in the 1980s, farming and consumer groups around the world came together and began seriously to pressure governments to regulate organic food production and create a common platform for communication between producers and consumers. This led to governments beginning to specify in legislation what constitutes organic food production, including certification standards. Most notably the first legislation in the USA (Organic Foods Production Act of 1990), followed by the 1991 EU Eco-regulation developed for twelve countries in the European Union

(Council Regulation EEC No 2092/91), and voluntary guidelines on sustainable agriculture issued by the Japanese Ministry of Agriculture, Forestry and Fisheries in 1992. These regulations were replaced by mandatory legislation in 2000 (Japanese Agricultural Standard of Organic Agricultural Products – MAFF Notification No. 59).

Defining organic food

Adoption of organic farming was initially driven by small, independent farmers and by consumers purchasing directly from the farms or through farmers' markets. However, the accelerating growth of the organic market led to the involvement of larger agribusiness interests threatening the viability of small-scale dedicated organic farms. This could have easily diluted and confused the meaning of organic farming as an agricultural method through an increasing commercial focus. It was thus necessary to agree on a fundamental set of principles for defining organic food production.

The fundamental driver of organic farming is to achieve optimum quantities of produce and food of high nutritional quality and superior taste without the use of artificial fertilisers or synthetic chemicals like herbicides and insecticides. Organic farming emphasizes the need to maintain appropriate land management and it aims to ecologically achieve the balance between animal life, the natural environment and food crops. The food that is produced through organic farming is thus supposed to be at its most natural form. Organic farming does not support the use of genetically modified (GM) foods, growth promoters or hormones. Organic farmers attempt to rear animals with care and attention to their welfare by letting them grow and develop in the most natural and humane way possible. Organic meat, poultry, eggs and dairy products should come from animals that are given no antibiotics or growth hormones (Kirchmann *et al.* 2008). It has been suggested that should it be relevant to consider the application of nanotechnology to food and agriculture in the future, nanotechnology should not be used within organic food production (Paull and Lyons 2008).

The organic movement represents a multitude of practices, attitudes and philosophies. On the one end of the spectrum, there are organic practitioners who would not use chemical fertilisers or pesticides under any circumstance. These producers follow a strictly purist philosophy. At the other end of the spectrum, there are organic farmers who follow a more flexible approach. They are still striving to avoid the use of chemical fertilisers and pesticides, but do not rule them out entirely. Instead, they might use fertilisers and herbicides very selectively and cautiously as a second line of defence when absolutely necessary. Nonetheless, this group of producers consider themselves also to be organic farmers.

In 2005, the IFOAM launched a set of four principles to inspire the organic movement, to create knowledge and to inform the wider world about the purpose of organic agriculture. The principles were intended to apply to agriculture in the broadest sense, including the way people tend to soil, water, plants and animals in order to produce, prepare and distribute goods. The principles concern the way people interact with living landscapes, relate to one another and shape the legacy for future generations.

The four principles of organic agriculture are (International Federation of Organic Agriculture Movements 2005):

- The *health principle* – organic agriculture should sustain and enhance the health of soil, plant, animal and human as one and indivisible;
- The *ecology principle* – organic agriculture should be based on living ecological systems and cycles, work with them, emulate them and help sustain them;
- The *fairness principle* – organic agriculture should build on relationships that ensure fairness with regard to the common environment and life opportunities; and
- The *care principle* – organic agriculture should be managed in a precautionary and responsible manner to protect the health and wellbeing of current and future generations and the environment.

Following the above principles typical organic farming practices can be defined as including:

- Wide crop rotation as a prerequisite for an efficient use of on-site resources;
- Complete avoidance of or very strict limits on chemical synthetic pesticide and synthetic fertiliser use, livestock antibiotics, food additives and processing aids and other inputs;
- Absolute prohibition of the use of genetically modified organisms;
- Use of on-site resources, such as livestock manure for fertiliser or feed produced on the farm;
- Choosing plant and animal species that are resistant to disease and adapted to local conditions;
- Raising livestock in free range, open-air systems and providing them with organic feed; and
- Using animal husbandry practices appropriate to different livestock species.

When implementing the guiding principles, specific practices will vary according to individual needs and ethical convictions. Marketing of produce defined as organic will thus require further description of the individual parameters adhered to by the particular production system used.

Certification of organic production systems

As mentioned before, in the early days of revitalised organic farming, consumers interested in organic food had to buy it directly from growers or from farmers' markets. This allowed for direct communication between the two groups. Consumers could ask about the background of products and the producer could inform them about future product lines. This opportunity for consumers to talk to farmers and see their farming activities and conditions first hand improved the consumers' knowledge and created interest in organic farming systems. The consumers could thus decide for themselves what constituted an acceptable organic production system. As the demand for organic food continued to increase, high-volume sales through supermarkets started to compete with the direct farmer connection. Consumers lost the opportunity for direct contact with farmers, and a system was needed to convey the practices used in producing the organic food. Official organic certification systems became essential tools to build trust to keep consumers' confidence in the organic product, to assure quality, to prevent fraud and to promote the organic commerce.

In countries where the government oversees organic certification, commercial use of the term organic is legally restricted. This is the case within the EU, the USA, Canada, Japan and many other countries where producers are required to obtain specific certification in order to market food as organic within their borders. In 2012, 88 countries had legislated requirements for organic production systems, with 12 countries in the process of drafting legislation (Willer and Lernoud 2014). As a common specification, organic food is defined as food produced in a way that complies with the respective national organic standards or adheres to standards set by international organisations. Some countries, such as Australia, have compulsory export standards to assure overseas customers of the authenticity of the organic food, while the standards are voluntary for food sold on the domestic market. In countries without specific legislation for organic food, third-party certification provides an alternative for consumers to rely on. Additionally, certified organic producers are subject to the same agricultural, food safety and other government regulations that apply to non-certified producers.

The need for clear and harmonised rules has not only been taken up by government authorities, but also by IFOAM, the Food and Agriculture Organization of the United Nations (FAO), the World Health Organization (WHO), the United Nations Conference on Trade and Development (UNCTAD) and private bodies. The Codex Alimentarius Commission approved plant production guidelines in June 1999 and animal production guidelines in July 2001. They also provide guidance to governments in developing national regulations for organic food (Huber and Schmid 2014). There are approximately 550 certification bodies that certify organic food in different parts of the world, each according to one of over 100 specific private organic standards that differ in detail and specificity; but all include similar minimum requirements (Gould 2014). The certification aims to assure consumers that they are buying genuinely organic food that can be traceable back to the farm. Although standards vary from country to country and between certification bodies, all involve a set of production standards for growing, storing, processing, packaging and shipping of the organic produce. The standards should comply, at a minimum, with existing government legislation. However, in several cases, the certification bodies set standards that exceed government regulations. In the EU, national governments cannot set more stringent standards than is in force in the EU as a whole, but private certifiers can. In general, any business directly involved in food production can be certified, including seed suppliers, farmers, food processors, retailers and restaurants. For each step of the food chain, certification identifies suppliers of products approved for use in their own certified operations.

The Soil Association in the UK is an example of a private organisation that introduced one of the earliest certification systems for organic farming with more stringent standards in certain areas than the minimum required (Sacert 2013). Their organic standards cover all aspects of organic food certification, including production and packaging, animal welfare, fish farming and wildlife conservation, and they ban unnecessary and harmful food additives in organically processed foods. Their standards exceed official government standards in areas concerning the environment and animal welfare. They inspect each of their licensed farms and businesses at least once a year with random spot checks in between. The Soil Association symbol is one of the most recognised organic insignia in the UK today (Gilbert and Bruszik 2005).

To achieve organic certification for food production and a product to be labelled as organic is a lengthy process. To qualify as organic, crops must be produced on farms that have excluded the use of synthetic pesticides, herbicides or fertiliser for three years before harvest and have a sufficient buffer zone to decrease contamination from adjacent lands. To be certified as an organic producer, farmers must know the relevant organic standards that apply, farm structures and production methods must comply with the details of the standards. Extensive documentation is required, detailing farm history and current setup, and it usually includes results of soil and water testing. An annual production plan must be documented and submitted, detailing everything from seed sources, field and crop locations, fertilization and pest control activities, harvest methods, storage locations, to the sale of the organic produce. Annual on-farm inspections are required, with a physical tour, examination of records and an oral interview. Diaries covering all activities of day-to-day farming and sales must be available for random inspection at any time.

The certification process for operations other than farms covers quality of ingredients and other inputs, as well as processing and handling conditions. A transport company, for example, would be required to detail the use and maintenance of its vehicles, storage facilities and containers. A restaurant would have its premises inspected and its suppliers verified as certified organic.

Use of the term organic is central to the certification process. Producers cannot use the word legally without certification where organic laws exist.

In countries without organic laws, government guidelines may exist to provide direction for certifying organisations that handle the actual certification. Internationally, official equivalency negotiations are underway, with some agreements already in place, to harmonise certification between countries and facilitating international trade. There are also international certification bodies, including members of the IFOAM, working on harmonisation efforts.

In 2011, IFOAM introduced a new programme with the aim to simplify coordination of guidelines under IFOAM's Family of Standards notion. It is a primary framework for guaranteeing that an organic standard adequately describes globally recognised expectations for what organic producers should do and their products represent. With over 50 approved standards included and growing, the Family of Standards is the model for multilateral recognition and equivalence agreements. The vision is to establish the use of one single global reference defining compulsory input standards to be applied to organic production systems rather than focusing on bilateral agreements (Gould 2014).

Quality of organic produce

From the risk society discourse perspective, organic food production systems provide clear benefits in relation to the environment, animal health and welfare. The European Commission (EC) states that organic farmers use a range of techniques that help sustain ecosystems and reduce overall pollution. They also explain how organic farming contributes to the protection of natural resources, to biodiversity and to animal welfare, and how it helps in the development of rural areas. In simple terms, organic farming is an agricultural system that seeks to provide fresh, original and natural food while respecting natural lifecycle systems. In addition, the EC states that the system and its products present the least damage to the environment and to the health of consumers; this creates a win–win situation and from a risk society perspective the most sustainable milieu for future generations (European Commission 2014a).

Food quality encompasses the public health aspects of nutritional quality, but also other intrinsic quality parameters like taste and appearance. Although input standards for organic production systems have been established, it is much more challenging to define the ultimate quality of the produced food. At first, the focus was mainly on quality as represented by quantifiable and measurable parameters, but attention has increasingly been paid to a more comprehensive holistic approach. For example, Luning *et al.* (2005) extended a model proposed by Evans and Lindsay in 1996 and named it the 'quality viewpoints' model. The model includes five different criteria:

- *assessment* – a comparison of a product's properties;
- *product-based* – a function of specified measurable variables/reflection of qualitative dependence between specified measurable parameters;

- *user-based* – determined by the consumer's needs;
- *value-based* – a proportion of price to satisfaction received; and
- *production-based* – quality as a desired result of production practices or compliance with standards.

By organising and developing this quality viewpoints model, the authors proposed a distribution of food quality features into *internal* – directly associated with a product, measurable, based on its physical and chemical characteristics; and *external* – connected with a product indirectly. The internal characteristics relates to the product's healthiness, sensory properties and durability, as well as product reliability and the convenience of use. The external quality characteristics include production characteristics, depending on the adopted production method, for example, organic versus conventional, environmental aspects and marketing. Furthermore, this comprehensive assessment model needs to correspond to the consumers' expected quality of organic products.

There is a public perception that organic production systems provide foods that have a better taste, are more nutritious and have added health benefits. Quite a number of studies are available examining the impact on amounts of certain nutritional compounds of organic crop cultivation practices. Several overviews, reports and meta-analyses have been conducted to analyse and summarise the results of previously carried out organic versus conventional food studies (Wööse *et al.* 1997; Worthington 2001; Bourn and and Prescott 2002; Winter and Davis 2006; Rembiałkowska 2007; Benbrook *et al.* 2008; Lairon 2009; Lima and and Vianello 2011). However, only a few studies have focused on a more holistic and comprehensive understanding as to whether organic production influences public health (Johansson *et al.* 2014). Findings have not been consistent, which is understandable when taking into account marked seasonal and geographical influences that might mask differences due to production methods.

It is suggested that consumption of organic fruits and vegetables have minor benefits over consumption of conventional foods in terms of improved health (Dangour *et al.* 2009). Dangour *et al.* found no consistent differences in vitamin content, and only phosphorus was significantly higher in organic versus conventionally grown produce, demonstrating only minor clinical significance. Others have found that organic plant products generally contained more vitamin C and significantly higher levels of total phenolic compounds, which have antioxidant properties (Matt *et al.* 2011). However, they pointed out that the level of carotenoids often was higher in conventional plant products. Some of the studies they reviewed showed a higher content of dry matter, total sugars and mineral components in organic plant products but, due to variable results, it is difficult to draw comprehensive conclusions from such findings in relation to the impact on human health.

Further comparisons demonstrated only minor differences in protein or fat content between organic and conventional milk, but found that organic grains had a lower amount, but a higher quality, of proteins compared to conventional grains (Zadoks 1989; Worthington 2001). There was also some evidence that organic milk and chicken contained higher levels of omega-3 fatty acids (Castellini *et al.* 2002; Benbrook *et al.* 2013).

There has been some focus on the amount of nitrate found in green leafy vegetables and tubers when grown organically compared to conventional varieties. While these vegetables and tubers, when grown organically, have been found to have lower nitrate levels, there is no consensus as to whether consumption translates into improved health (Magkos *et al.* 2006).

Most of the research has looked at differences in nutrient availability while other health impact parameters have barely been studied. Some results indicate that carrots grown under strict organic conditions improved immune status by inducing changes in lymphocyte populations, including an increase in regulatory T cells, when fed to laboratory mice. Such findings will still need to be scientifically evaluated in human trials (Roselli *et al.* 2012).

Many studies that have compared the taste and organoleptic quality of organic and conventional foods report no consistent or significant differences between organic and conventional produce (Fillion and Arazi 2002; Zhao *et al.* 2007; Talaver-Bianchi *et al.* 2010). However, a few rigorously designed scientific studies of fruits and vegetables have found minor differences, the majority in favour of organic produce (Canavari 2009). This might be because some organic fruit seems to be drier than conventionally grown fruit. A slightly drier fruit may have a more intense flavour due to the higher concentration of nutrients and as a result may be preferred by the consumer. Organic farmers are also known for using a larger variety of plant and livestock species in their operations (Bengtsson *et al.* 2005). This provides consumers with the opportunity to enjoy new tastes and eating experiences. However, taste advantages for organic produce are very much subjective and difficult to differentiate from inherent sensory attributes (Sörqvist *et al.* 2013).

Furthermore, there is evidence that some organically grown fruits have a higher resistance to deterioration and better keeping quality, attributed to the lower moisture content. Others espouse the view that organic fruits and vegetables may spoil faster because they are not treated with waxes or preservatives. Some organic produce may look less than perfect with odd shapes, varying colours or smaller sizes (Spellman and Bieber 2012:388). However, consumers expect that organic foods should meet the same quality standards as those of conventional foods.

Due to increasing anthropogenic environmental pollution, it has been claimed that more and more people suffer from so-called lifestyle diseases, which include allergies, diabetes, obesity, atherosclerosis and some cancers. One of the reasons for the development of lifestyle diseases might be improper and unhealthy eating habits, but it is also claimed to be a cumulative effect of artificial food additives and pesticides in producing conventional food (Johansson *et al.* 2014).

Safety of organic produce

An anticipated positive impact on human health is one among several key reasons why a number of governments have set goals for the expansion of organic agriculture in their respective countries. In the USA, the Food, Conservation and Energy Act of 2008 includes a mandatory five-fold funding increase for organic research programmes and cost share assistance for farmers and handlers (Greene *et al.* 2009). Similarly, the 2014 European Action Plan for Organic Farming strengthens information and research, as well as improving production standards and streamlining public support (European Commission 2014b). In Africa, the African Union has taken a decision to support and develop frameworks and strategies for organic policies (Willer and Lernoud 2014).

There is a widespread public belief that consumption of organic food is beneficial to health and significantly safer than food grown conventionally. This view is based mainly on anecdotal evidence and testimonials of organic food as more 'natural' rather than scientific evidence. Reviews of the available body of scientific literature on public health found that the number of studies are limited and only a few of those performed confirm positive public health benefits from consuming organic food (Matt *et al.* 2011; Johansson *et al.* 2014). However, the reviewers suggested that positive effects on animals from consumption of organically produced food could be regarded as an indication of favourable effects also on humans. Effects of organic or conventional animal feed have mainly been studied in relation to parameters such as immune status, fertility rate, and the survival rate of the young, where in some studies, but not all, a positive impact was found for animals fed with organic compared to conventionally grown feed. Positive results from organic feed were found for reproductive performance in rabbits and fruit flies (Paci *et al.* 2003; Chhabra *et al.* 2013), and immune status in rats and chicken (Huber *et al.* 2010; Finamore *et al.* 2004). Organic feed stimulated proliferation of lymphocytes, gave higher levels of immunoglobulin G in blood serum, increases in regulatory T cells and enhanced immune reactivity after challenge (Lauridsen *et al.* 2008; Huber *et al.* 2010; Roselli *et al.* 2012).

Most claims of improved safety of organic food have focused on pesticide residues. Organic food should carry no synthetic pesticide residues. Studies show that consumption of organic foods can reduce exposure to pesticide residues by at least 30 per cent depending on their share of the total food basket (Smith-Spangler *et al.* 2012). Although studies have shown that organically grown fruits and vegetables have significantly lower pesticide residue levels, the importance of this finding in relation to actual health risk reduction is debatable as both conventional foods and organic foods generally have pesticide levels well below government guidelines for what is considered safe. It is not possible at this stage to estimate potential health benefits associated with reducing pesticide exposure through switching to organic food (Barański *et al.* 2014).

There is a potential that organic food consumption systems might be affected by increases in some environmental contaminants. There are indications that free range eggs might carry slightly higher levels of dioxins, because the land they roam have previously been contaminated by dioxin through conventional production methods, but this would be expected to have little consequence for the overall dioxin burden (European Food Safety Authority 2012).

Other possible sources of increased safety risk from organic food consumption, like use of biological pesticides or the risk from mycotoxins produced by fungi grown on products due to the lack of effective organic compliant fungicides, have likewise not been confirmed by rigorous studies published in the scientific peer reviewed literature. In most cases occurrence of mycotoxins in organic products have shown to be at the same level or in some cases even lower than in conventional products (Matt *et al.* 2011). In fact, the preventive measures used in organic systems, despite the non-use of fungicides, appear generally able to maintain contamination at a low level (Lairon 2009).

It has been noted that the risks from microbiological sources are likely to be much more significant than short-term or chronic risks from pesticide residues. There is an anticipated increased risk from microbiological contamination. This is due to increased manure use during organic produce production, as fertiliser from animal sources can contain organisms like *Escherichia coli* O157:H7. However, such contamination risks do not differ significantly between organic and conventional crop production systems (Lairon 2009). In addition, bacterial contamination of retail chicken and pork was common, but unrelated to farming method. Nonetheless, the risk of carrying bacteria showing antibiotic resistance was higher in conventional than in organic chicken and pork production (Smith-Spangler *et al.* 2012).

Organic regulations ban or severely restrict the use of food additives, processing aids – that is, substances used during processing, but not added directly to the food product – and fortifying agents commonly used in non-organic foods. These include preservatives, artificial sweeteners, colourings, flavourings and monosodium glutamate (Beck *et al.* 2006). The American Cancer Society (ACS) has noted that interest in organic food is partly derived from the perceived risk of cancer caused by additives not found in organic foods. However the ACS has officially stated that 'whether organic foods carry a lower risk of cancer because they are less likely to include compounds that might cause cancer is largely unknown' (Kushi *et al.* 2012).

In summary, it is difficult to draw precise conclusions regarding the impact of organic food on animal and human health status. The increased amounts of nutritionally highly valued individual compounds, such as the higher antioxidant capacity in organic foods, do not seem to be the key for improved public health from organic food consumption. Instead, synergistic effects of several constituents might be the reason for the possible positive effects of organic food, as well as absence of pesticide residues. However, firm conclusions about the relative safety of organic foods have been hampered by the difficulty in scientifically grounded research design and a relatively small number of studies directly comparing organic food to conventional food (Johansson *et al.* 2014).

Public perception

There is a declining trust in the safety of food among some members of the public in response to intensive farming systems that is seen to have negative impacts not only on the environment, but also on food quality and safety. Research by Jackson (2010) found a variety of anxieties about food including ethical and moral concerns about animal welfare, the increasingly industrial scale of modern agriculture, and fears about food safety and contamination, often expressed in terms of the health and wellbeing of family and friends. He explored how anxieties were framed, mediated and institutionalised, and how they spread or were eventually contained. Jackson pointed out that anxieties move between social fields like public health to environmental sustainability, and vary historically, geographically and social. They proliferate predominantly in conditions of uncertainty such as in the gap between expert knowledge and lay understanding.

Anxiety following recent crises concerning food safety at different stages of the agricultural and food chain has prompted consumers to look for safer and more authentic food, contributing to an increased demand for organic products (Matt *et al.* 2011). According to Ulrich Beck's risk society thesis, modern anxieties are particularly oppressive because of the way that they travel invisibly through the conduits of everyday life. Beck warns of the invisible risks associated with air pollution, radiological hazards and food contamination: the 'stowaways of normal consumption' that 'travel on the wind and in the water', passing through 'all the otherwise strictly controlled protective areas of modernity' (Beck 1992:40–41).

There are numerous factors that lead organically minded consumers to buy organic food products, including availability, price, perceived quality, family considerations, political, ethical and health concerns (Hjelmar 2011). Many studies have found health and nutritional concerns to be the most important factors influencing organic food purchase (Honkanen *et al.* 2006; Magnusson *et al.* 2003). Superior taste, environmental concerns, food safety, animal welfare and supporting the local economy have also been found to be important factors in explaining consumer attitudes towards organic food (Hughner *et al.* 2007). In addition, studies have identified several factors that restrain consumers from buying organic food. An insufficient availability of organic products, a lack of awareness of organic food, and the higher prices of organic compared with conventional products are considered major barriers to further the development of the organic food market (Ritson and Oughton 2007; Padel and Foster 2005). Consumption of organic food is assumed to depend on whether the consumer perceives it as providing higher health benefits and better taste, which compensate for its higher prices and possible shorter shelf life.

The volume of research in recent years directed at trying to understand organic consumers and their behaviour has been immense (Hughner *et al.* 2007). This can largely be explained by the fact that organic foods are occupying an ever more central position in the global food market and in global consumption patterns. The global production of organic food is expected to grow further, and the organic market is frequently regarded as one of the biggest growth markets in the food industry, although it is still small compared with the global food market (Baker 2004; Gifford and Bernard 2005).

Despite the difficulty to clearly demonstrate possible benefits associated with organic food production, a majority of food shoppers (albeit in so-far limited surveys) associate organic foods with positive words (Raab and Grobe 2005). 'Chemical-free' was the word most commonly mentioned in association with organic food, by about 40 per cent of respondents, followed by specific types of food, mentioned by about 15 per cent of the respondents. In decreasing frequency were 'natural', 'home grown', 'healthier', 'more nutritious', 'earth friendly', 'clean', and 'pure and fresh'. Similarly, a study of 21,261 consumers in 38 countries reported that consumers nominated their main reasons for purchasing organic food as: 'healthier for me'; 51 per cent, 'healthier for my children'; 17 per cent, 'better for the environment'; 15 per cent, 'kinder to animals'; 7 per cent, and 'other', 10 per cent (AC Nielsen 2005).

A comprehensive literature review of the public perception of organic foods found that the majority of studies covered design and labelling issues (Schleenbecker and Hamm 2013). A trend towards the so called 'organic plus' positioning was noted, with many consumers expecting an extensive orientation towards sustainability. The diversity of certification labels featured prominently, as well as the low degree of awareness of the meaning of the many labels amongst consumers. In July 2010, a mandatory European Union logo for organic food was introduced to make the identification of organic products easier for consumers. The public perception of the logo was tested in five EU countries using focus groups and a survey of 2,042 participants (Janssen and Hamm 2012). While the introduction of a mandatory EU logo for organic food was generally welcomed in all countries, trust in the underlying production standards and the inspection system, although generally positive, was not very pronounced, except in Italy.

The media can play an influential role in contemporary food choice. The existence of an inter-relationship between media meanings and social life, whereby mass media provides a subject and a vocabulary for social interaction, includes wider processes of cultural transmission (Abercrombie and Longhurst 1998). Food is a particularly good vehicle for the expression of a wide range of social sentiments, its powerful symbolic qualities deriving from the way that, as we eat it, it is literally incorporated within the body (Jackson *et al.* 2013). A Danish survey of 3,200 households investigated the effects of health-related media information on the demand for organic fruit and vegetables (Smed 2012). Smed found that negative information about pesticides contained in conventional fruit and vegetables was the main influence on a consumer entering the organic market, not the quantities consumed by households already purchasing organic foods. On the other hand, positive information that linked health and the consumption of organic food influenced both steps of the decision process. Research results suggest that directly obtained information through media is the main type of information influencing consumers, a 'reason for this might be due to that indirectly obtained information is disseminated through the population and takes time to spread' (Smed 2012:44).

Studies suggest that families with children and adolescents or younger consumers in general are more likely to buy organic fruits and vegetables than other consumer groups (Thompson and Kidwell 1998; Loureiro *et al.* 2001; Magnusson *et al.* 2003). However, according to Dettmann and Dimitry (2010), the factor most consistently associated with the increased propensity to purchase organic food is level of formal education. Higher education levels led to higher likelihoods of purchasing organic vegetables, and spending a greater share of household income on these products. They also found that higher income households were more likely to try organic vegetables, but unlikely to consistently devote a large share of their expenditures toward organic vegetables, while lower income families spent more on organic vegetables proportionate to their overall expenditures on vegetables.

Extensive studies have been conducted to associate the source of food-related risk with consumer risk perception. It appears, however, that consumer risk perception of food safety is determined not so much by the risk per se, as by the social, cultural and psychological characteristics of the perceived food danger. Research demonstrates that much of the public's reaction to risks is attributed to sensitivity, not only to the technical, but also to the social and cultural aspects of risk (Slovic, 1993). This is the reason that consumer behaviour during periods of a food scare is often judged by scientists and industrialists to be due to irrationality or to ignorance of the true facts (Lofstedt and Frewer 1998) and the fact that social perception of risk is out of line with the technical assessment of risk.

Conclusion

Organic food production and the consumption of organic food can be seen as the anti-risk and the least risk adverse way to produce food and the healthiest food to eat. Organic food production is the traditional way to grow food. The problem is that it is an expensive method of growing and producing food. It is work intensive and this increases the cost of the products. This restricts the consumer base as organic food products become too expensive for a large part of the population, especially people on low income and people outside the labour market. The people who can afford the perceived healthy food can thus avoid risking their health and wellbeing while others cannot. This divides people not only according to social class, but also on health and possible life expectancy grounds. It will increase the divide between people who have and people who have not.

To develop a dominating market of organic food might not be feasible at present, and it might create resistance from investors in commercial non-organic production. Nonetheless, there could be specific demands for aspects of organic production, for example, less use of artificial enhancements, pesticides and better conditions for animals.

The proponents of commercial production of food will stress that there is a very small amounts of hormones, antibiotics and pesticides in the conventional products when ready for consumption, and that these amounts pose no danger to the consumer. The issue is rather the compounded effects of multiple residues and the long-term effects of eating food, which has potentially harmful inputs.

This leads to the question of what people can do when they are concerned about the food they eat, but cannot buy the food they perceive as being good for them. However, it is not that simple to change whole production systems, to clean the soil from pesticides and other artificial inputs, to change animal husbandry so that use of antibiotics and hormones can be avoided, and to naturally breed resistant crops with high yields that can feed a growing global population. This is also a question that is significant when introducing genetically modified crops for short term gain (see Chapter 9), where irreparable damage can be caused to other species with long-term environmental implications. Issues not always considered in the regulatory decision-making process.

Part IV

The governmentality risk perspective

The third sociological risk discourse covers the governmentality risk perspective derived from Foucault's (1991), Ewald's (1991) and Dean's (1999, 2009) discussions about government's role in regulating citizens. A central focus of Foucault's discourse is that power is facilitated through socio-cultural assumptions, which extends to institutional authority. This includes government's use of different strategies to manage the citizens and to maintain the preferred social order within society (Rose 1990:ix). The created social order aims to instill trust and prosperity among the citizens, create an atmosphere of acceptance of the rule of law, democratic traditions and transparent political institutions. Governments' regulation of food production and manufacturing of food should deliver food suitable for consumption. Citizens would logically assume that safe food would be foremost on the government's mind. However, the question of what constitutes a risk is subjective and a dependent on who is defining it, as '[n]othing is a risk in itself; there is no risk in reality ... anything can be a risk; it all depends on how one analyses the danger, considers the event' (Ewald 1991:199).

Regulation of the whole food chain is nothing new, as governments have regulated food based on different criteria over time, controlling production for social, cultural and religious, but also for political and economic reasons. The governmentality risk perspective persuades citizens to voluntary adopt practices and behaviours that are classified as 'good citizen' conduct, to adhere to regulations and social norms and to accept the government's power to govern and enforce laws, as well as instil in the citizens the moral duty to self-regulate their behaviour to become good citizens. With increasingly intensive debates and questions about food safety, governments' concerns about people's health – that they eat the right food and not indulge in food products high in sugar and fat – have gained priority. However, it is also a balancing act in deciding what risks are acceptable and what can be classified as safe food without damaging existing food production. The commercialisation of food, and governments' priority in creating sustainable industries, create conflicts or disagreements between governments' and experts' advice about what can be classified as safe food both in the short and long term. Here the public sometimes voice a different opinion.

Chemicals are essential for the efficiency of production and processing of food, but their use should be balanced in a way that the food is fit for consumption and that residue contamination is within the official food standards guidelines (see Chapter 11). Nonetheless, the main risk issue is not limited to hazardous chemicals remaining in food because of production and processing; chemical contamination can also occur during household preparation of food.

Government action through information campaigns and warning labels on the food is one way to minimise risks to public health, although it is difficult to control this last phase of food handling before consumption, when the risk management responsibility depends on the individual household members. It becomes the individual's responsibility to be aware and follow the guidelines (Foucault 2007).

The governmentality risk discourse uses prohibition with imposed fines, advice and social control to influence accepted food production, processing and consumption behaviour. As discussed in section I (Chapter 5), this is strongly enforced in relation to drugs, such as alcohol and the growing of illegal crops like hemp and poppies. Attitudes to alcohol and its governance are based on social and cultural traditions, but also on faith. It is commonly accepted that overindulgence in alcohol and other drugs, legal or not within the society, will have negative effects on people's health, similar to overconsumption of food high in fat and sugar.

However, the influence of government recommendations, the urging of experts' advice and public dissemination of scientific knowledge will not necessarily change people's food consumption priorities, as cultural and social belonging and their long-established traditions will have more influence on their food consumption habits (Bourdieu 1984). This is very much reflected in consumers putting themselves at risk by not heeding governments' and scientists' advice to eat more fruits and vegetables that protect against a range of maladies (see Chapter 12).

In the following two chapters, food production, processing and consumption habits are analysed from the governmentality risk perspective. However, since the governmentality risk discourse is all-encompassing in relation to the food chain, the governmentality discourse underpins most of the prior sections as well.

11 Tasty and toxic – a culinary risk dilemma

Introduction

Risks are part of any society, and even when risks are considered to be occasional events, this is not the situation with food as it is consumed daily. Food can cause and create risks throughout the whole food chain, from production to consumption, including the formation of harmful chemicals during food preparation in the kitchen, which is the focus of this chapter.

Except for specific food groups, preparation of food for consumption is most likely to involve forms of heating: grilling, roasting, frying, boiling, baking, toasting or heating by microwave ovens. Heating improves the palatability of food, changes its physical structure and reduces the microbial load. Heat-induced chemical reactions change numerous existing substances, but also generate a range of new chemical compounds that influence the quality and safety of the food. Some heat-induced reactions can be beneficial, like the breakdown of a natural legume toxin known as phytohaemagglutinin (Liu *et al.* 2013), while others can produce hazardous chemical compounds detrimental to health (Rietjens and Alink 2003). The latter substances are commonly called process-induced contaminants, and they include carcinogens, genotoxins, neurotoxins and anti-nutrients. They are compounds that can cause cancer, damage people's genetic code, destroy nerve tissue or interfere with the absorption of nutrients. All these activities can be harmful to people's health.

People strive to create and consume tasty food, and in countries with an abundance of food, consumers are spoilt for choices in preparing appetising cuisine. There are plenty of cookbooks available presenting ever more tasty dishes and a proliferation of cooking shows filling television programming schedules with teams competing to please judges' taste buds. It is all about taste and presentation to satisfy diverse culinary senses.

Over the last few decades, the sensory impact of food on the mechanisms of human appetite regulation has been extensively studied. Not surprisingly, results suggest that the impression people get from the sensory properties of food plays a very important role in the way food is selected and on how much we eat (Sørensen *et al.* 2003). However, sensory properties of food are complex and involve not only taste buds, but also smell or aroma, and the texture during chewing as well as the sight of food.

Research indicates that there is evidence of an interaction of sensory characteristics of food, as individuals combine the sensory components to assess the food's overall quality. In particular, the sensations of taste and smell interact with aroma and rises with increasing taste compound concentrations, and taste rating is rising with increasing aroma compound concentrations. Smell, in particular, seems to affect mood – by reviving positive memories – and influence expectations about food quality, food choice and intake. Even food the eaten previously and the current hunger state will affect the individual's perception of overall food palatability (Stroebele and De Castro 2004).

Although nutritional satisfaction is a basic requirement of food intake, food has also become a form of aesthetic gratification. The development of high cuisine represents an attempt to enrich life and produce culinary pleasures, as nutritional fulfilment alone does not require artistic presentations of the dish or the use of elaborate spice mixtures (Rozin 2006).

Even the simple use of heat to process food ensured considerable improvements to food palatability in early human life. Through evolutionary history, the adoption of cooking should probably be regarded as one of the most significant improvements in dietary quality, and one of the leading changes in food distribution and availability, in that storage deterioration could be at least partly nullified. Cooking had particularly dramatic effects on the food supply, including softening food difficult to ingest, increasing the amount of food suitable for consumption, and food handling such as preparing manageable batches of meat around fires (Wrangham and Conklin-Brittain 2003).

Many meat cuts are rich in collagen, making them tough to chew when raw (Bailey 1972), while cooking above 80°C (176°F) coagulates the connective tissue collagen and hydrolyses it to soluble gelatine. This allows muscle fibres to be easily separated, and give them a short, brittle texture facilitating easy mastication (Birch *et al.* 1986). Further, browning of meat at high surface temperatures induces a range of complex chemical reactions giving it flavours that are more desirable. Cooked meat is therefore much more enjoyable to eat than raw meat, but unfortunately with improved taste comes the risks presented by potentially toxic chemicals induced by the cooking process.

As consumer, it is difficult to comprehend the chemical processes and easy to ignore the risks created by these contaminants, despite being studied extensively by scientists (Lineback and Stadler 2008). Public perception of risk is not necessarily based on fact, as has been discussed in previous chapters. Rather, it can depend on a fear of the unknown and a feeling of not being in control. Children are taught not to talk to strangers outside parents' control, but a threat to a child's safety is statistically more likely to come from a person known to or acquainted with the child and the family, rather than from a total stranger. Equally, flying is often perceived as riskier than driving a car that we can control, although car accidents are much more common than aeroplane crashes and cause more annual fatalities than flying accidents. Hence, this risk perception anomaly can be seen as related to the ability to personally control a situation. Thus, public risk perception becomes inversely related to the amount of control exerted by the individual. Governments' role is to ensure safe food in the whole food chain through regulating the different process stages and instil in the consumer the 'right' food handling procedures.

Consumers have control over food preparation at home and do not necessarily see it as a risky process, while agricultural production and industrial processing are seen as part of a 'black box' and inherently more risky. Beck (1992) has highlighted the difficulties for the general population, which includes experts, to be knowledgeable about all stages of modern industrialisation, the manufactured risks in modern society, as information is not effortlessly available in a straightforwardly digestible format for the public. Conversely, individuals are more confident in their ability to control what is happening in their own kitchen, despite a similar lack of knowledge about the numerous invisible chemical reactions occurring during food preparation.

The rapid pace of change in science and technology, and in food legislation, and the improved socio-economic status and growing middle class, as well as socio-demographic realities with concentration of populations to urban areas, have all had a marked impact on food supply and food production. Modern industrialisation, which is proposed by some sectors of the society as a necessity to feed a growing world population, creates uncertainty about production procedures and harmful effects of the production. Modern industrialisation has alienated people's ability directly to influence their living environment and life choices (Beck 1992:35–36). The need for continuous risk assessment and management, to respond to manufactured known and emerging risks in order to protect consumers, have become essential tasks for governments and regulators. However, since little regulatory influence is possible on consumer behaviour in the kitchen, governments have to focus on raw material inputs that can diminish risks as well as issuing public advice.

The rapid change in food innovation has made the public circumspect about novel additives and processing aids used by the food industry, but little consideration is given to toxic compounds formed during home processing for which the public actually has some control. For example, despite repeated public warnings, meat is often charred in the barbecue generating a range of toxic polycyclic aromatic hydrocarbons. Gravy is made from pan drippings containing toxic heterocyclic amines formed during high temperature frying, and bread is partly burnt in the toaster causing excess acrylamide to be formed. Coffee is brewed in closed circuit espresso machines causing high levels of toxic furan to be retained. The preferred taste can be in conflict with health warnings, and this causes culinary risk dilemmas, as there is a direct correlation between the intensity of the chemical reactions that enhance taste and the amount of toxic compounds formed in the heated food.

Development of process-induced contaminants

Industrial food processing make use of many techniques, predominantly heating, drying, smoking, curing, fermentation, or the use of preservatives in order to produce the desired taste and to ensure that food products are free from spoilage and disease-causing microorganisms. Some of these processing methods create new health risks, as they can produce chemical compounds that are harmful to human health. The health risks are compounded by a range of processing contaminants that can be formed during home cooking because of modification of or interactions between compounds that are natural components of the food.

Process-induced contaminants are not new, as they have existed in foods since the first discovery that cooking food over a fire improved its taste and overall palatability. Applying high temperatures to food generates a host of new chemical compounds, some of which may have a beneficial effect, while others can be toxic. This has been known for many years, with some widely studied process contaminants including polycyclic aromatic hydrocarbons, a large group of potentially carcinogenic chemicals (Knize *et al.* 1999), and a range of carcinogenic heterocyclic amines (Kizil *et al.* 2011). Polycyclic aromatic hydrocarbons consist of multiple aromatic rings of only carbon and hydrogen, while heterocyclic amines include at least two other compounds, such as nitrogen, oxygen or sulphur, in their rings. While many food contaminants have been known for decades, the formation and presence of some chemicals in food have been discovered relatively recently. These are the so-called emerging food contaminants like acrylamide and furan (Lineback and Stadler 2008; Kantiani *et al.* 2010).

The presence of process-induced contaminants in food is difficult to avoid completely, but an understanding of how the contaminants are formed can allow changes to food preparation methods, recipes or processes to reduce the formation of such chemicals. Replacing dry heat cooking with moist heat cooking is one example, which allows for lower cooking temperatures to be used and thus reduces the formation of heat-induced process contaminants in industrial as well as in home settings. From the consumer perspective, a balanced diet without overindulgence in particular foods, such as deep fried, barbecued or toasted foods, can contribute to reducing exposure to process contaminants and lower potential health risks.

The following sections cover four of the most common process-induced contaminants, namely polycyclic aromatic hydrocarbons formed in particular during barbecuing, heterocyclic amines produced when pan frying at high temperatures, acrylamide developing as part of high-temperature browning reactions, and furan emerging during roasting of coffee. These are settings where the governmentality discourse can be applied, governments having regulations in place to protect consumers, but also deciding where regulations are warranted and effective.

Polycyclic aromatic hydrocarbons

Polycyclic aromatic hydrocarbons form a class of diverse organic compounds, each of them containing two or more aromatic ring structures, so named after their benzene-like closed rings. They are primarily formed by incomplete combustion or pyrolysis of oil, coal and organic matter and during various industrial or home cooking processes. They generally occur as complex mixtures, which may consist of hundreds of compounds. A range of polycyclic aromatic hydrocarbons was initially isolated from coal tar deposits (Culp *et al.* 1998). The problem is that a number of them can be found in food and some have been shown to be genotoxic carcinogens – the most toxic carcinogen (International Agency for Research on Cancer 1973, 1987; United States Environmental Protection Agency 1984; Montizaan *et al.* 1989; International Programme on Chemical Safety 1998). The most widely studied is benzo[a]pyrene. The International Agency for Research on Cancer (IARC) (1987) concluded in 1987 that benzo[a]pyrene is a probable human carcinogen.

The natural and anthropogenic sources of polycyclic aromatic hydrocarbons in the environment are numerous, as they are emitted from processing of coal, crude oil, petroleum, and natural gas, from production of aluminium, iron and steel, from heating in power plants and homes – oil, gas, charcoal-fired stoves, wood stoves, burning of refuse, forest fires and motor vehicle exhausts (Scientific Committee on Food 2002). Humans are exposed to polycyclic aromatic hydrocarbons in various ways. While for non-smokers the major route of exposure is consumption of food, for smokers the contribution from smoking may be significant. Food can be contaminated by environmental particles present in air, soil or water, through industrial food processing methods, and through home food preparation.

The compounds have been detected in a variety of foods, notably vegetables, due to the deposition of airborne particles, and in fish and mussels from contaminated waters (Edwards 1983; Nielsen *et al.* 1996). Polycyclic aromatic hydrocarbons can also contaminate food during industrial smoking, heating and drying processes that allow combustion products to come into direct contact with food. Contamination of cereals and of vegetable oils, including seed oils and olive residue oils, usually occurs during technological processes like direct fire drying, where combustion products may be exposed to the grain, oil seeds or the final oil (Speer *et al.* 1990; Standing Committee on Foodstuffs 2001).

At home, polycyclic aromatic hydrocarbons are formed as a result of certain food preparation methods, such as grilling, roasting and smoking. The highest concentrations are usually found in charcoal grilled/barbecued foods, foods processed by traditional smoking techniques, fish in particular, and in mussels and other seafood from polluted waters (Guillen *et al.* 1997; Phillips 1999). Several studies have been undertaken to determine the levels of exposure to polycyclic aromatic hydrocarbons from representative human diets. In its assessment of exposure to polycyclic aromatic hydrocarbons, the European Food Safety Authority (2008a) found that the two largest contributors were cereals and cereal products, and seafood and seafood products. Vegetable oils used for seasoning and cooking, as well as those incorporated into biscuits and cakes, and fruits and vegetables, can be significant dietary sources of polycyclic aromatic hydrocarbons as well (Butler *et al.* 1993). However, smoked and grilled food may contribute considerably to the intake of polycyclic aromatic hydrocarbons, if they are a large part of the usual diet (Phillips 1999).

Barbecuing as a cooking method is entrenched in many parts of the world. The modern word barbecue derives from the word *barabicu* found in the language of the Taíno people of the Caribbean and the Timucua of Florida and translates as 'sacred fire pit' (Hale 2000). The word describes a grill for cooking meat, consisting of a wooden platform resting on sticks over a hole in the ground. The word barbecue was first recorded in the English language in the mid-seventeenth century (Oxford Dictionaries Online 2013).

Although barbecuing was used to cook whole pigs in the United States of America in the nineteenth century, the modern barbecue tradition can be credited to the carmaker Henry Ford, who ignited America's passion for outdoor cooking. In the 1920s, Ford was determined to find a use for the growing piles of wood scraps from the production of his Model T car. He learned the process of converting the wood scraps into charcoal briquettes and soon quickly built a charcoal plant known as 'Ford Charcoal' (Slater 2014).

Cooking meat on an open flame is also an Australian institution. Customary Aboriginal cooking always involved the use of a traditional barbecue – outdoor cooking over a fire or hot coals. Aborigines would also use the earth to create ovens (O'Dea 1991). Although Australians think of themselves as the great barbecue nation, barbecuing as a social habit only dates to about just after the Second World War. Lately, supported by a range of celebrity cooking shows, people have become more sophisticated. The initial burnt sausages and chops are competing with gourmet sausages, marinated steaks and fresh seafood, which are increasingly cooked to perfection and served with complementing gourmet salads, wines and boutique beer.

Government attempts to reduce polycyclic aromatic hydrocarbons contamination

Governments in several countries have set maximum levels for polycyclic aromatic hydrocarbons in certain commercial foods. In 2005, the European Commission introduced harmonised maximum levels for benzo[a]pyrene in oils and fats, smoked meats and smoked meat products, smoked fish and smoked fish products, meat of fish other than smoked, crustaceans, cephalopods, bivalve molluscs and infant foods. The legislation was amended in 2011 to include a composite measure of four compounds.

Because of the EU legislation, there are some problems with certain traditional products. Smoked sprats, a small fish found in the Baltic Sea, are part of the Latvian culture and considered a delicacy across many parts of the former Soviet Union. High levels of benzo[a]pyrene have consistently been found in the smoked sprats, but because of their cultural significance, smoked sprats remain a highly sought after food. Latvian authorities have asked for a derogation from European limits, despite common health warnings. Drabova *et al.* (2013) found that 67 per cent of the samples of smoked sprats in oil exceeded the maximum level of 5 μg/kg benzo[a]pyrene established for smoked fish by European Union legislation.

Canadian authorities have set a regulatory limit for benzo[a]pyrene in olive pomace oils. In the USA, the Environment Protection Agency has set regulatory limits for benzo[a]pyrene in drinking water, but the Food and Drug Administration has not set regulatory limits for food. Equally, there are no set limits in Australia. However, regulations are used worldwide to control residential exposure to surface soil contamination and rulings have been issued by 44 United Nations member states plus four territories or administrative regions, to control exposure to seven polycyclic aromatic hydrocarbons generally considered to be carcinogenic or mutagenic (Jennings 2012).

Governments regularly issue warnings of the dangers of polycyclic aromatic hydrocarbons. Although the dangers of barbecuing and smoking of meat and fish should be well known among the public, it is such an entrenched part of the culture that most warnings are being ignored (American Institute for Cancer Research 2014; Klein 2013; Edgar 2014).

Warnings about the risks inherent in barbecuing food are not aimed at preventing barbecuing, but at encouraging that it be done in the least harmful way, as the amount of polycyclic aromatic hydrocarbons formed during cooking or processing of food depends markedly on how the food is cooked (Lijinsky and Ross 1967; Lijinsky 1991; Knize *et al.* 1999). Simple methods, such as selecting lean meat and fishes, avoiding contact between foods and flames when barbecuing, using less fat for grilling and, in general, cooking at a lower temperature for a longer time. Fat dripping down onto an open flame and sending up a column of smoke coating the food with polycyclic aromatic hydrocarbons should be avoided. The use of medium to low heat, and placement of the meat further from the heat source, can greatly reduce formation of the compounds. The intensity of flavour is not necessarily associated with the depth of the brown colour of grilled foods, hence overcooking the food does not improve the flavour. Nonetheless, food must be cooked in accordance with recommendations to avoid possible bacteria, for example, chicken and hamburgers need to be cooked through to be safe, while most other whole meat cuts can be red in the middle.

Heterocyclic amines

In 1977, Japanese scientists found cancer causing compounds in food following normal household cooking processes at temperatures over 150°C (Nagao *et al.* 1977). Over 25 different compounds, now known as heterocyclic amines, have since been isolated and identified to date in fried meat, fish and poultry (Sanz Alaejos *et al.* 2008). These compounds are found in foods that are cooked to 'well done', in pan drippings and on food surfaces that show a crispy brown crust. The compounds have been divided into two groups. First, the thermic group with compounds that are formed at conventional temperatures of 150–300°C by reactions between creatine or creatinine and sugars called Maillard reactions. Second, the pyrolytic group with compounds that are formed at temperatures above 300°C by pyrolysis of amino acids and proteins. The formation of either group of compounds during cooking depends on the type of food used, the temperature of the cooking surface, the degree of browning and the length of cooking time. Foods that are lower in fat and water content show higher concentrations of heterocyclic amines after cooking. Beef, chicken and fish have higher concentrations than pork. Sausages are high in fat and water and show lower concentrations of heterocyclic amines after cooking (Augustsson *et al.* 1999; Kizil *et al.* 2011).

Numerous heterocyclic amines have been shown to be genotoxic carcinogens in animal experiments and have been classified by the International Agency for Research on Cancer (1993) as probable or even possible carcinogens in humans. Although several classes of carcinogens are present in red meat and processed meat, and multiple mechanisms of carcinogenesis are likely to be involved, the exposure and causal role of heterocyclic amines in cancer development through eating meat cooked well done has been an area of intense research interest (Ferguson 2010). Some epidemiological investigations examining the connection between consumption of meat and the potential cancer causing role of heterocyclic amines have shown a clear dose response relationship between cancer risk and well done meat consumption, while others have showed no such association (Zheng and Lee 2009).

Government attempts to reduce heterocyclic amines contamination

There seem to be no government regulations or guidelines relevant to reduction of exposure to heterocyclic amines. However, although there is no general agreement on the role of heterocyclic amines in relation to human health, authorities in many countries consider the risk high enough to recommend that their presence in our diet should be minimised. This can be achieved through several means. One way could be to follow the recommendations of World Cancer Research Fund International and reduce overall meat consumption (Ferguson 2010). If this is not feasible, changes in cooking techniques have been shown to reduce the level of heterocyclic amines in meat. Differences in heterocyclic amine levels can be more than 100-fold depending on the time and temperature combination used for cooking the meat (Sinha *et al.* 1998). More heterocyclic amines are formed when pan surface temperatures are higher than 220°C, so reducing the surface temperature is beneficial in avoiding the creation of burnt crust. The pan drippings and meat residue that remain after meat is fried also have high concentrations of heterocyclic amines and using them for making gravy might best be avoided (Augustsson *et al.* 1999). Ground beef patties show lower levels of heterocyclic amines if they are flipped every minute until cooked through (Knize and Felton 2005).

Again, frying of meat products is an entrenched part of human culture and a culinary improvement that is not easy to change, but public warnings about the formation of heterocyclic amines (National Cancer Institute 2010; Worth 2010; Chilkov 2012) have also been less frequent compared to warnings about polycyclic aromatic amines.

Acrylamide

Acrylamide is yet another toxic compound formed during industrial food processing or home cooking. It came to prominence in 2002 when it was first reported to be formed in certain starchy foods during high tempera- tures by researchers at Stockholm University and the Swedish National Food Administration (Tareke *et al.* 2002; Swedish National Food Administration 2002). Acrylamide has long been used as an industrial chemical in water treat- ment and in the manufacture of adhesives, dyes and fabrics. To find it in food was a surprise, but presumably it had been present in some heated foods for hundreds, if not thousands of years without detection. The finding sparked a renewed interest in the area of process contaminants.

The concern is that acrylamide's presence in heated foods is widespread and that it has been demonstrated to be genotoxic and carcinogenic in animal testing. Acrylamide has been classified as probably carcinogenic to humans, and it can have toxic effects on neurological and reproductive systems at high doses (International Agency for Research on Cancer 1994; Friedman 2003). Currently, epidemiological studies, with a few exceptions, have not been able to prove associations between acrylamide in food and human cancer (Hogervorst *et al.* 2010; Lipworth *et al.* 2012). This is no surprise since it is difficult to find an unexposed control group because of pervasive population exposure. In addition, large variations in acrylamide levels, even in foods of the same type, make it impossible to estimate accurately acrylamide expos- ure from simple consumption tools used in most epidemiological studies. In research, using a blood biomarker for acrylamide exposure, a positive associ- ation between biomarker levels and an oestrogen receptor positive to breast cancer was identified (Olesen *et al.* 2008). Despite the general lack of asso- ciation between estimated dietary acrylamide exposure and human cancer, a number of official organisations worldwide recommend that exposure to acrylamide should be limited to the lowest possible level. Among others, the Joint FAO/WHO Expert Committee on Food Additives expressed its con- cern for human health based on the currently available scientific information (World Health Oganization 2011b).

Since the initial discovery, acrylamide has been found at varying levels in a wide range of cooked foods, especially potato crisps and French fries, bread and baked cereal products, and roasted and ground coffee (European Food

Safety Authority 2012b). Swiss scientists also detected considerable levels of acrylamide in dried fruits (Amrein *et al.* 2007). Acrylamide is rapidly metabolised in the human body to the even more toxic glycidamide (Gamboa da Costa *et al.* 2003; Vikström *et al.* 2011).

Three major sources of human acrylamide exposure have been identified: industrial workplaces, tobacco smoking and cooked food. Human exposure from industrial sources has mainly occurred because of workplace accidents. Smoking releases acrylamide and tobacco smoke is the major source of acrylamide exposure among smokers (Urban *et al.* 2006). Because of its ubiquity in food after high temperature processing, such as in cooking, frying, roasting and baking, it is almost impossible to avoid some exposure (Dybing *et al.* 2005).

The principal route of formation is currently considered to be reactions between carbohydrates and amino acids, particularly the non-essential amino acid asparagine and reducing sugars, such as glucose and fructose. The reactions occur during browning of food at high temperatures by Maillard reactions (Zhang and Zhang 2007). These reactions, named after the French chemist Louis-Camille Maillard, are responsible for a range of complex chemical events during browning giving foods their desirable flavours, but unfortunately also giving rise to toxic compounds (Lineback *et al.* 2012).

When, on 24 April 2002, the Swedish National Food Administration announced that acrylamide had been found in baked and fried starchy foods, it was followed by a strong, but short-lived interest in mass media. Subsequently, published research findings over the years have sparked a renewed interest by the popular press. As an example, more than one hundred articles were written in 2007 according to Nexis and Factiva in newspapers like the *LA Times*, *Boston Globe*, *Guardian* and *Wall Street Journal*, among many others. Irrespective of the publicity, the public seems to have taken little notice, probably because of entrenched dining habits, with French fries at fast food restaurants as popular as ever.

Governments attempts to reduce acrylamide contamination

There are currently no maximum permissible limits in the US or Europe governing the amount of acrylamide in food and beverages. However, acrylamide has been on the watch list for government authorities for some time since the 2002 discovery of its presence in many foods. In February 2011, acrylamide was added to the State of California's Proposition 65 list. Any products sold in California that contain a Proposition 65 listed compound must carry a label warning the purchaser that the substance is present in the product. Acrylamide warning signs have been posted at many coffee shops in that state. Acrylamide is also on the European Union's Substances of Very High Concern list following a unanimous decision by an expert EU health panel and indicative values for testing of different food categories have been issued by the European Commission.

There are some risk reduction strategies available that can be adopted by the public when made aware of the potential health hazards of burning food. Calls for reducing the formation of acrylamide during cooking have been directed both at the manufacturers of carbohydrate-rich foods and consumers who prepare, for instance, potatoes or cereal products at home. As a rule of thumb, temperatures during roasting, baking and frying should be kept below 175°C to produce a golden instead of charred surface. Since reducing sugars, so named because they are oxidised by mild oxidising compounds while in turn reducing the compound, can be formed during cold storage of potatoes, they should not be stored at temperatures below 8°C. Finally, bread and other foods should be toasted to the lightest colour possible to produce an acceptable taste, noting that the crust will have higher levels of acrylamide.

There are several current studies of the severity of the harmful effects that are potentially caused by acrylamide exposure. In June 2015, the European Food Safety Authority issued a scientific opinion following a thorough risk assessment of the public health risks of acrylamide in food, and concluded that it potentially increases the risk of developing cancer for consumers in all age groups. Since acrylamide is present in a wide range of everyday foods, this concern applies to all consumers with children the most exposed age group on a body weight basis. Ingredients, storage, and commercial processing conditions, as well as home cooking choices can have a substantial impact on the level of acrylamide humans are exposed to through the diet (European Food Safety Authority 2015b).

Furan

Furan is a simple organic compound widely used in various industrial processes, including in the manufacturing of lacquers and resins, and for the production of pharmaceuticals and agricultural chemicals. Furan can be found in the environment as a constituent of cigarette smoke, wood smoke, and exhaust gas from diesel and petrol engines (International Agency for Research on Cancer 1995).

Similar to acrylamide, furan is also a process contaminant, which forms during the heating of food, but in this case the process is far more complex, with a range of possible natural components intrinsic to food serving as precursors. So far, reducing sugars like fructose and glucose, amino acids such as serine and cysteine, ascorbic acid, unsaturated fatty acids and carotenoids have been identified as possible precursors, which transforms into furan under the influence of heat (Yaylayan 2006; Moro *et al.* 2012).

Furan was subject to a comprehensive toxicological evaluation in 1993 and proven to be toxic to the liver. Animal studies showed furan to be carcinogenic in rats and mice with a dose dependant increase in hepatocellular adenomas and carcinomas (National Toxicology Program 1993). As a result, furan has been classified as possibly carcinogenic for humans (International Agency for Research on Cancer 1995).

Furan and its derivatives have long been known to occur in heat-treated foods and contribute to the sensory properties of food (Merritt *et al.* 1963; Maga and Katz 1979). Additionally, furan has been found at low levels in some heat-treated foods, such as coffee, canned meat, bread, cooked chicken, sodium caseinate, hazelnuts, soy protein isolate, hydrolysed soy protein, rapeseed protein, fish protein concentrate and caramel, without getting much attention (Stoffelsma *et al.* 1968; Persson and von Sydow 1973; Maga and Katz 1979). Concern over furan in foods dates back only to 2004 when a Food and Drug Administration survey of heat processed foods in the USA revealed that furan could be found in a number of products processed in closed containers, such as cans and jars (United States Food and Drug Administration 2004). The fact that it occurred in baby food processed in jars was alarming, and it has since been confirmed that a relatively high level of furan contamination can be found in processed baby foods, although it is so volatile that levels fall quickly when containers are opened.

Coffee is another product with a high level of furan contamination. Not surprisingly, estimates of exposure were highest in toddlers eating jarred baby foods and among adults drinking coffee. These two sources are the major contributors to furan ingestion; other age groups seemed to have lower furan exposure (European Food Safety Authority 2011b).

Since coffee is a major contributor to furan exposure, scientists have looked at the impact of coffee roasting and brewing methods. It was found that formation of furan during roasting was dependent on roasting conditions and directly linked to achieving targeted flavour profiles. Modifications in process conditions to reduce furan levels had the opposite effect on other undesired reaction products like acrylamide. Even if furan concentrations are lower if coffee is roasted at low temperatures over a longer time – 140°C for 20 minutes – than in coffee roasted under usual conditions – 200–220°C for 10–15 minutes – much of the flavour was also lost (Guenther *et al.* 2010). However, it was estimated that only approximately 10 per cent of the initially generated furan during roasting is consumed by drinking a cup of coffee. The highest concentrations were found in coffee from espresso machines and of them, the highest was in coffee made from capsules. Capsules are hermetically sealed which prevents the highly volatile furan from being released. Since the capsule coffee machines use hot water at higher pressures, much of the furan is extracted into the cup (Altaki *et al.* 2011). The health risks can be minimised, as furan will start to evaporate when the cup of coffee is exposed to air so a slight delay before drinking the coffee might help. Furan levels also decreased in most canned and jarred foods after heating in a saucepan, but less so when heated in a microwave. Additionally, furan decreased slightly if foods were left to stand before consumption, but did so more rapidly on stirring (Roberts *et al.* 2008). The volatility of furan, means it is possible that some of it can be inhaled during food preparation and contribute to overall exposure (Crews 2009).

Governments attempts to reduce furan contamination

Acrylamide and furan in food have both become significant issues for the US Food and Drug Administration, with one or both compounds appearing on programme priority research lists since 2003. More information is considered necessary before any specific regulatory action can be considered. Equally, the European Commission prescribed in March 2007 further monitoring of the presence of furan in food to gain a better knowledge for eventual regulatory action. The European Food Safety Authority is currently collecting Europe-wide data with monitoring results collected between 2004 and 2010 published so far. Health Canada continues to conduct toxicological studies in laboratory animals in order to better understand the potential human health risks posed by levels of furan and its derivatives that humans are exposed to through the diet.

Disconnection between cooking habits and cancer risk

The four process contaminants described here are all suspected of being involved in the complex process of human cancer development. However, since this is a long-term chronic event there are few signs recognisable by the public connecting particular cooking habits with the progression of cancer later in life. Although cancer is a feared disease, the disconnection between food preparation methods used and the risk of future cancer formation in the minds of the public favours culinary aspects over absolute safety. Although public warnings have been issued numerous times covering the potential risks associated with certain food preparation methods, there is not surprisingly little evidence available that cooking habits have changed to any significant extent. Barbecuing seems to be as popular as ever and coffee capsule sales are steadily increasing.

The choice of food preparation method is complex and involves cultural and social aspects, economic issues as well as important culinary attributes. The latter include taste preference, sensory attributes, cognitive restraint and cultural familiarity. Research has found that sensory responses to the taste, smell and texture of foods in particular help determine food preferences and eating habits (Drewnowski 1997). However, sensory responses alone do not predict food consumption, as there are multiple links between taste perceptions, taste preferences, food preferences, food choices and the ultimate food consumption pattern.

A range of socio-cultural, genetic, physiological, and metabolic variables influence taste responses. The impact of taste factors on food intake further depends on gender, age, education level and exposure to diverse foods. Taste is also modulated by obesity, eating disorders and other pathologies of eating behaviour. Food preferences and food choices of populations are further linked to attitudinal, social, cultural, educational and economic variables (Drewnowski 1997).

Nonetheless, the actual behaviour of consumers is often inconsistent with their reported attitudes or concerns. This is particularly true with regard to health risks. Although consumers often express concern about food safety, few appear to change their food consumption behaviour in view of their concern (Lane and Bruhn 1991). In evaluating the gap between consumer attitudes and behaviour, it was found that people expressing concern about health risks associated with the consumption of French fries rose by 39 per cent between 1985 and 1990, yet the number eating them at least once in a fortnight declined by just 7 per cent (Townsend 1991).

Mass media promote hedonistic food values. There is a wide range of food-related programming offered by TV networks, ranging from instructional or aspirational, to experiential (Pope *et al.* 2015). These shows tend to provide instruction on how to make meals that will please others and often try to make food appear attractive, innovative or fun to improve the culinary experience (Caraher *et al.* 2000; Ketchum 2005; Meister 2001). There are indications that TV chefs' recipes are high in fat and sodium supporting palatability in contravention to World Health Organization guidelines (Howard *et al.* 2012). These shows might influence people to more frequently indulge in cooking with more fat, sugar and salt than they normally would do, hence adopting the culinary messages given in television shows for 'party' food as everyday food (Jones *et al.* 2013).

Given tradition and the populist influence of mass media on food preparation and culinary preferences, there is an uphill battle for risk communicators to spread the message of the potential health threats posed by heat-induced process contaminants, although good communication practices seek to bridge the divide between scientific experts, policy makers and consumers (Barnett *et al.* 2011). Nonetheless, scientifically supported messages might still be ignored by the public. Effective communication requires clear identification and thorough understanding of the target audience's needs, and appropriate management of the information provision so that it optimally addresses particular needs and interests for people at the right time – for example, at the time of shopping or through an attached label on the food product which can be read before preparation of the food. Palatability is clearly an important parameter that must be integrated into any risk messages trying to influence food preparation habits. The balance between taste and toxicity remains a culinary conundrum.

Conclusion

The most common household food preparation methods involve some form of heating. While heating improves palatability, heat-induced chemical reactions can generate a range of hazardous chemical compounds detrimental to health. Such substances are commonly called process-induced contaminants, and they include compounds that can cause cancer, damage the genetic code, destroy nerve tissue or interfere with the absorption of nutrients, all activities harmful to health.

Despite repeated public warnings, meat is often charred in the barbecue, generating a range of toxic polycyclic aromatic hydrocarbons; gravy is made from pan drippings containing toxic heterocyclic amines formed during high temperature frying. Bread that is partly burnt in the toaster will cause excess acrylamide to be formed, and coffee brewed in closed circuit espresso machines will cause high levels of toxic furan to be retained. This creates a culinary risk dilemma, as there is a direct correlation between the intensity of the chemical reactions, which enhances the tastiness of the food, but also makes it more risky to eat.

Public food safety information and food scares published in the popular press might help people to become aware of health issues in regard to some products. Nonetheless, it is questionable if it will have long-term effects, particularly in relation to traditional activities such as barbecue. Having knowledge about burning food might not extend to applying that knowledge, hence meat and sausages are most likely to continue to be burnt, as the barbecuing tradition is a social activity, not necessarily aimed at producing high quality healthy dinners, but an opportunity to talk and have a beer, where the food is often forgotten. Hence, it is likely that process contaminants will continue to be an emerging food safety issue.

Thus, nutrition education and intervention strategies aimed at improving population diets ought to consider sensory pleasure response to foods, in addition to a wide range of demographic and socio-cultural variables.

12 Unbalanced diet – a public health risk issue

Introduction

Science clearly points to the health benefits of eating a balanced diet including fruits and vegetables to reduce the risk of developing several maladies. However, public advice to eat a balanced diet, and especially to increase fruit and vegetable consumption (World Health Organization 2004b), seems largely to be ignored by sections of the populace in many parts of the world. The reasons for the low intake of vegetables in particular and the public ignorance of food and health advice are predictably multifaceted. It is not only about food preferences, but also about societal inequality in affording healthy food low in sugar, fat and salt, as well as accessibility to a diverse range of foods the whole year round. The enduring power of public preferences has so far meant that scientists' recommendations and governments' attempt to influence consumers' eating habits have come to nothing. This is especially true in relation to vegetables, but the problem also extends to fruit.

Food choice is based on a number of physiological, nutritional, financial, socio-cultural and environmental factors internal or external to the individual. As has been discussed in several of the preceding chapters, perhaps the most essential internal factor that influences people's food intake is habits and the sensory qualities of food, as these are critical to dietary preferences, and taste in particular may be the most immediate determinant important when choosing food (Drewnowski and Rock 1995). Foremost among the external barriers in eating a healthy diet is cost. Research has repeatedly shown that limited availability and the relatively high cost of fruit and vegetables are barriers to healthy eating for people on low incomes (Cassady et al. 2007; Drewnowski and Eichelsdoerfer 2010). A fast food meal, for example a McDonald's hamburger with accoutrements, can be seen as much better value for money: it is cheaper and it immediately satisfies hunger.

Concern about food choices that may have adverse effects on health has been at the forefront of public health for decades (Pollard et al. 2002). A diet incorporating several servings of fruits and vegetables hardly seems to be a risk issue, but there is an inverse problem, in that large parts of the public ignore the benefits of plant foods and in doing so create risks to their health and wellbeing. In some instances, people have aversions to eating vegetables that started in early childhood.

It has been postulated that the loathing of vegetables can be linked to a negative childhood experience. Research shows that dietary behaviours follow from childhood to adolescence (Resnicow *et al.* 1998), and food choices established in childhood or adolescence may significantly spread into adulthood (Mikkila *et al.* 2004). Environmental, habitual and socio-cultural factors are important, with the family environment strongly influencing dietary behaviour of young people. Accordingly, parental food consumption, availability of healthy food at home and convenient accessibility of vegetables and fruit for purchase all year around have proven to be some of the most consistently supported determinants of fruit and vegetable consumption in young people (Rasmussen *et al.* 2006). From this perspective, food habits evolve from learned experience – especially the foods to which children are exposed. Habitual access to healthy or unhealthy food leads to the development of persistent attitudes towards preferred foods. Hence, socially and culturally derived food habits and traditions are very difficult to change (Pollard *et al.* 2002).

Food is not just a necessity for survival; it also provides one of the most significant social interaction and networking occasions. Many eating occasions occur in social company and this social and cultural setting may affect the types and amounts of foods eaten. Research focusing on married heterosexual couples indicates that marriage is positively associated with fruit and vegetable intake among older men, as the presence of a female in the household is associated with higher fruit and vegetable intake of male household members. However, the benefits of partnership for fruit and vegetable intake are difficult to separate from the benefits related to companionship and eating meals together (Donkin *et al.* 1998; Davis *et al.* 2000; Payette and Shatenstein 2005).

It is generally agreed that the social and cultural environment and habitus influence people's eating habits and choice of food, especially those of young people and children (Bourdieu 1984:177–200). Health professionals identify food provision in the home as a key stimulus for children's food preferences, while parents often perceive children's food preferences to be inherited and difficult to influence. Nonetheless, research has noted a genetic connection to some people's sensitivity to bitter, sweet, umami (a savoury taste associated with monosodium glutamate), and, more recently, fat. This suggests an influence on taste beside the family meal experience (Garcia-Balio *et al.* 2009). It has been noted that there are innate physiological reasons to why some people have an aversion to certain vegetables. A genetic trait has been identified that seems to provide some people with extra sensitive receptors for bitter tastes. The vegetables that taste bitter for some people include cruciferous vegetables like broccoli and cauliflower, some leafy greens, and eggplant (Drewnowski 1997).

Research involving three-year-old twins living in the same household was undertaken to assess the relative importance of socio-cultural, environmental and inherited influences on preferences for 114 foods (Fildes *et al.* 2014). It was found that both socio-cultural and genetic influences were significant for all food groups. Genetic influences seemed to dominate for nutrient-dense foods, such as for certain vegetables, fruits and high protein foods, whereas for snacks, dairy and starch-based foods both socio-cultural factors and genetics influenced the choices. They also noted that all food preferences involved socio-cultural factors influencing the choice of food. The age of the participants might have had an impact on the outcome of the study. The study did not include other age groups where individual decisions of food choice could be ascertained. The researchers concluded that health professionals were right, in that the home environment is the main determinant of the food that children prefer, especially in their liking for energy-dense foods. To link a genetic influence to food intake and weight gain was not supported, except partly in relation to the liking of the food (Fildes *et al.* 2014).

From a risk society point of view, consuming too few portions of fruits and vegetables is a critical factor in the development of several non-communicable diseases; this fact is disregarded by some consumers, but the impact is also due to limited access in parts of the world, where seasonal patterns still determine the availability of fruit and vegetables. There might also be a slight downside in consuming the wrong fruit and vegetable products with the potential risks of concomitant ingestion of natural toxins, pesticides or high levels of nitrate.

Some plants contain natural constituents that are known to be toxic to both animals and humans. Some of these chemicals have evolved in plants to protect them against insects, plant pathogens and other organisms (Kessler and Baldwin 2002). A toxin may also be formed to protect the plant from spoilage when damaged by weather, handling, UV light or microbes. In most cases, humans have learnt by experience what plants to eat and how to prepare them to avoid becoming poisoned; hence, plants normally do not pose a threat to the local population, but could be harmful when introduced to new global customers unfamiliar with the product.

Pesticides, which are regulated by government agencies in most countries, are used to protect the produce from insect attacks and other diseases, and to control the growth of weeds. Pesticide residues may remain on or in the food after they are applied to food crops. Nonetheless, most producers of fruits and vegetables meet the requirements set for use and pesticide residues are often not found at all or with residues 10 to 100 times below set safety limits. The latest available European Union report of pesticide residues in food found that over 97 per cent of samples contained residue levels that fell within permissible limits (European Food Safety Authority 2014b), while in the USA more than 95 per cent complied with set limits (United States Department of Agriculture 2014). Still, pesticide residues are high up on the list of food safety threats quoted by consumers.

Nitrate is a naturally occurring inorganic compound. It plays an important role in the nutrition and function of plants. Higher levels of nitrate tend to be found in green leaves whereas lower levels occur in seeds or roots and tubers. The highest levels of nitrate have been found in green leafy vegetables like rucola, also called roquette or rocket salad, followed by different varieties of lettuce and spinach. Nitrate in itself is relatively non-toxic (European Food Safety Authority 2008b). However, part of the swallowed and absorbed nitrate is transported in the blood stream and excreted back into the saliva. In the saliva, it is converted to nitrite by bacteria in the mouth and subsequently swallowed as nitrite. While nitrite on its own does not cause cancer (Bryan *et al.* 2012), it can be a precursor in the formation of nitrosamines, a class of compounds that are carcinogenic in a wide range of animals (Bogovski and Bogovski 1981) and have been classified as probably causing human cancer (International Agency for the Research on Cancer 1978). On the contrary, research over the past 15 years has led to the view that nitrate and its metabolites might be indispensible nutrients essential for cardiovascular health by promoting nitric oxide production (Bryan *et al.* 2012). The science is still undecided on the effects of nitrate, although this is not an issue high on the consumer agenda.

Despite some negative aspects, increased consumption of fruits and vegetables is widely recommended, because of the generally agreed beneficial health effects; the benefits are judged more important than minor negative effects (European Food Safety Authority 2008b). The choice seems evident from all the promotion of increased consumption of fruit and vegetables as part of a healthy lifestyle issued by public and private organisations (World Health Organization 2003; World Cancer Research Fund/American Institute for Cancer Research 2007; Nordic Nutrition Recommendations 2012). The potentially negative health issues can be easily managed with the correct preparation methods, consideration given to the choice of vegetables consumed and sometimes their country of origin.

Then why do so many consumers put themselves at risk by not heeding the authorities' advice to eat more fruit and vegetables? There are obvious discrepancies between recommendations based on science and consumer behaviour. The public has developed an apprehension about changing eating habits, and public health recommendations are not transcending to choice of food products.

The health benefits of fruit and vegetable consumption

The science is unambiguous, with increasing evidence of the health benefits that consumption of fruit and vegetables provide. In this respect, fruit and vegetables are frequently considered as a dietary category that provides a variety of biologically active substances. These substances are classified as phytochemicals, and they include a range of essential nutrients. In addition, most fruits and vegetables lack saturated fat and trans fatty acids and are low in sodium, which is beneficial from a nutritional point of view. Although it has proven difficult to pinpoint beneficial effects of individual compounds, there are several reports that demonstrate a relationship between fruits and vegetables in the diet and the overall effect on health (Verhagen *et al.* 2006).

The World Health Organization has concluded, based on published research, that fruit and vegetables, if consumed daily in sufficient amounts, could help prevent major non-communicable diseases such as cardiovascular diseases, cancer, obesity and type 2 diabetes (Bazzano 2005).

Research findings from both intervention and observational studies indicate that the consumption of fruits and vegetables may play an important role in the prevention of ischaemic heart disease and stroke. An estimate of the potential contribution of an increased intake of fruits and vegetables is the prevention of 26,000 deaths before the age of 65 annually in the European Union (World Health Organization 2005).

Furthermore, it has been estimated that approximately one in ten cancers in western populations are due to an insufficient intake of fruits and vegetables. The clearest evidence of a cancer-protective effect of eating more fruits is for stomach and oesophageal cancers. Similarly, a higher intake of vegetables is likely to reduce the incidence of colon-rectum cancers (International Agency for Research on Cancer 2003; World Cancer Research Fund/American Institute for Cancer Research 2007).

Short term intervention studies and studies with dietary advice to increase consumption of fruits and vegetables, show that in general a diet high in fruits and vegetables and low in fat, accomplishes significant weight loss for both females and males (World Health Organization 2005). A small but growing body of evidence links a diet rich in fruits and vegetables with a lower risk of type 2 diabetes. The available studies support a role for fruit and vegetables, independent of other diet and lifestyle factors in the prevention of type 2 diabetes (Bazzano 2005).

Currently it is unclear what exactly should be consumed, and it is not easy for consumers to understand, since the definitions of fruits and vegetables are somewhat arbitrary and ambiguous. All parts of herbaceous plants eaten as food by humans are normally considered vegetables. Mushrooms belong to the biological kingdom fungi, but they are commonly considered vegetables. Potatoes and other starchy tubers are included in the definition of vegetables in some countries, but not in others, which creates confusion. Nuts, grains, herbs, spices and culinary fruits are normally not considered as vegetables. Botanically, fruits are reproductive organs, while vegetables are vegetative organs, which sustain the plant. Nevertheless, several fruits, e.g. cucumbers and tomatoes, are also included in the term vegetables.

The following is the formal definition of fruits and vegetables by the World Health Organization (International Agency for Research on Cancer 2003):

- Fruit and vegetables are edible plant foods excluding cereal grains, nuts, seeds, tealeaves, coffee beans, cocoa beans, herbs and spices.
- Fruits are edible parts of plants that contain the seeds and pulpy surrounding tissue; have a sweet or tart taste and are generally consumed as breakfast beverages, breakfast and lunch side dishes, snacks or desserts.

- Vegetables are edible plant parts including stems and stalks, roots, tubers, bulbs, leaves, flowers, and some fruits; they usually include seaweed and sweet corn and may or may not include pulses or mushrooms; they are generally consumed raw or cooked with a main dish, in a mixed dish, as an appetiser, or in a salad.

Adherence to official advice

The international health adviser, the World Health Organization (WHO), recommended in 1990 that the minimum daily intake of fruit and vegetables should be 400 g a day. This advice excludes consumption of potatoes and other starchy tubers (World health Organization 1990). The aim of the recommendation was to prevent chronic diseases, such as heart disease, cancer, diabetes and obesity, and to reduce several micronutrient deficiencies, especially in less developed countries. To promote the recommendations, WHO and the Food and Agriculture Organization of the United Nations (FAO) started a joint worldwide initiative in 2004 to educate the global population about the health benefits of eating fruit and vegetables (World Health Organization 2004b).

Countries have taken up the advice and they have attempted to translate the recommended consumption of fruit and vegetables by weight into portions to help customers calculate the number of portions they ought to consume. In the United Kingdom the recommendation is to eat five fruit and vegetable portions a day with each portion equivalent to 80 g. Research has shown that only about 30 per cent of the population manage to consume the recommended amount (Bates *et al.* 2012). This demonstrates that social and cultural habits have more influence over people's eating preferences than government recommendations and scientists' advice. This gap in eating perceptions has implications for the public health status of a society, but it is also a serious social inequality issue, where affordability becomes a dividing barrier between a 'healthy' long life or a life exposed to lifestyle health risks. Here social and cultural habits are interlinked with socio-economic realities.

Australia has gone one step further, with the public health authorities recommending two fruit and five to six vegetable portions a day with the fruit portion at 150 g and vegetable portion at 75 g. This equates to a total of 675 to 750 g, which is an ambitiously high target. Close to 50 per cent of Australians reported that they usually ate two or more servings of fruit per day, while 8 per cent usually ate five or more serves of vegetables per day. Considering both guidelines, only 5.5 per cent of Australian adults had a compliant daily average intake of fruit and vegetables (Australian Bureau of Statistics 2013).

Canada previously recommended five to ten portions for all, but changed this in 2007 to specific recommendations for each age and gender group. They now recommend a minimum of four portions for young children up to a minimum of eight portions for adult males. Only 26 per cent of the population, aged from two years consumed the minimum number of daily servings recommended for their respective age and gender group (Black and Billett 2013).

France and Germany also recommend five portions a day like the United Kingdom, while portion numbers vary in other European countries. The United States partly abandoned the number of recommended portions in favour of a generic fruit and vegetable campaign in 2007 indicating that the more you eat the better it is. In Europe, the average consumption of fruit and vegetables is only 220 g per person per day. A survey of European females with children showed that just 27 per cent consumed over 400 g (Anon 2011). The French did not reach the recommended amounts consuming fruit only 1.3 times per day and vegetables 2.3 times per day despite all the support for the beneficial Mediterranean diet based on an abundance of fruit and vegetables (Anon 2011). Still this was better than the Americans. Adults in the United States consume fruit about 1.1 times per day and vegetables about 1.6 times per day (Centers for Disease Control and Prevention 2013a). This is comparatively on the low side, but not breaking any non-existent quantified recommendations.

Even if compliance with the recommended fruit and vegetable consumption is dismal, a further caveat is in place. Given our notorious dishonesty when confronted by pollsters with questions that touch on our self-regarded healthy living and consumption, there might even be far more eaters of less than five-a-day than indicated in the presented research figures.

With a majority of populations in many countries struggling to reach the current recommended consumption of fruit and vegetables, new research points to the importance to increase the recommendations even further. Researchers at University College London analysed information from more than 65,000 adults aged 35 years and older, who responded to the annual Health Survey for England in the years 2001 to 2008. They then followed up participants for a median period of 7.7 years after their initial participation. The study found that people who ate seven or more portions of fruit or vegetables a day had a 33 per cent reduced risk of death from any cause, compared to people who ate less than one portion per day. In the high fruit and vegetable eating group, there was a 25 per cent reduced risk of death from cancer, and a 31 per cent reduced risk of death from cardiovascular disease, (Oyebode *et al.* 2014).

This research demonstrates that not even five portions of fruit and vegetables a day may be sufficient, after all, to optimise health and longevity. There was a surprise finding in that eating canned or frozen fruit, did not prove to be helpful at all and drinking juice did not add to health benefits. This seems contradictory, but the authors point out that people eating canned fruit might have influenced the findings. People eating canned fruit might not live in areas with easily available and affordable fresh fruit, which could indicate a generally poorer diet. Further, to merge canned and frozen fruit might not be fair to the frozen produce. Juice, although providing some of the benefits of whole fruits and vegetables, contains plenty of energy from sugar, partly offsetting any benefit.

The findings indicate that eating more fresh fruit and vegetables, including salads, is linked to living a longer life generally, and in particular as a strategy to lower the risk of death from heart disease, stroke and cancer. Overall, vegetables have shown to be significantly more protective against disease than eating fruit. This is if the reduced risk of disease is entirely attributable to fruit and vegetable consumption, or it acts as markers of a broader dietary pattern associated with improved health.

From these findings, it is evident that governments' recommendations should include targeted health advice, but also facilitate access to these food groups for people living in areas currently poorly served by affordable fresh vegetable and fruits to make it possible to have a year round supply. This strategy, might provide long term health benefits for socio-economically disadvantaged population groups, but also alleviate ever increasing public health expenditure.

The inertia in changing dietary habits

Dietary habits evolve during the first years of the individual's life or earlier: there are even suggestions that the food choices a female makes during her pregnancy may set the stage for an infant's later acceptance of solid foods (Savage *et al.* 2007). In Western societies the abundance and variety of foods to choose from are extensive, allowing children's eating habits to develop under unprecedented conditions where palatable, inexpensive, ready-to-eat foods are easily available. However, human food choices are complex phenomena influenced by a wide range of factors. Food is not just eaten for its nutrient value; food intake extends well beyond physiological needs as a source of pleasure, as it is an enjoyable experience, and even a comforting activity (Clark 1998). Anthropological and sociological research has highlighted the value of food and eating in self designation and cultural definition, playing a role in identity expression, communication and social interactions, as well as in delineating status and gender roles (Counihan 1999; Murcott 1983). Eating behaviour is therefore likely to be vulnerable to various social influences, including aspirations to respond in a socially desirable manner (Herman *et al.* 2003). However, the social norms about foods and meal composition, and the familiarity with how to prepare food that guided previous generations appear to be eroding, leaving people with a lack of knowledge about essential food composition and eating behaviour (Fischler 1980).

Food selection is influenced by numerous interrelating factors, ranging from social and cultural factors to biological mechanisms and genetic profiles. Factors influencing food choice relate to individual circumstances, external economic factors and social context in which the choice is made (Shepherd *et al.* 1995). These influencing food choice factors include social, cultural, religious or demographic variables. In relation to the food itself, there are chemical components and physical properties that are likely to have an impact on choice through sensory perception. The individual's predilection for a specific attribute will most likely influence the choice of a particular food (Gibson 2006). Psychological differences between people, such as personality, may also influence food choice. Contemporary consumers have fears and conflicts involving food and health (Mennell *et al.* 1992; Rozin *et al.* 1999).

People prioritise food in response to their social and cultural environment and their financial circumstances, as well as based on faith and personal likes and dislikes. Balancing food consumption with availability, likes and habits is a process that people negotiate every day, and these choices are not necessarily improving their wellbeing. In addition, the balance involves time and the knowledge of how to prepare food, eating occasions, places or eating partners (Connors *et al* 2001). The personal food system is the way that individuals construct food choices, considering values and employing other cognitive processes for selecting foods. Individual food systems may be particularly important to recognise in societies where many options for eating are available and few rules exist to guide how and what is consumed (Murcott 1998).

Some studies suggest that food choice is a way to express individual philosophy of life with the current emphasis on dieting and being slim being the preferred body shape. Such considerations suggest that food choice has important implications for social judgments. Contemporary food choice obstacles include social change such as extended work-hour commitments as well as increased participation in the workforce of females, who traditionally have been the main contributor to purchase and prepare food. These factors have led to people having reduced time available for food selection and meal preparation (Monsivais *et al.* 2014). The limited time that has become available for cooking may be one of the barriers to the possible adoption of a more healthy diet. Time scarcity was especially highlighted among working parents earning low wages in the United States of America (Jabs *et al.* 2007). Lack of time was also a leading barrier to adopting dietary guidance cited by European adults (Lappalainen *et al.* 1997).

In relation to fruit and vegetable consumption, affordability and availability are important considerations. Although the supply chains in many countries now offer year round availability of many seasonal crops, in some cases the price can be exorbitant for out-of-season products imported from far away countries. Thus, there is a consistently positive association between household income and fruit and vegetable consumption (Johansson *et al.* 1999; Giskes *et al.* 2002; Laaksonen *et al.* 2003). Individuals with a smaller household budget, or who are living in a disadvantaged area, consume fewer fruits and vegetables, and this may be due to a perception that fresh fruits and vegetables are expensive (Mooney 1990; Sooman *et al.* 1993; Kamphuis *et al.* 2007), have a short shelf life, or are difficult to store in the home (Giskes *et al.* 2002). People in low socio-economic areas in particular pay a relatively higher premium for healthy compared with less healthy foods (Mooney 1990; Sooman *et al.* 1993).

Cooking skills can also be an important variable. An Australian study found that families purchased a greater variety of vegetables on a regular basis when the main food preparer had confidence in preparing these foods (Winkler and Turrell 2010). Similarly, another study found that females who planned meals ahead of time and enjoyed trying new recipes were more likely to consume two or more servings of fruit per day whereas females who found cooking a chore and spent little time cooking were less likely to consume fruit (Crawford *et al.* 2007). Advanced cooking skills were associated with healthier food consumption patterns, characterised by people consuming more fruits and vegetables, spending less money on food away from home, and having fewer visits to fast food restaurants. All factors that have shown to be significantly associated with more time spent preparing, cooking and cleaning up from meals (Monsivais *et al.* 2014).

There is also a gender difference in the selection of healthier food. It has been shown that males favour taste and convenience over health in making their food choices (Steptoe *et al.* 2002), and males show more vacillation when challenged to make healthy dietary choices (Sparks *et al.* 2001). As a result, males eat fewer fruits and vegetables and low-fat foods, they select fewer high-fibre foods, and consume more soft drink than females (Beardsworth *et al.* 2002; Pollard *et al.* 2002). The consistent interconnection between gender and food and the similarity of gender patterning in population subgroups point to the stability of masculine versus feminine food habits (Prättälä *et al.* 2007). Other studies have confirmed the health concerned attitudes of females, and their inclination to comply with dietary recommendations (Roininen *et al.* 2001; Wadolowska *et al.* 2008), while males demonstrate little conscious efforts to eat a healthy diet (Hearty *et al.* 2007).

Impact of sociological risk discourses

Within the socio-cultural risk perspective certain foods have become the habitual norm that often has been developed over generations influenced by environmental and religious considerations, hence the need to have convincing arguments to make dietary changes. If increasing fruit and vegetable consumption to safeguard health and wellbeing are not part of the tradition, it will hardly be adjusted through generalised government health policy. Social values and cultural traditions strongly affect individual risk awareness as pertains to food choice (Bourdieu 1984). Social and cultural food traditions also signify people's social identity demonstrating the relationship between social interaction and food and as emphasised by Germov and Williams (1999 [cited in Pollard *et al.* 2002:379]):

> [P]eople can seek to differentiate themselves from others, or alternatively, convey their membership of a particular social group through their food consumption. Ordering a vegetarian meal, eating a meat pie, dining at a

trendy café, or eating an exotic cuisine may be used and interpreted as social 'markers' of the individual's social status and group membership.

From the socio-cultural risk discourse perspective, we have covered issues surrounding obesity and excessive energy intake, dieting and the urge to use dietary supplements to avert perceived nutritional deficiencies, as well as caffeine and alcohol consumption as psychoactive substances, all areas influenced by socio-cultural customs and social status positions. For many people, health is an important consideration when choosing what food to eat, but not for all. There are indications that consumers who eat few portions of fruits and vegetables are less interested in food in general and what they eat (Thompson *et al.* 1999). However, there is an 'optimism bias' in that people habitually believe they are less at risk to suffer lifestyle illnesses than other people in the society might be. Exacerbating the situation is the fact that people often rate their own intake of fruit and vegetables as much higher than their estimated objective intake (Lechner *et al.* 1997).

The risk society perspective of modern industrialisation focuses on the strong aversion among many consumers to the use of genetically modified organisms in food production, the food industries' reluctance to embrace detailed labelling of ingredients for all products and declaring GM content. Additionally, the increasing movement to embrace organic food, which reflects the trust in traditional food production methods, and the ignorance of the upsurge in food pathogens is partly triggered by modern factory farming. Fruit and vegetable consumption is less influenced by the modern industrialisation perspective, albeit the food industry has attempted to introduce some convenience food products, like pre-prepared fruit salads and leafy vegetables, and snacks like processed apple slices and bite size carrots. Pre-packaged leafy vegetables have been embraced by consumers and are now common in many supermarkets. Apple wedges with a shelf life of 21 days have seen some success; however, there has been a reaction to the chemical treatment necessary to prevent browning of the slices and there has even been a recall in USA and Canada in 2015 due to listeria contamination (Centers for Disease Control and Prevention 2015). Natural apples are perfectly fine. Similarly, producing convenient baby carrots involves industrial peelers in which ordinary carrots are cut down to size. Peeled and polished to get the round appearance, while generating a large amount of waste. On balance, convenience may encourage consumption, but there is a price to pay for the excessive handling. A further disadvantage with the processed baby carrots is that they lose their thick protective skins and become more vulnerable to microbial growth.

The governmentality risk perspective proposes environmental and policy interventions as strategies for creating population wide improvements in health behaviour. Throughout this book we have presented the considerable efforts governments have dedicated to try to limit the impact of heat-induced process contaminants, by avoiding to barbeque meat to a burnt stage and to toast bread until dark brown. Governments have a central role in encouraging healthy food consumption including sufficient levels of fruit and vegetables in the diet to enhance overall public health. Consideration of the food choice process in relation to fruit and vegetables is particularly important when trying to implement coherent and practical dietary advice for the public. Any advice has to be realistic and must take into account social and cultural habits that influence personal choices of food to buy and consume. People need to be made aware of government health standards relevant for their life situation and measure it against their personal consumption levels of fruit and vegetables, in order for health promotion messages to be considered personally relevant.

Overall, all three risk discourse perspectives can be applied to most food consumption issues. The socio-cultural risk perspective is concerned with the impact of status quo driven by traditions and expectations and the difficulty in achieving behavioural change. The risk society perspective of modern industrialisation is at the other end of the spectrum concerned with novel risks from the adoption of radical change in food production methods. Finally, the governmentality risk perspective is focused on assessing traditional as well as novel risks in attempts to influence industry processes and public behaviour through legislation and policy interventions. Independently, mass media play a crucial role in influencing cultural change and conveying suitable health messages to the public, but frequently focuses on issues that are attention grabbing and induce 'moral panic'.

Conclusion

There is no question about the beneficial effects of eating substantial amounts of a variety of fruits and vegetables. The list of potentially beneficial compounds found in these food categories is long and diverse, including vitamins, minerals and fibre, as well as antioxidants and other phytochemicals. There are certainly some negative aspects to consider as well, including the presence of natural toxins, pesticide residues, and high nitrate levels in certain vegetables. On balance, science is adamant that the beneficial effects on health of eating plenty of fruits and vegetables clearly dwarf any detrimental consequences.

Still, recommendations to increase the consumption of fruits and vegetables seem to be less than successful judging from worldwide consumption studies. Research demonstrates that there are discrepancies between recommendations based on science and consumer behaviour. The public appears to be apprehensive when trying to change socially and culturally ingrained eating habits. There might be a healthy scepticism creeping into the public mind about the multitude of diet warnings issued by nutrition scientists, but also by government interventions, which advocate unachievable food recommendations in the number of servings required. Generalising food recommendation that do not take into account availability and the personal cost involved if following scientists advice and government recommendations, will have limited adherence.

Nonetheless, public scepticism about epidemiological findings and concomitant dietary recommendations might be justified. Science is not always right and the advice given can be confusing; sometimes common sense might be more accurate and should prevail.

13 Concluding remarks and the future

Introduction

In this book, we have tried to demonstrate from three risk discourses – the socio-cultural, the risk society and the governmentality risk discourse, that production, processing and consumption of food is not without considerable risks to consumer health and wellbeing, to the environment and to animals, but also sometimes to the people involved in the industry. We have contrasted expert views of specific food safety risk issues with the concomitant public perception, which often deviate from scientific and official assessment.

Although not universally agreed as factual by experts, a common belief expressed by both social and political observers is that society is becoming more risk cognisant. This belief has been supported over the last 30 years by social science research, which has consistently called attention to a considerable gap between how risk assessment experts reason about, define and evaluate risks in comparison with members of the public. Food risks have become particularly salient in light of several recent food scares, with a number of researchers arguing that there is a diminishing public confidence in the food supply, which has damaged trust in actors in the food chain (Berg 2004, Berg et al. 2005, Kjaernes et al. 2007, Bildtgård 2008). Both cultural and socio-economic trends in conjunction with intensive media coverage have interacted to prompt acute episodes of widespread public anxiety (Frewer et al. 1993; Fitzgerald and Campbell 2001; De Boer et al. 2005). The emotional response toward food safety incidents has been shown to be a stronger predictor of both food safety risk perception and prevention, than factual awareness (Mou and Lin 2014).

The rapid pace of change in science and technology, changes in legislation and the current social, cultural, socio-economic and socio-demographic realities as well as market globalisation have all had a marked impact on the food we buy today (Urry 2014b:ix; Beck 1992). Intensified farming, with an extensive use of pesticides and monocultures, and industrialisation of food production, with an increased use of additives and preservatives to improve taste, appearance and shelf life, are causes for concern for many consumers. New technologies such as genetic engineering are altering agriculture and food production in a way that is seen as unnatural. Globalisation is a driver of change, with products brought to us from all corners of the world and, as a result, food safety knows no boundaries. Ageing populations and lifestyle changes, due in part to modern working life and urbanisation, and the rise in obesity, have led to health, nutrition and diet becoming areas of greater concern.

However, risk should be neither overstated nor underestimated; uncertainty prevails, due to the fact that it might take several years to understand the real impact that new technologies, new pesticides and newly discovered process contaminants can have on people and the environment, as emphasised by Beck in the trend-setting book the *Risk Society* (1992). Still, there is an industry urge to introduce novel approaches rapidly into food production, with unknown effects lingering due to protracted timeframes for epidemiological research to establish links between potentially hazardous food products and people's health. As a result, it seems that consumers are generally uncertain about the safety and quality of their food, and they display behavioural patterns and make choices that seem irrational or illogical – or at least inconsistent with expert opinion and scientific knowledge (Hilgartner 1990).

What conclusions can be drawn about food from a sociological risk discourse perspective?

Food is intrinsic to the social and cultural environment. In this book, risks have been analysed from socio-cultural, societal, and regulatory contexts. There are obviously other perspectives possible that have not been discussed in the book. What is presented is research, analyses, and discussions of food within a risk discourse perspective across disciplinary boundaries, which makes the book unique. The book explores the gap between the views of scientific food expertise and scientific social expertise in understanding the societal and cultural fabric of communities and its inhabitants in influencing food choice – a gap that is one of several reasons why the populace often ignores expert advice.

As continuous access to food is vital to life as we know it, it is essential that risks around food be minimised to the extent possible. Nevertheless, as discussed, knowledge and action are two very different things, as demonstrated by the gap between consumers, scientific experts and governments' regulatory activities, especially the difference in consumer food preferences and consumption in contrast to expert advice.

The challenge is to bridge the gap between the different disciplines in understanding each other, presenting information in the appropriate way, at the relevant time, to the affected population group, and in a suitable format for the target group. Any attempts to manage food-related risks therefore need to be based on both technical risk assessments and assessment of public perception of risk.

Multiple factors contribute to explaining consumers' resistance towards information processing and rational decision-making. Information may be irrelevant or useless to consumers if it fails to target particular needs or interests (Verbeke 2005). The ability to explain this distinction between experts' and the lay public's view of risk has been one of the main aims of risk perception research to date.

However, the need to understand this discrepancy and act upon its repercussions is a message only slowly being embraced by hazard managers in both the public and private sectors. In the meantime, the social and economic costs incurred because of this difference in perception are high. In the longer term, changes in dietary habits, as a result of increasing public attention to potential food risks, may in themselves have public health implications (Cade *et al.* 1998).

What to expect in the future food risk society?

Public awareness is growing, and the interest in food, where it comes from and how it has been manufactured, is snowballing. Especially the growing middle class has become interested in food, as demonstrated by the increased number of television programmes and books about food and food preparation. The establishment of traceability and labelling, segmented communication approaches and public involvement in risk management decision-making are some examples of strategies that might be used to restore consumer confidence.

Quality labels or other safety assurances, accompanied by simple disclosures of source and treatment, could provide appropriate information for the product to be valued by at least some consumers. A quality label can function as a cue to reducing consumer uncertainty and facilitating decision-making, including potential product avoidance in cases of heightened risk perception. However, to improve consumer confidence, there must be a trustworthy system behind any quality structure. The current organic certification system that works well in many countries can serve as a template for improving trust in the food supply.

A generic approach, involving the provision of vast amounts of information to the general public, stands a real risk of leading to information overload, bewilderment and lack of interest among mainstream consumers. A more effective approach to change consumer food buying and consumption behaviour, is to focus on segmenting the population according to their information needs, and developing information with high levels of personal relevance to specific groups of respondents who may be at greater risk than the rest of the population. Such information is more likely to create attitudinal change and subsequent behavioural change as the perceived personal relevance is high (Petty and Cacioppo 1996). The problem with such an approach is that it is resource intensive, as social science research firstly needs to be conducted in order to identify individual differences with respect to people's perceptions and behaviours and then tailored information has to be designed and delivered. The particular challenge lies in identifying and effectively researching market segments. In many cases this is feasible, though it may be problematic when variables such as involvement in making decisions about food consumption, social and cultural traditions, personal and family motivations or attitudes to food come into play.

In response to growing consumer uncertainty about food safety and the perceived decline in consumer trust, regulatory bodies have increasingly stressed the importance of transparency in policy decision making processes, as well as attempting to better understand the concerns, attitudes and values of the general public (Frewer *et al.* 2005). Current risk management efforts try to restore public confidence by involving laypeople early in decision processes when policy options include varying degrees of human exposure to potential risks. This could include proactive participatory processes that engage citizens in a debate before the development of technologies and products for which public acceptance is questionable (Frewer *et al.* 2004). Although examples of participatory democracy as a trust building activity are scarce (Einsiedel *et al.* 2001), it is assumed by many decision makers that this approach will have a positive effect on consumer confidence in the long term.

Unfortunately, public perception of risk is not uniform in any given population. Demographic differences in risk perception might relate to regional, ethnic, religious, socio-economic, age or gender distinctions, which have important implications for risk communication practices. Thus, risk perceptions associated with technological and environmental hazards cannot be rectified and assessed independently of the social and cultural context in which they are embedded. If the public are to respond in a positive way to scientific developments, it is not enough to try to influence risk perceptions through communication alone. Increasing public trust in the risk management process itself and the responsible authorities is essential for any risk mitigation strategy to be effective.

References

Abercrombie, N. and Longhurst, B. (1998). *Audiences: towards a theory of performance and imagination.* London, United Kingdom: Sage.

Abhilash, P.C., Jamil, S. and Singh, N. (2009). Transgenic plants for enhanced biodegradation and phytoremediation of organic xenobiotics. *Biotechnology Advances*, 27(4): 474–88.

Abramson, J.L., Williams, S.A., Krumholz, H.M. and Vaccarino, V. (2001). Moderate alcohol consumption and risk of heart failure among older persons. *JAMA*, 285(15): 1971–7.

AC Nielsen (2005). *Consumer attitudes towards organic foods, a global consumer survey.* Oxford, United Kingdom: AC Nielsen.

Acheson, D.W. (1999). Foodborne infections. *Current Opinion in Gastroenterology*, 15: 538–45.

Adams, C.E., Greenway, F.L. and Brantley, P.J. (2011). Lifestyle factors and ghrelin: critical review and implications for weight loss maintenance. *Obesity Review*, 12(5): e211–e218.

Adams, C.J. (1987). The sexual politics of meat. *Heresies*, 21: 51–5.

Adams, C.J. (1995). On Beastliness and a politics of solidarity. In Adams C.J. (ed.), *Neither man nor beast: feminism and the defense of animals.* New York, NY and London, United Kingdom: Continuum, Chapter 4: 71–84.

Adams, C.J. (2010). The sexual politics of meat. In Adams, C.J. (ed.), *20th Anniversary edition. The sexual politics of meat. A feminist vegetarian critical theory.* London, United Kingdom: Bloomsbury Academic, Chapter 2: 47–63.

Adams, M. (2003). The reflexive self and culture: a critique. *British Journal of Sociology*, 54(2): 221–38.

Adams, M. and Raisborough, J. (2010). Making a difference: ethical consumption and the everyday. *The British Journal of Sociology*, 61(2): 256–74.

Adewale, A. and Ifudu, O. (2014). Kidney injury, fluid, electrolyte and acid-base abnormalities in alcoholics. *Nigerian Medical Journal*, 55(2): 93–8.

Adler, N.E. and Newman, K. (2002). Socioeconomic disparities in health: pathways and policies. *Health Affairs*, 21(2): 60–76.

Ahmed, S.M., Hall, A.J., Robinson, A.E., Verhoef, L., Premkumar, P., Parashar, U.D., Koopmans, M. and Lopman, B.A. (2014). Global prevalence of norovirus in cases of gastroenteritis: a systematic review and meta-analysis. *The Lancet Infectious Diseases*, 14(8): 725–30.

Akbari, O.S., Bellen, H.J., Bier, E. *et al.* (2015). Safeguarding gene drive experiments in the laboratory. *Science*, 349(6251): 927–929.

Alberts, B., Johnson, A., Lewis, J., Raff, M., Roberts, K. and Walter, P. (2015). *Molecular biology of the cell* (Sixth ed.). New York, NY: Garland Science.

Alexander, J. (1996). Critical reflections on 'reflexive modernisation'. *Theory, Culture and Society*, 13(4): 133–8.

Altaki, M.S., Santos, F.J. and Galceran M.T. (2011). Occurrence of furan in coffee from Spanish market: contribution of brewing and roasting. *Food Chemistry*, 126(4): 1527–32.

Aluko, R.E. (2012). *Functional foods and nutraceuticals*. New York, NY: Springer.

American Institute for Cancer Research [AICR] (2014). Guide to healthy grilling. *AICR eNews*, 94. Accessed on 9 July 2015 at: www.aicr.org/enews/2014/05-may/enews-guide-to-healthy-grilling.html.

Amrein, T.M., Andres, L., Escher, F. and Amadò, R. (2007). Occurrence of acrylamide in selected foods and mitigation options. *Food Additives and Contaminants*, 24(Suppl. 1): 13–25.

Anon (2008). Channel check. *Beverage Spectrum*, 6: 10–2.

Anon (2010). Govt says no to Bt brinjal for now. *The Times of India*, 9 February. Accessed on 6 March 2015 at: http://timesofindia.indiatimes.com/india/Govt-says-no-to-Bt-brinjal-for-now/articleshow/5552403.cms.

Anon (2011). How can the consumption of vegetables in Europe be increased? Louis Villeneuve-d'Ascq, France: Bonduelle Foundation. Accessed on 4 August 2015 at: www.fondation-louisbonduelle.org/uploads/tx_flbnews/how-can-the-consumption-of-vegetables-in_europe-be-increased-file-louis-bonduelle-foundation-2011_05.pdf.

Anon (2012). NBJ's global supplement & nutrition industry report 2012. *Nutrition Business Journal*. New York, NY: Penton Media.

Arab, J.B. and Blumberg, L. (2008). Introduction to the proceedings of the fourth international scientific symposium on tea and human health. *Journal of Nutrition*, 138: 1526–8.

Arendash, G.W. and Cao, C. (2010). Caffeine and coffee as therapeutics against Alzheimer's disease. *Journal of Alzheimer's Disease*, 20(Suppl 1): S117–S126.

Arendash, G.W., Schleif, W., Rezai-Zadeh, K., Jackson, E.K., Zacharia, L.C., Cracchiolo, J.R., Shippy, D. and Tan, J. (2006). Caffeine protects Alzheimer's mice against cognitive impairment and reduces brain beta-amyloid production. *Neuroscience*, 142(4): 941–52.

Argan, M., Akyildiz, M., Ozdemir, B., Bas, A., Akkus, E. and Kaya, S. (2015). Leisure aspects of Turkish coffee consumption rituals: an exploratory qualitative study. *International Journal of Health and Economic Development*, 1(1): 26–36.

Arganini, C., Saba, A., Comitato, R., Virgili, F. and Turrini, A. (2012). Gender differences in food choice and dietary intake in modern Western societies. In Maddock, J. (ed.), *Public Health – Social and Behavioral Health*. Rijeka, Croatia: InTech: 83–102.

Arnaud, M.J. (1993). Metabolism of caffeine and other components of coffee. In Garattini, S. (ed.), *Caffeine, coffee, and health*. New York, NY: Raven Press: 43–96.

Arnaud, M.J. (2011). Pharmacokinetics and metabolism of natural methylxanthines in animal and man. *Handbook of Experimental Pharmacology*, 200: 33–91.

Arranz, S., Chiva-Blanch, G., Valderas-Martínez, P., Medina-Remón, A., Lamuela-Raventós, R.M. and Estruch, R. (2012). Wine, beer, alcohol and polyphenols on cardiovascular disease and cancer. *Nutrients*, 4(7): 759–81.

Arya, L.A., Myers, D.L. and Jackson, N.D. (2000). Dietary caffeine intake and the risk for detrusor instability: a case-control study. *Obstetrics and Gynecology*, 96: 85–9.

Ashihara, H. and Suzuki, T. (2004). Distribution and biosynthesis of caffeine in plants. *Frontiers in Bioscience*, 9: 1864–76.

Astrup, A., Larsen, T.M. and Harper, A. (2004). Atkins and other low-carbohydrate diets: hoax or an effective tool for weight loss? *The Lancet*, 364(9437): 897–9.

Atkins, R.C. (2004). *Atkins for life: the complete controlled carb program for permanent weight loss and good health*. New York, NY: St. Martin's Press.

Augustsson, K., Lindblad, J., Overik, E. and Steineck, G. (1999). A population-based dietary inventory of cooked meat and assessment of the daily intake of food mutagens. *Food Additives and Contaminants*, 16: 215–25.

Austin, C. and Lo, H. (1999). *Oral evidence to House of Commons Science & Technology Committee Scientific Advisory System: genetically modified food*. London, United Kingdom: TSO.

Australian Bureau of Statistics [ABS] (2013). *Profiles of Health, Australia, 2011–13. Daily intake of fruit and vegetables*. Canberra, Australia: Australian Bureau of Statistics. Accessed on 4 August 2015 at: www.abs.gov.au/ausstats/abs@.nsf/Lookup/by Subject/4338.0~2011–13~Main Features~Daily intake of fruit and vegetables~10009.

Aven, T. and Renn, O. (2009). On risk defined as an event where the outcome is uncertain. *Journal of Risk Research*, 12(1): 1–11.

Aven, T. and Renn, O. (2010). Response to Professor Eugene Rosa's viewpoint to our paper. *Journal of Risk Research*, 13(3): 255–9.

Axelrod, J. and Reisenthal, J. (1953). The fate of caffeine in man and a method for its estimation in biological material. *The Journal of Pharmacology and Experimental Therapeutics*, 107: 519–23.

Baan, R., Straif, K., Grosse, Y., Secretan, B., El Ghissassi, F., Bouvard, V., Altieri, A. and Cogliano, V. (2007). Carcinogenicity of alcoholic beverages. *Lancet Oncology*, 8: 292–3.

Babor, T. (1986). *Alcohol: customs and rituals*. New York, NY: Chelsea House.

Babor, T., Caetano, R., Casswell, S., Edwards, G., Giesbrecht, N., Graham, K., Grube, J.W., Hill, L., Holder, H., Homel, R., Livingston, M., Österberg, E., Rehm, J., Room, R. and Rossow, I. (2010). *Alcohol: no ordinary commodity-research and public policy*. Oxford, United Kingdom: Oxford University Press.

Babu, K.M., Church, R.J. and Lewander, W. (2008). Energy drinks: the new eye-opener for adolescents. *Clinical Pediatric Emergency Medicine*, 9(1): 35–42.

Backett-Milburn, K., Wills, W.J., Gregory, S. and Lawton, J. (2006). Making sense of eating, weight and risk in the early teenage years: views and concerns of parents in poorer socio-economic circumstances. *Social Science and Medicine*, 63(3): 624–65.

Bacon, L. and Aphramor, L. (2011). Weight science: evaluating the evidence for a paradigm shift. *Nutrition Journal*, 10: 9–12.

Bailey, A.J. (1972). The basis of meat texture. *Journal of the Science of Food and Agriculture*, 23(8): 995–1007.

Baker, A.H. and Wardle, J. (2003). Sex differences in fruit and vegetable intake in older adults. *Appetite*, 40(3): 269–75.

Baker, D.A., Stevenson, D.W. and Little, D.P. (2012). DNA barcode identification of black cohosh herbal dietary supplements. *Journal of AOAC International*, 95(4): 1023–34.

Baker, S. (2004). Mapping the values driving organic food choice. Germany vs. the UK. *European Journal of Marketing*, 38(8): 995–1012.

Bangcuyo, R.G., Smith, K.J., Zumach, J.L., Pierce, A.M., Guttman, G.A. and Simons, C.T. (2015). The use of immersive technologies to improve consumer testing: the role of ecological validity, context and engagement in evaluating coffee. *Food Quality and Preference*, 41: 84–95.

Banks, T. (2009). Using tapeworms to lose weight. Accessed on 14 October 2014 at: www.sidereel.com/The_Tyra_Banks_Show/season-5/episode-45.

Barański, M., Średnicka-Tober, D., Volakakis, N., Seal, C., Sanderson, R., Stewart, G.B., Benbrook, C., Biavati, B., Markellou, E., Giotis. C., Gromadzka-Ostrowska, J., Rembiałkowska, E., Skwarło-Sońta, K., Tahvonen, R., Janovská, D., Niggli, U., Nicot, P. and Leifert, C. (2014). Higher antioxidant and lower cadmium concentrations and lower incidence of pesticide residues in organically grown crops: a systematic literature review and meta-analyses. *British Journal of Nutrition*, 112(5): 794–811.

Barber, M. and Nefer, R. (2014). Fast food facts. *Michigan Citizen,* 36(26): 10.

Barker, J., Vipond, I.B. and Bloomfield, S.F. (2004). Effects of cleaning and disinfection in reducing the spread of norovirus contamination via environmental surfaces. *Journal of Hospital Infection*, 58(1): 42–9.

Barnett, J., McConnor, A., Kennedy, J., Raats, M., Shepherd, R., Verbeke, W., Fletcher, J., Kuttschreuter, M., Lima, L., Wills, J. and Wall, P. (2011). Development of strategies for effective communication of food risks and benefits across Europe: design and conceptual framework of the FoodRisC project. *BMC Public Health*, 11: 308–17.

Baron, J.H. (1997). Byron's appetites, James Joyce's gut, and Melba's meals and mésalliances. *BMJ*, 315(7123): 1697–703.

Barone, J.J. and Roberts, H.R. (1996). Caffeine consumption. *Food and Chemical Toxicology*, 34(1): 119–29.

Barr, S.I. and Chapman, G.E. (2002). Perceptions and practices of self-defined current vegetarian, former vegetarian, and nonvegetarian women. *Journal of the American Dietetic Association*, 102(3): 354–60.

Bates, B., Lennox, A., Prentice, A., Bates, C. and Swan, G. (2012). National diet and nutrition survey: headline results from years 1, 2 and 3 (combined) of the rolling programme 2008/09-2010/11. Accessed on 4 August 2015. Archived at: webarchive.nationalarchives.gov.uk/20130402145952/http://transparency.dh.gov.uk/2012/07/25/ndns-3-years-report.

Batista, R. and Oliveira, M.M. (2009). Facts and fiction of genetically engineered food. *Trends in Biotechnology*, 27(5): 277–86.

Bauer, M. (1995). *Resistance to new technology: nuclear power, information technology and biotechnology*. Cambridge, United Kingdom: Cambridge University Press.

Bauman, Z. (1998). *Work, consumerism and the new poor*. Buckingham, United Kingdom: Open University Press.

Bauman, Z. (2007). *Liquid times. Living in an age of uncertainty*. Cambridge, United Kingdom: Polity Press.

Bawa, A.S. and Anilakumar, K.R. (2013). Genetically modified foods: safety, risks and public concerns – a review. *Journal of Food Science and Technology*, 50(6):1035–46.

Bazzano, L.A. (2005). Dietary intake of fruit and vegetables and risk of diabetes mellitus and cardiovascular diseases. Background paper for the Joint FAO/WHO Workshop on Fruit and Vegetables for Health, 1–3 September 2004, Kobe, Japan.

Accessed on 15 December 2014 at: www.who.int/dietphysicalactivity/publications/ f&v_cvd_diabetes.pdf.

BBC News (2004). China 'fake milk' scandal deepens. BBC 22 April. Accessed on 27 November 2013 at: http://news.bbc.co.uk/go/pr/fr/-/2/hi/asia-pacific/3648583.stm.

Beardsworth, A., Bryman, A., Keil, T., Goode, J., Haslam, C. and Lancashire, E. (2002). Women, men and food: the significance of gender for nutritional attitudes and choices. *British Food Journal*, 104: 470–91.

Beck, A., Kretzschmar, U. and Schmid, O. (eds) (2006). *Organic food processing – principles, concepts and recommendations for the future. Results of a European research project on the quality of low input foods.* Frick, Switzerland: Research Institute of Organic Agriculture (FiBL).

Beck, U. (1992[2007]). *Risk society. Towards a new modernity.* London, United Kingdom: Sage Publications.

Beck, U. (1995). *Ecological politics in an age of risk.* Cambridge, United Kingdom: Polity Press.

Beck, U. (1997a). *The reinvention of politics.* Cambridge, United Kingdom: Polity Press.

Beck, U. (1997b). *Democracy without enemies.* Cambridge, United Kingdom: Polity Press.

Beck, U. ([1999]2007). *World risk society.* Cambridge, United Kingdom: Polity Press.

Beck, U. (2003). Risk society. In Slattery, M. (ed.), *Key ideas in sociology.* New York, NY: Nelson Thornes.

Beck, U. and Beck-Gernsheim, E. (2009). Global generations and the trap of methodological nationalism for a cosmopolitan turn in the sociology of youth and generation. *European Sociological Review*, 25(1): 25–36

Beck, U., Bonß, W. and Lau, C. (2003). The theory of reflexive modernization. Problematic, hypotheses and research programme theory. *Culture & Society*, 20(2): 1–33.

Beck, U. and Holzer, B. (2007). Organizations in world risk society. In Pearson C.M., Roux-Dufort, C. and Clair, J.A. (eds), *International handbook of organizational crisis management.* Thousand Oaks, CA: Sage Publications: 3–24.

Beck-Gernsheim, E. (1996). Life as a planning project. In Scott, L., Szerszynski, B. and Wynne, B. (eds), *Risk, environment and modernity. Towards a new ecology.* London, United Kingdom: Sage Publications: 139–53.

Becker, H. (1963). *Outsiders. Studies in the sociology of deviance.* New York, NY: The Free Press.

Bekin, C., Carrigan, M. and Szmigin, I. (2007). Communities and consumption. *International Journal of Sociology and Social Policy*, 27(3/4): 101–5.

Bellavia, A., Bottai, M., Wolk, A. and Orsini, N. (2014). Alcohol consumption and mortality: a dose-response analysis in terms of time. *Annals of Epidemiology*, 24(4): 291–6.

Bellows-Riecken, K.H. and Rhodes, R.E. (2008). A birth of inactivity? A review of physical activity and parenthood. *Preventive Medicine*, 46(2): 99–110.

Benbrook, C.M. (2012). Impacts of genetically engineered crops on pesticide use in the US – the first sixteen years. *Environmental Sciences Europe*, 24: 24–37.

Benbrook, C.M., Butler, G., Latif, M.A., Leifert, C. and Davis, D.R. (2013). Organic production enhances milk nutritional quality by shifting fatty acid composition: a United States–wide, 18-month study. *PLoS One,* 8(12): e82429: 1–13.

Benbrook, C.M., Zhao, X., Yanez, J., Davies, N. and Andrews, P. (2008). *New evidence confirms the nutritional superiority of plant-based organic foods. State of science review.* Foster, RI: The Organic Center.

Bengtsson, J., Ahnström, J. and Weibull, A-C. (2005). The effects of organic agriculture on biodiversity and abundance: a meta-analysis. *Journal of Applied Ecology*, 42(2): 261–9.

Bennett, W. and Gurin, J. (1982). *The dieter's dilemma*. New York, NY: Basic Books.

Berg, L. (2004). Trust in food in the age of mad cow disease. A comparative study of consumers' evaluation of food safety in Belgium, Britain and Norway. *Appetite*, 42: 21–32.

Berg, L., Kjaernes, U., Ganskau, E., Minina, V., Voltchkova, L., Halkier, B. and Holm, L. (2005). Trust in food safety in Russia, Denmark and Norway. *European Societies*, 7(1): 103–29.

Bergman, Å., Heindel, J.J., Jobling, S., Kidd, K.A. and Zoeller, R.T. (eds) (2013). *State of the science of endocrine disrupting chemicals – 2012*. Geneva, Switzerland: World Health Organization. Accessed on 7 May 2015 at: www.who. int/iris/bitstream/10665/78101/1/9789241505031_eng.pdf?ua=1.

Berry, I. (2011). Bayer to pay rice farmers for gene contamination. *The Wall Street Journal*, 1 July. Accessed on 2 July 2015 at: www.wsj.com/articles/SB100014240527 02304450604576420330493480082.

Besharov, D.J. (2002). We're feeding the poor as if they're starving. *The Washington Post*, 8 December. Accessed on 2 March 2015 at: www.aei.org/article/society-and-culture/ poverty/were-feeding-the-poor-as-if-theyre-starving/.

Bhalla, P.L., Swoboda, I. and Singh, M.B. (1999). Antisense-mediated silencing of a gene encoding a major ryegrass pollen allergen. *Proceedings of the National Academy of Sciences*, 96(20): 11676–80.

Bhatt, S.R., Lokhandwala, M.F. and Banday, A.A. (2011). Resveratrol prevents endothelial nitric oxide synthase uncoupling and attenuates development of hypertension in spontaneously hypertensive rats. *European Journal of Pharmacology*, 667: 258–64.

Bildtgård, T. (2008). Trust in food in modern and late-modern societies. *Social Science Information*, 47: 99–128.

Birch, G.G., Cameron, A.G. and Spencer, M. (1986). *Food science*. Oxford, United Kingdom: Pergamon Press.

Birch, L.L. (1992). Children's preferences for high-fat foods. *Nutrition Reviews*, 50(9): 249–55.

Birch, L.L. (1999). Development of food preferences. *Annual Review of Nutrition*, 19: 41–62.

Bjelakovic, G., Nikolova, D., Gluud, C. (2013). Antioxidant supplements to prevent mortality. *JAMA*, 310: 1178–9.

Black, J.L. and Billette, J-M. (2013). Do Canadians meet Canada's Food Guide's recommendations for fruits and vegetables? *Applied Physiology, Nutrition, and Metabolism*, 38: 234–42.

Blackburn, G.L. (2011). Medicalizing obesity: individual, economic, and medical consequences. *Virtual Mentor*, 13(12): 890–95.

Blair, S.N., Shaten, J., Brownell, K.D., Collins, G. and Lissner, L. (1993). Body weight fluctuation, all-cause mortality, and cause-specific mortality in the Multiple Risk Factor Intervention Trial. *Annals of Internal Medicine*, 119: 747–57.

Blaser, M.J. and Newman, L.S. (1982). A review of human salmonellosis: I. Infective dose. *Reviews of Infectious Diseases*, 4: 1096–106.

Blass, E.M., Anderson, D.R., Kirkorian, H.L., Pempek, T.A., Price, I. and Koleini, M.F. (2006). On the road to obesity: television viewing increases intake of high-density foods. *Physiology & Behavior*, 88(4–5): 597–604.

Blauch, J.L. and Tarka, S.M. (1983). HPLC determination of caffeine and theobromine in coffee, tea, and instant hot cocoa mix. *Journal of Food Science*, 48: 745–7.

Blendon, R.J., Des Roches, C.M., Benson, J.M., Brodie, M. and Altman, D.E. (2001). Americans' views on the use and regulation of dietary supplements. *Archives of Internal Medicine*, 161(6): 805–10.

Blix, G. (2001). Religion, spirituality, and a vegetarian dietary. In Sabaté, J. (ed.), *Vegetarian nutrition*, Boca Raton, FL: CRC Press: 507–32.

Blocker, J.S., David, M., Fahey, D.M., Ian, R. and Tyrrell, I.R. (eds) (2003). *Alcohol and temperance in modern history: an international encyclopedia*. Santa Barbara, CA: ABC-CLIO.

Blum, L.N., Nielsen, N.H. and Riggs, J.A. (1998). Alcoholism and alcohol abuse among women: report of the Council on Scientific Affairs. *Journal of Women's Health*, 7(7): 861–71.

Bock, R. (2010). The give-and-take of DNA: horizontal gene transfer in plants. *Trends in Plant Science*, 15(1): 11–22.

Bogovski, P. and Bogovski, S. (1981). Animal species in which N-nitroso compounds induce cancer. *International Journal of Cancer*, 27: 471–4.

Bond, T.J. (2011). The origins of tea, coffee and cocoa as beverages. In Crozier, A., Ashihara, H. and Barbéran, F.T. (eds), *Tea, cocoa and coffee: plant secondary metabolites and health*. Oxford, United Kingdom: Wiley-Blackwell Publishing: 1–24.

Bondarianzadeh, D., Yeatman, H. and Condon-Paoloni, D. (2007). Listeria education in pregnancy: lost opportunity for health professionals. *Australian and New Zealand Journal of Public Health*, 31: 468–74.

Boone-Heinonen, J., Gordon-Larsen, P., Kiefe, C.L., Shikany, J.M., Lewis, C.E. and Popkin, B.M. (2011). Longitudinal associations with diet in young to middle-aged adults: the CARDIA Study. *Archives of Internal Medicine*, 171(13): 1162–70.

Bourdieu, P. ([1979]1984). *Distinction: a social critique of the judgement of taste*. London, United Kingdom: Routledge.

Bourn, D. and Prescott, J. (2002). A comparison of the nutritional value, sensory qualities, and food safety of organically and conventionally produced foods. *Critical Reviews in Food Science and Nutrition*, 42: 1–34.

Bowman, S.A., Gortmaker, S.L., Ebbeling, C.B., Pereira, M.A. and Ludwig, D.S. (2004). Effects of fast-food consumption on energy intake and diet quality among children in a national household survey. *Pediatrics*, 113(1 Pt 1): 112–8.

Boyne, R. (2003). *Risk*. Milton Keynes, United Kingdom: Open University Press.

Branca, F., Nikogosian, H. and Lobstein, T. (eds) (2007). *The challenge of obesity in the WHO European region and the strategies for response*. Copenhagen, Denmark: World Health Organization Regional Office for Europe. Accessed on 2 March 2015 at: http://apps.who.int/bookorders/anglais/detart1.jsp?codlan=1&codc ol=34&codcch=70.

BrandRepublic (2005). Superbrands case studies: Lucozade. Accessed on 2 March 2015 at: www.brandrepublic.com/news/232378/Superbrands-case-studies-Lucozade/.

Bray, G.A. and Popkin, B.M. (1998). Dietary fat intake does affect obesity! *American Journal of Clinical Nutrition*, 68(6): 1157–73.

Breda, J.J., Whiting, S.H., Encarnação, R., Norberg, S., Jones, R., Reinap, M. and Jewell, J. (2014). Energy drink consumption in Europe: a review of the risks, adverse health effects, and policy options to respond. *Frontiers in Public Health*, 14 October.

Breithaupt, H. (2003). Blame game. *EMBO Reports*, 4(9): 819.

Brenton, J. (2014). Gendered health discourse. In Cockerham, W.C., Dingwall, R. and Quah, S.R. (eds), *The Wiley Blackwell encyclopedia of health, illness, behavior, and society*. Hoboken, NJ: John Wiley & Sons: 648–50.

Britten, P., Marcoe, K., Yamini, S. and Davis, C. (2006). Development of food intake patterns for the MyPyramid Food Guidance System. *Journal of Nutrition Education and Behavior*, 38(6): S78–S92.

Bruening, G. and Lyons, J.M. (2000). The case of the FLAVR SAVR tomato. *California Agriculture*, 54(4): 6–7.

Bryan, N.S., Alexander, D.D., Coughlin, J.R., Milkowski, A.L. and Boffetta, P. (2012). Ingested nitrate and nitrite and stomach cancer risk: an updated review. *Food and Chemical Toxicology*, 50(10): 3646–65.

Budd, G.M. and Peterson, J.A. (2014). The obesity epidemic. Part 1: Understanding the origins. *American Journal of Nursing*, 114(12): 40–46.

Buiatti, S. (2009). Beer composition: an overview. In Preedy, V.R. (ed.), *Beer in health and disease prevention*. Burlington, MA: Elsevier: 213–6.

Bull, A.T., Holt, G. and Lilly, M.D. (1982). *Biotechnology: international trends and perspectives*. Paris, France: Organisation for Economic Co-operation and Development.

Burchell, G., Gordon, C. and Miller, P. (eds) (1991). *The Foucault effect: studies in governmentality*. London, United Kingdom: Harvester/Wheatsheaf.

Burnett, D. (2007). Fast-food lawsuits and the cheeseburger bill: critiquing Congress's response to the obesity epidemic. *Virginia Journal of Social Policy and the Law*, 14(3): 357–418.

Butler, J.P., Post, G.B., Lioy, P.J., Waldman, J.M. and Greenberg, A. (1993). Assessment of carcinogenic risk from personal exposure to benzo[a]pyrene in the total human environmental exposure study (THEES). *Journal of the Air and Waste Management Association*, 43: 970–77.

Butt, M.S. and Sultan, M.T. (2011). Coffee and its consumption: benefits and risks. *Critical Reviews in Food Science and Nutrition*, 51(4): 363–73.

Caballero, B. (2001). Early nutrition and risk of disease in the adult. *Public Health Nutrition*, 4(6A): 1335–6.

Cadden, I.S., Partovi, N. and Yoshida, E.M. (2007). Review article: possible beneficial effects of coffee on liver disease and function. *Alimentary Pharmacology and Therapeutics*, 26: 1–8.

Cade, J., Thomas, E. and Vail, A. (1998). Case-control study of breast cancer in south east England: nutritional factors. *Journal of Epidemiology & Community Health*, 52: 105–10.

Cady, R.J. and Durham, P.L. (2010). Cocoa-enriched diets enhance expression of phosphatases and decrease expression of inflammatory molecules in trigeminal ganglion neurons. *Brain Research*, 1323: 18–32.

Calzada, C., Bruckdorfer, R. and Rice-Evans, C.A. (1997). The influence of antioxidant nutrients on platelet function in healthy volunteers. *Atherosclerosis*, 128: 97–105.

Cameron, E., Pauling, L. and Leibovitz, B. (1979). Ascorbic acid and cancer: a review. *Cancer Research*, 39: 663–81.

Campbell, S.B., Macfarlane, D.J., Fleming, S.J. and Khafagi, F.A. (1994). Increased skeletal uptake of Tc-99m methylene diphosphonate in milk-alkali syndrome. *Clinical Nuclear Medicine*, 19(3): 207–11.

Canavari, M. (2009). *Summary report on sensory-related socio-economic and sensory science literature about organic food products*. Deliverable No. 1.2, ECROPOLIS Project (No. 218477-2). Bologna, Italy and Frick, Switzerland: Dipartimento di Economia e Ingegneria agrarie, Alma Mater Studiorum-University of Bologna and Research Institute of Organic Agriculture (FiBL).

Caraher, M., Lange, T. and Dixon, P. (2000). The influence of TV and celebrity chefs on public attitudes and behavior among the English public. *Journal for the Study of Food and Society*, 4(1): 27–46.

CARE Study Group (2008). Maternal caffeine intake during pregnancy and risk of fetal growth restriction: a large prospective observational study. *BMJ*, 337: a2332–40.

Cargiulo, T. (2007). Understanding the health impact of alcohol dependence. *American Journal of Health-System Pharmacy*, 64(5), Supplement 3: S5–S11.

Carroll, M.E. (1998). Acquisition and reacquisition (relapse) of drug abuse: modulation by alternative reinforcers. *NIDA Research Monograph*, 169: 6–25.

Casey, R., Oppert, J.-M., Weber, C., Charreire, H., Salzed, P., Badariotti, D., Banos, A., Fischler, C., Giacoman Hernandez, C., Chaix, B. and Simon, C. (2014). Determinants of childhood obesity: what can we learn from built environment studies? *Food Quality and Preference*, 31: 164–72.

Casey, T.R. and Bamforth, C.W. (2010). Silicon in beer and brewing. *Journal of the Science of Food and Agriculture*, 90(5): 784–8.

Cassady, D., Jetter, K.M. and Culp, J. (2007). Is price a barrier to eating more fruits and vegetables for low-income families? *Journal of the American Dietetic Association*, 107(11): 1909–15.

Castaneda, R., Sussman, N., Westreich, L., Levy, R. and O'Malley, M. (1996). A review of the effects of moderate alcohol intake on the treatment of anxiety and mood disorders. *Journal of Clinical Psychiatry*, 57(5): 207–12.

Castel, R. (1991). From dangerousness to risk. In Burchell, G., Gordon, C. and Miller, P. (eds), *The Foucault effect: studies in governmentality*. London United Kingdom: Harvester/Wheatsheaf.

Castellini, C., Mugnai, C. and Dal Bosco, A. (2002). Effect of organic production system on broiler carcass and meat quality. *Meat Science*, 60: 219–25.

Castells, M. (2000). *The rise of the network society* (Second ed.). Hoboken, NJ: Wiley-Blackwell.

Castells, M. (2001). *The Internet galaxy*. Oxford, United Kingdom: Oxford University Press.

Castells, M., Fernandez-Ardevol, M., Linchuan Qiu, J. and Araba Sey, A. (2009). *The mobile communication society: a cross-cultural analysis of available evidence on the social uses of wireless communication technology*. Los Angeles, CA: Annenberg Research Network on International Communication, University of Southern California.

Caulfield, L.E., Richard, S.A., Rivera, J.A., Musgrove, P. and Black, R.E. (2006). Stunting, wasting, and micronutrient deficiency disorders. In Jamison, D.T., Breman, J.G., Measham, A.R., Alleyne, G., Claeson, M., Evans, D.B., Jha, P., Mills, A. and Musgroveet, P. (eds), *Disease control priorities in developing countries* (Second ed.) Washington, DC: World Bank. Accessed on 20 March 2015 at: www.ncbi.nlm.nih.gov/books/NBK11761/.

Cavadini, C., Siega-Riz, A.M. and Popkin, B.M. (2000). US adolescent food intake trends from 1965 to 1996. *Archives of Disease in Childhood*, 83: 18–24.

Cavalieri, D., McGovern, P.E., Hartl, D.L., Mortimer, R. and Polsinelli, M. (2003). Evidence for *S. cerevisiae* fermentation in ancient wine. *Journal of Molecular Evolution*, 57(1): S226–S232.

Cavin, C., Marin-Kuan, M., Langouët, S., Bezençon, C., Guignard, G., Verguet, C., Piguet, D., Holzhäuser, D., Cornaz, R. and Schilter, B. (2008). Induction of Nrf2-mediated cellular defenses and alteration of phase I activities as mechanisms of chemoprotective effects of coffee in the liver. *Food and Chemical Toxicology*, 46(4): 1239–48.

Cawley, J. and Meyerhoefer, C. (2012). The medical care costs of obesity: an instrumental variables approach. *Journal of Health Economics*, 31(1): 219–30.

Celimli-Inaltong, I. (2014). You are what you eat. In Thompson, P.B. and Kaplan, D.M. (eds), *Encyclopedia of food and agricultural ethics*. Dordrecht, The Netherlands: Springer: 1–6.

Center for Behavioral Health Statistics and Quality (2013). *The DAWN report: update on emergency department visits involving energy drinks: a continuing public health concern*. Rockville, MD: Substance Abuse and Mental Health Services Administration.

Center for Food Safety (2013). Genetically engineered food labeling laws map. Accessed on 11 Novemer 2014 at: www.centerforfoodsafety.org/issues/976/ge-food-labeling/reports/1413/genetically-engineered-food-labeling-laws-map.

Center for Food Safety and Applied Nutrition Adverse Event Reporting System [CAERS] (2012). *Adverse events reports allegedly related to energy drinks*. Washington, DC: US Food and Drug Administration. Accessed on 20 June 2015 at: www.fda.gov/downloads/AboutFDA/CentersOffices/OfficeofFoods/CFSAN/CFSANFOIAElectronicReadingRoom/UCM328270.pdf.

Centers for Disease Control and Prevention [CDC] (2004). Trends in intake of energy and macronutrients – United States, 1971–2000. *Morbidity and Mortality Weekly Report*, 53(04): 80–82.

Centers for Disease Control and Prevention [CDC] (2013). State indicator report on fruits and vegetables. Accessed on 4 August 2015 at: www.cdc.gov/nutrition/downloads/State-Indicator-Report-Fruits-Vegetables-2013.pdf.

Centers for Disease Control and Prevention [CDC] (2015). Multistate outbreak of listeriosis linked to commercially produced, prepackaged caramel apples made from Bidart Bros. Apples. Accessed on 1 August 2015 at: www.cdc.gov/listeria/outbreaks/caramel-apples-12-14/.

Chadbourn, B.C. (2014). Asceticism in the modern world: the religion of self-deprivation. *Student Pulse*, 6(3): 2–4.

Chapman, N., Gordon, A.R. and Burghardt, J.A. (1995). Factors affecting the fat content of National School Lunch Program lunches. *American Journal of Clinical Nutrition*, 61(1 Suppl): 199S–204S.

Chapple, C.K. (2011). Roots, shoots, and Ahimsa: the Jain yoga of vegetarianism. In: Rosen, S.J. (ed.), *Food for the soul: vegetarianism and yoga traditions*. Santa Barbara, CA: Praeger: 117–28.

ChartsBin (2011). Current worldwide annual coffee consumption per capita. ChartsBin Statistics Collector Team. Accessed on 25 June 2015 at: http://chartsbin.com/view/581.

Chen, H. and Lin, Y. (2013). Promise and issues of genetically modified crops. *Current Opinion in Plant Biology*, 16(2): 255–60.

Cherrington, E.H. (ed.) (1925–1930). *Standard encyclopedia of the alcohol problem* (6 vols). Westerville, OH: American Issue Publishing.

Chhabra, R., Kolli, S. and Bauer, J.H. (2013). Organically grown food provides health benefits to Drosophila melanogaster. *PLoS One*, 8(1): e52988 (1–8).

Chilkov, N. (2012). The link between grilled foods and cancer. *Huffington Post*, 23 April. Accessed on 23 April 2015 at: www.huffingtonpost.com/nalini-chilkov/grilling-health_b_1796567.html.

Chin, J.M., Merves, M.L., Goldberger, B.A., Sampson-Cone, A. and Cone, E.J. (2008). Caffeine content of brewed teas. *Journal of Analytical Toxicology*, 32(8): 702–4.

Chiolero, A., Faeh, D., Paccaud, F. and Cornuz, J. (2008). Consequences of smoking for body weight, body fat distribution, and insulin resistance. *American Journal of Clinical Nutrition*, 87(4): 801–9.

Christen, A.G. and Christen, J.A. (1997). Horace Fletcher (1849–1919): the great masticator. *Journal of the History of Dentistry*, 45(3): 95–100.

Clark, J.E. (1998). Taste and flavour: their importance in food choice and acceptance. *Proceedings of the Nutrition Society*, 57: 639–43.

Codex Alimentarius Commission [CAC] (2003). *Principles for risk analysis and guidelines for safety assessment of foods derived from modern biotechnology* (CAC/GL 44–46). Rome, Italy: Codex Alimentarius Commission.

Codex Alimentarius Commission [CAC] (2007). *Working principles for risk analysis for food safety for application by governments* (CAC/GL 62–2007). Rome, Italy: Codex Alimentarius Commission.

Cohen, S. ([1997]2002). *Folk devils and moral panics* (Third ed.). New York, NY: Routledge.

Colagiuri, S., Lee, C.M.Y., Colagiuri, R., Magliano, D., Shaw, J.E., Zimmet, P.Z. and Caterson, I.D. (2010). The cost of overweight and obesity in Australia. *Medical Journal of Australia*, 192(5): 260–64.

Combs, G.F. (2008). *The vitamins: fundamental aspects in nutrition and health* (Third ed.) Burlington, MA: Elsevier Academic Press.

Connors, M.M., Bisogni, C.A., Sobal, J. and Devine, C. (2001). Managing values in personal food systems. *Appetite*, 36: 189–200.

Contento, I. (2007). *Nutrition education: linking research, theory, and practice*. Sudbury, MA: Jones and Bartlett Publishers.

Corder, R., Mullen, W., Khan, N.Q., Marks, S.C., Wood, E.G., Carrier, M.J. and Crozier, A. (2006). Oenology: red wine procyanidins and vascular health. *Nature*, 444(7119): 566.

Cordova, A.C. and Sumpio, B.E. (2009). Polyphenols are medicine: is it time to prescribe red wine for our patients? *The International Journal of Angiology*, 18(3): 111–17.

Corrao, G., Bagnardi, V., Zambon, A. and La Vecchia, C. (2004). A meta-analysis of alcohol consumption and the risk of 15 diseases. *Preventive Medicine*, 38: 613–19.

Corrao, G., Rubbiati, L., Zambon, A. and Arico, S. (2002). Alcohol-attributable and alcohol-preventable mortality in Italy. A balance in 1983 and 1996. *European Journal of Public Health*, 12: 214–23.

Costanzo, S., Di Castelnuovo, A., Donati, M.B., Iacoviello, L. and de Gaetano, G. (2011). Wine, beer or spirit drinking in relation to fatal and non-fatal cardiovascular events: a meta-analysis. *European Journal of Epidemiology*, 26(11): 833–50.

Counihan, C.M. (1999). *The anthropology of food and body*. New York, NY: Routledge.

Cova, B. (1997). Community and consumption: towards a definition of the linking value of products and services. *European Journal of Marketing*, 31(3/4): 297–316.

Cowan, B. (2001). What was masculine about the public sphere? Gender and the coffeehouse milieu in post-restoration England. *History Workshop Journal*, 51, 127–57.

Cravotto, G., Boffa, L., Genzini, L. and Garella, D. (2010). Phytotherapeutics: an evaluation of the potential of 1000 plants. *Journal of Clinical Pharmacy and Therapeutics*, 35(1): 11–48.

Crawford, D., Ball, K., Mishra, G., Salmon, J. and Timperio, A. (2007). Which food-related behaviours are associated with healthier intakes of fruits and vegetables among women? *Public Health Nutrition*, 10(3): 256–65.

Crerar, D.O. (2013). An inquiry into the death of Natasha Marie Harris, findings of Coroner D. O. Crerar, New Zealand Coroner's Court at Invercargill.

Crescente, M., Jessen, G., Momi, S., Holtje, H.D., Gresele, P., Cerletti, C. and de Gaetano, G. (2009). Interactions of gallic acid, resveratrol, quercetin and aspirin at the platelet cyclooxygenase-1 level. Functional and modelling studies. *Thrombosis and Haemostasis*, 102: 336–46.

Crews, C. (2009). Consumer exposure to furan from heat-processed food and kitchen air (Scientific/technical report submitted to EFSA). Accessed on 10 December 2014 at: www.efsa.europa.eu/en/supporting/doc/30e.pdf.

Crim, S.M., Iwamoto, M., Huang, J.Y., Griffin, P.M., Gilliss, D., Cronquist, A.B., Cartter, M., Tobin-D'Angelo, M., Blythe, D., Smith, K., Lathrop, S., Zansky, S., Cieslak, P.R., Dunn, J., Holt, K.G., Lance, S., Tauxe, R. and Henao, O.L. (2014). Incidence and trends of infection with pathogens transmitted commonly through food – Foodborne Diseases Active Surveillance Network, 10 US sites, 2006–2013. *Morbidity and Mortality Weekly Report*, 63(15): 328–32.

Crothers, L. (2011). *Australia – agricultural biotechnology annual* (Global Agricultural Information Network Report AS1120). Washington, DC: USDA Foreign Agricultural Service.

Crum Cianflone, N.F. (2008). Salmonellosis and the GI tract: more than just peanut butter. *Current Gastroenterology Reports*, 10(4): 424–31.

Culp, S.J., Gaylor, D.W., Sheldon, W.G., Goldstein, L.S. and Beland, F.A. (1998). A comparison of the tumours induced by coal tar and benzo[a]pyrene in a 2-year bioassay. *Carcinogenesis*, 19: 117–24.

Cusumano, D.L. and Thompson, J.K. (1997). Body image and body shape ideals in magazines: exposure, awareness, and internalization. *Sex Roles*, 37: 701–21.

D'Souza, D.H., Sair, A., Williams, K., Papafragkou, E., Jean, J., Moore, C. and Jaykus, L. (2006). Persistence of caliciviruses on environmental surfaces and their transfer to food. *International Journal of Food Microbiology*, 108(1): 84–91.

Daee, A., Robinson, P., Lawson, M., Turpin, J.A., Gregory, B. and Tobias, J.D. (2002). Psychologic and physiologic effects of dieting in adolescents. *Southern Medical Journal*, 95(9): 1032–41.

Dake, K. (1992). Myths of nature: culture and the social construction of risk. *Journal of Social Issues*, 48(4): 21–37.

Dangour, A.D., Dodhia, S.K., Hayter, A., Allen, E., Lock, K. and Uauy, R. (2009). Nutritional quality of organic foods: a systematic review. *American Journal of Clinical Nutrition*, 90(3): 680–85.

Darmon, N. and Drewnowski, A. (2008). Does social class predict diet quality? *American Journal of Clinical Nutrition*, 87: 1107–17.

Davis, M.A., Murphy, S.P., Neuhaus, J.M., Gee, L. and Quiroga, S.S. (2000). Living arrangements affect dietary quality for US adults aged 50 years and older: NHANES III 1988–1994. *Journal of Nutrition*, 130: 2256–64.

Davison, J. (2010). GM plants: science, politics and EC regulations. *Plant Science*, 178(2): 94–8.

de Boer, M., McCarthy, M., Brennan, M., Kelly, A.L. and Ritson, C. (2005). Public understanding of food risk issues and food risk messages on the island of Ireland: the views of food safety experts. *Journal of Food Safety*, 25(4): 241–65.

de Ruyter, J.C., Olthof, M.R., Seidell, J.C. and Katan, M.B. (2012). A trial of sugar-free or sugar-sweetened beverages and body weight in children. *New England Journal of Medicine*, 367: 1397–406.

de Schutter, O. (2010). *Rapporteur on the right to food*. Geneva, Switzerland: United Nations Human Rights. Accessed on 8 December 2014 at: www2.ohchr.org/english/issues/food/docs/A-HRC-16–49.pdf.

de Silva, A.P., de Silva, S.H.P., Haniffa, R., Liyanage, I.K., Jayasinghe, K.S.A., Katulanda, P., Wijeratne, C.N., Wijeratne, S. and Rajapakse, L.C. (2015). A cross sectional survey on social, cultural and economic determinants of obesity in a low middle income setting. *International Journal for Equity in Health*, 14: 6–15.

de Wit, M.A.S., Koopmans, M.P.G., Kortbeek, L.M., Wannet, W.J.B. Vinjé, J., van Leusden, F., Bartelds, A.I.M. and van Duynhoven, Y.T.H.P. (2001). Sensor, a population-based cohort study on gastroenteritis in the Netherlands: incidence and aetiology. *American Journal of Epidemiology*, 154: 666–74.

Dealer, S.F. and Lacey, R.W. (1990). Transmissible spongiform encephalopathies: the threat of BSE to man. *Food Microbiology*, 7: 253–79.

Dean, M. (1999). Risk, calculable and incalculable. In Lupton, D. (ed.), *Risk and sociocultural theory: new directions and perspectives*. Cambridge United Kingdom: Cambridge University Press.

Dean, M. (2009). *Governmentality: power and rule in modern society* (Second ed.). London, United Kingdom: Sage Publications.

Deloitte (2010). Deloitte 2010 food survey – genetically modified foods. Accessed on 6 November 2014 at: www.deloitte.com/assets/Dcom-UnitedStates/Local Assets/Documents/ConsumerBusiness/us_cp_2010FoodSurveyFactSheetGeneticallyModifiedFoods_05022010.pdf.

Delormier, T., Frohlich, K.L. and Potvin, L. (2009). Food and eating as social practice – understanding eating patterns as social phenomena and implications for public health. *Sociology of Health & Illness*, 31(2): 215–28.

Dennis, M.J., Howarth, N., Key, P.E., Pointer, M. and Massey, R.C. (1989). Investigation of ethyl carbamate levels in some fermented foods and alcoholic beverages. *Food Additives and Contaminants*, 6: 383–9.

Dettmann, R.L. and Dimitri, C. (2010). Who's buying organic vegetables? Demographic characteristics of U.S. consumers. *Journal of Food Products Marketing*, 16(1): 79–91.

Devipriya, N., Srinivasan, M., Sudheer, A.R. and Menon, V.P. (2007). Effect of ellagic acid, a natural polyphenol, on alcohol-induced prooxidant and antioxidant imbalance: a drug dose dependent study. *Singapore Medical Journal*, 48(4): 311–18.

Diamanti-Kandarakis, E., Bourguignon, J-P., Giudice, L.C., Hauser, R., Prins, G.S., Soto, A.M., Zoeller, R.T. and Gore, A.C. (2009). Endocrine-disrupting chemicals: an Endocrine Society scientific statement. *Endocrine Reviews*, 30(4): 293–342.

Dickson, P.G.M. (1960). *The Sun Insurance Office 1710–1960: the history of two and a half centuries of British insurance*. London, United Kingdom: Oxford University Press.

Dietler, M. (1990). Driven by drink: the role of drinking in the political economy and the case of early Iron Age France. *Journal of Anthropological Archaeology*, 9(4): 352–406.

Dixon, J. and Broom, D. (eds) (2007). *The 7 deadly sins of obesity: how the modern world is making us fat*. Sydney, Australia: University of New South Wales Press.

Dolinoy, D.C. (2008). The agouti mouse model: an epigenetic biosensor for nutritional and environmental alterations on the fetal epigenome. *Nutrition Review*, 66 (Suppl 1): S7–S11.

Donkin, A.J., Johnson, A.E., Morgan, K., Neale, R.J., Page, R.M. and Silburn, R.L. (1998). Gender and living alone as determinants of fruit and vegetable consumption among the elderly living at home in Urban Nottingham. *Appetite*, 30: 39–51.

Douglas, M. ([1966]1969). *Purity and danger: an analysis of the concepts of pollution and taboo*. London, United Kingdom: Routledge.

Douglas, M. (1982). Cultural bias. In Douglas, M. (ed.), *The active voice*. London, United Kingdom: Routledge & Kegan Paul: 183–254.

Douglas, M. (1984). *Food in the social order: studies of food and festivities in three American communities*. New York, NY: Russell Sage Foundation.

Douglas, M. (1985). *Risk acceptability according to the social sciences*. New York, NY: Russell Sage Foundation.

Douglas, M. (1992). *Risk and blame: essays in cultural theory*. London, United Kingdom: Routledge.

Douglas, M. and Wildavsky, A.B. (1982). *Risk and culture: an essay on the selection of technical and environmental dangers*. Berkeley, CA: University of California Press.

Drabova, L., Pulkrabova, J., Kalachova, K., Tomaniova, M., Kocourek, V. and Hajslova, J. (2013). Polycyclic aromatic hydrocarbons and halogenated persistent organic pollutants in canned fish and seafood products: smoked versus non-smoked products. *Food Additives and Contaminants. Part A, Chemistry, Analysis, Control, Exposure and Risk Assessment*, 30(3): 515–27.

Drewnowski, A. (1995). Energy intake and sensory properties of food. *American Journal of Clinical Nutrition*, 6 (suppl): 1081S–1085S.

Drewnowski, A. (1997). Taste preferences and food intake. *Annual Review of Nutrition*, 17: 237–53.

Drewnowski, A. (1999). Intense sweeteners and energy density of foods: implications for weight control. *European Journal of Clinical Nutrition*, 53: 757–63.

Drewnowski, A. and Eichelsdoerfer, P. (2010). Can low-income Americans afford a healthy diet? *Nutr Today*, 44(6): 246–9.

Drewnowski, A. and Rock, C.L. (1995). The influence of genetic taste markers on food acceptance. *American Journal of Clinical Nutrition*, 62: 506–11.

Drewnowski, A. and Specter, S.E. (2004). Poverty and obesity: the role of energy density and energy costs. *American Journal of Clinical Nutrition*, 79(1): 6–16.

Drici, M-D. (2014). Energy drinks cause heart problems. Accessed on 20 June 2015 at: www.escardio.org/about/press/press-releases/esc14-barcelona/Pages/energy-drink-cardiac-safety.aspx.

Driessen, H. (1992). Drinking on masculinity: alcohol and gender in Andalusia. In Gefou-Madianou, D. (ed.), *Alcohol, gender and culture*. London, United Kingdom: Routledge.

Duchan, E., Patel, N.D. and Feucht, C. (2010). Energy drinks: a review of use and safety for athletes. *The Physician and Sportsmedicine*, 38(2): 171–9.

Durkheim, E. (1933). *Division of labour in society*. Translation: Simpson, G., New York, NY: Macmillan.

Durkheim, E. (1951). *Suicide: a study in sociology*. London, United Kingdom: Routledge.

Durnin, J.V.G.A. and Womersley, J. (2007). Body fat assessed from total body density and its estimation from skinfold thickness: measurements on 481 men and women aged from 16 to 72 years. *British Journal of Nutrition*, 32(1): 77–97.

Dworkin, M.S., Shoemaker, P.C., Goldoft, M.J. and Kobayashi, J.M. (2001). Reactive arthritis and Reiter's syndrome following an outbreak of gastroenteritis caused by *Salmonella* enteritidis. *Clinical Infectious Diseases*, 33: 1010–4.

Dybing, E., Farmer, P.B., Andersen, M., Fennell, T.R., Lalljie, S.P.D., Müller, D.J.G., Olin, S., Petersen, B.J., Schlatter, J., Scholz, G., Scimeca, J.A., Slimani, N., Törnqvist, M., Tuijtelaars, S. and Verger, P. (2005). Human exposure and internal dose assessments of acrylamide in food. *Food and Chemical Toxicology*, 43: 365–410.

Ebbeling, C.B., Feldman, H.A., Chomitz, V.R., Antonelli, T.A., Gortmaker, S.L., Osganian, S.K. and Ludwig, D.S. (2012). A randomized trial of sugar-sweetened beverages and adolescent body weight. *New England Journal of Medicine*, 367: 1407–16.

Ebbeling, C.B., Feldman, H.A., Osganian, S.K., Chomitz, V.R., Ellenbogen, S.J. and Ludwig, D.S. (2006). Effects of decreasing sugar-sweetened beverage consumption on body weight in adolescents: a randomized, controlled pilot study. *Pediatrics*, 117: 673–80.

Eckardt, M., File, S., Gessa, G., Grant, K., Guerri, C., Hoffman, P., Kalant, H., Koop, G., Li, T. and Tabakoff, B. (1998). Effects of moderate alcohol consumption on the central nervous system. *Alcoholism, Clinical and Experimental Research*, 22: 998–1040.

Edgar, J. (2014). How beer with your BBQ could save your life. *The Telegraph*, 28 March. Accessed on 10 July 2015 at: http://www.telegraph.co.uk/foodanddrink/foodanddrinknews/10727624/How-beer-with-your-BBQ-could-save-your-life.html.

Edwards, N.T. (1983). Polycyclic hydrocarbons (PAHs) in the terrestrial environment. A review. *Journal of Environmental Quality*, 12: 427–41.

Einsiedel, E., Jelsøe, E. and Breck, T. (2001). Publics at the technology table. Consensus conference in Denmark, Canada and Australia. *Public Understanding of Science*, 10(1): 83–98.

Ekberg, M. (2007). The parameters of the risk society. A review and exploration. *Current Sociology*, 55(3): 343–66.

Elliott, A. (2002). Beck's sociology of risk: a critical assessment. *Sociology*, 36(2): 293–315.

Ellis, J.D. and Tucker, M. (2009). Factors influencing consumer perception of food hazards. *CAB Reviews: Perspectives in Agriculture, Veterinary Science, Nutrition and Natural Resources*, 4: 1–8.

Engs, R.C., Slawinska, J.B. and Hanson, D.J. (1991). The drinking patterns of American and Polish university students: a cross-national study. *Drug and Alcohol Dependence*, 27(2): 167–75.

Ernsberger, P. (2012). BMI, body build, body fatness, and health risks. *Fat Studies*, 1(1): 6–12.

Eskelinen, M.H. and Kivipelto, M. (2010). Caffeine as a protective factor in dementia and Alzheimer's disease. *Journal of Alzheimer's Disease*, 20 (Suppl 1): S167–S174.

Eskelinen, M.H., Ngandu, T., Tuomilehto, J., Soininen, H. and Kivipelto, M. (2009). Midlife coffee and tea drinking and the risk of late-life dementia: a population-based CAIDE study. *Journal of Alzheimer's Disease*, 16(1): 85–91.

Eurobarometer (2010). *Biotechnology* (Special Eurobarometer 341). Brussels, Belgium: TNS Opinion & Social. Accessed on 1 July 2015 at: http://ec.europa.eu/public_opinion/archives/ebs/ebs_341_en.pdf.

Eurobarometer (2010). *Food-related risk.* (Special Eurobarometer 354). Brussels, Belgium: TNS Opinion & Social. Accessed on 2 July 2015 at: www.efsa.europa.eu/sites/default/files/assets/sreporten.pdf.

European Commission [EC] (2011). 4th report on the implementation of the "community strategy for endocrine disrupters" a range of substances suspected of interfering with the hormone systems of humans and wildlife. Brussels, Belgium: European Commission. Accessed on 7 May 2015 at: http://ec.europa.eu/environment/chemicals/endocrine/pdf/sec_2011_1001.pdf.

European Commission [EC] (2014a). *What is organic farming*. Brussels, Belgium: European Commission. Accessed on 3 December 2014 at: http://ec.europa.eu/agriculture/organic/organic-farming/what-is-organic-farming/index_en.htm.

European Commission [EC] (2014b). *European action plan for organic farming*. Brussels, Belgium: European Commission. Accessed on 7 December 2014 at: http://ec.europa.eu/agriculture/organic/eu-policy/action-plan_en.

European Environment Agency (2012). *The impacts of endocrine disrupters on wildlife, people and their environments – the Weybridge+15 (1996–2011) report* (Technical Report No. 2/2012). Copenhagen, Denmark: European Environment Agency.

European Food Safety Authority [EFSA] (2007). Ethyl carbamate and hydrocyanic acid in food and beverages. *EFSA Journal*, 551: 1–44

European Food Safety Authority [EFSA] (2008a). Polycyclic aromatic hydrocarbons in food. *EFSA Journal*, 724: 1–114.

European Food Safety Authority [EFSA] (2008b). Scientific risk assessment on nitrate in vegetables. *EFSA Journal*, 689: 1–79.

European Food Safety Authority [EFSA] (2011a). Scientific opinion on *Campylobacter* in broiler meat production: control options and performance objectives and/or targets at different stages of the food chain. *EFSA Journal*, 9(4): 2105–246.

European Food Safety Authority [EFSA] (2011b). Update on furan levels in food from monitoring years 2004–2010 and exposure assessment. *EFSA Journal*, 9(9): 2347–380.

European Food Safety Authority [EFSA] (2012a). Update of the monitoring of dioxins and PCBs levels in food and feed. *EFSA Journal*, 10(7): 2832–914.

European Food Safety Authority [EFSA] (2012b). Update on acrylamide levels in food from monitoring years 2007–2010. *EFSA Journal*, 10(10): 2938–76.

European Food Safety Authority [EFSA] (2014a). *Salmonella*. Parma, Italy: European Food Safety Authority. Accessed on 25 November 2014 at: www.efsa.europa.eu/en/topics/topic/salmonella.htm?wtrl=01.

European Food Safety Authority [EFSA] (2014b). The 2012 European Union report on pesticide residues in food. *EFSA Journal*, 12(12): 3942–4098.

European Food Safety Authority [EFSA] (2015a). Scientific opinion on the safety of caffeine. *EFSA Journal*, 13(5): 4102–214.

European Food Safety Authority [EFSA] (2015b). Scientific opinion on acrylamide in food. *EFSA Journal*, 13(6): 4104–425.

European Parliament (1996). Research on Islam and alcohol. Luxembourg: Directorate General for Research. Accessed on 18 February 2015 at: www.radioradicale.it/exagora/ep-research-on-islam-and-alcohol.

Evans, B. and Lupescu, M. (2012). *Canada – agricultural biotechnology annual* (Global Agricultural Information Network Report CA12029). Washington, DC: USDA Foreign Agricultural Service.

Ewald, F. (1991). Insurance and risk. In Burchell, G., Gordon, C. and Miller, P. (eds), *The Foucault effect: studies in governmentality*. London United Kingdom: Harvester Wheatsheaf: 197–210.

Ewald, F. (1993). Two infinities of risk. In Massumi, B. (ed.), *The politics of everyday fear*. Minneapolis, MN: University of Minnesota Press: 221–228.

Fabiansson, C. (1998). *Management and employee attitudes towards quality systems*. Sydney, Australia: Meat Research Corporation, MRC-Project MSRE.001: 1–36.

Fabiansson, C. (2010). *Pathways to excessive gambling: a societal perspective on youth and adult gambling pursuits*. Farnham, England: Ashgate.

FAOSTAT (2014). FAOSTAT databases. Accessed on 20 June 2015 at: faostat.fao.org.

Featherstone, M. (2010). Body, image and affect in consumer culture. *Body & Society*, 16(1): 193–221.

Feinman, L. and Lieber, C.S. (1998). Nutrition and diet in alcoholism. In Shils, M.E., Olson, J.A., Shike, M. and Ross, A.C. (eds), *Modern nutrition in health and disease* (Ninth ed.). Baltimore, MD: Williams & Wilkins: 1523–42.

Felt, U., Felder, K., Öhler, T. and Penkler, M. (2014). Timescapes of obesity: coming to terms with a complex socio-medical phenomenon. *Health (London)*, 18(6): 646–64.

Ferguson, L.R. (2010). Meat and cancer. *Meat Science*, 84: 308–13.

Fernandez-Cornejo, J., Wechsler, S., Livingston, M. and Mitchell, L. (2014). *Genetically engineered crops in the United States* (ERR-162). Washington, DC: US Department of Agriculture, Economic Research Service. Accessed on 1 July 2015 at: www.ers.usda.gov/publications/err-economic-research-report/err162.aspx.

Fiddes, N. (1991). *Meat: a natural symbol*. London, United Kingdom: Routledge and Kegan Paul.

Fife-Schaw, C. and Rowe, G. (1996). Public perceptions of everyday food hazards: a psychometric study. *Risk Analysis*, 16: 487–500.

Fildes, A., van Jaarsveld, C.H.M., Llewellyn, C.H., Fisher, A., Cooke, L. and Wardle, J. (2014). Nature and nurture in children's food preferences. *American Journal of Clinical Nutrition*, 99(4): 911–17.

Fillion, L. and Arazi, S. (2002). Does organic food taste better? A claim substantiation approach. *Nutrition & Food Science*, 32(4): 153–7.

Finamore, A., Britti, M.S., Roselli, M., Bellovino, D., Gaetani, S. and Mengheri, E. (2004). Novel approach for food safety evaluation. Results of a pilot experiment to evaluate organic and conventional foods. *Journal of Agricultural and Food Chemistry*, 52(54): 7425–31.

Fischer, A.R.H. and Frewer, L.J. (2009). Consumer familiarity with foods and the perception of risks and benefits. *Food Quality and Preference*, 20(8): 576–85.

Fisone, G., Borgkvist, A. and Usiello, A. (2004). Caffeine as a psychomotor stimulant: mechanism of action. *Cellular and Molecular Life Sciences*, 61(7–8): 857–72.

Fitzgerald, R. and Campbell, H. (2001). Food scares and GM: movement of the nature/culture faultline. *The Drawing Board: An Australian Journal of Public Affairs*. Accessed on 5 June 2015 at: www.australianreview.net/digest/2001/10/fitzgerald_campbell.html.

Flegal, K.M., Troiano, R.P., Pamuk, E.R., Kuczmarski, R.J. and Campbell, S.M. (1995). The influence of smoking cessation on the prevalence of overweight in the United States. *New England Journal of Medicine*, 333: 1165–75.

Flynn, J., Peters, E., Mertz, C.K. and Slovic, P. (1998) Risk media and stigma at rocky flats. *Risk Analysis*, 18: 715–27.

Food Safety and Inspection Service [FSIS] (2010). *Refrigeration and food safety*. Washington, DC: Food Safety and Inspection Service. Accessed on 26 November 2014 at: www.fsis.usda.gov/shared/PDF/Refrigeration_and_Food_Safety.pdf.

Food Safety News (2015). European Union expands COOL requirements beyond beef. Accessed on 22 July 2015 at: www.foodsafetynews.com/2015/04/european-un ion-expands-cool-requirements-beyond-beef/#.Va8czXjUE7R.

Ford, G. (1988). *The benefits of moderate drinking: alcohol, health and society*. San Francisco, CA: Wine Appreciation Guild.

Forman, J. and Silverstein, J. (2012). Organic foods: health and environmental advantages and disadvantages. *Pediatrics*, 130(5): e1406–e1415.

Fortmann, S.P., Burda, B.U., Senger, C.A., Lin, J.S. and Whitlock, E.P. (2013). Vitamin and mineral supplements in the primary prevention of cardiovascular disease and cancer: An updated systematic evidence review for the U.S. Preventive Services Task Force. *Annals of Internal Medicine*, 159: 824–34.

Foucault, M. (1983). On the genealogy of ethics: an overview of work in progress. In Dreyfus, H. and Rabinow, P. (eds), *Michel Foucault: beyond structuralism and hermeneutics*. Chicago, IL: University of Chicago Press.

Foucault, M. (1991). Governmentality. In Burchell, G., Gordon, C. and Miller, P. (eds), *The Foucault effect: studies in governmentality*. London, United Kingdom: Harvester Wheatsheaf: 87–104.

Foucault, M. (2007). *Security, territory, population*. Basingstoke, United Kingdom: Palgrave Macmillan.

Fox, G.P., Wu, A., Yiran, L. and Force, L. (2013). Variation in caffeine concentration in single coffee beans. *Journal of Agricultural and Food Chemistry*, 61(45): 10772–78.

Fox, J.L. (2012). First plant-made biologic approved. *Nature Biotechnology*, 30: 472.

Foxcroft, L. (2012). *Calories and corsets: a history of dieting over two thousand years*. London, United Kingdom: Profile Books.

Frary, C.D., Johnson, R.K. and Wang, M.Q. (2005). Food sources and intakes of caffeine in the diets of persons in the United States. *Journal of the American Dietetic Association*, 105(1): 110–13.

Fredholm, B.B., Bättig, K., Holmén, J., Nehlig, A. and Zvartau, E.E. (1999). Actions of caffeine in the brain with special reference to factors that contribute to its widespread use. *Pharmacological Review*, 51(1): 83–133.

French, S.A. (2003). Pricing effects on food choices. *Journal of Nutrition*, 133(3): 841S–843S.

French, S.A., Lin, B.H. and Guthrie, J.F. (2003). National trends in soft drink consumption among children and adolescents age 6 to 17 years: prevalence, amounts, and sources, 1977/1978 to 1994/1998. *Journal of the American Dietetic Association*, 103: 1326–31.

French, S.A., Story, M., Neumark-Sztainer, D., Fulkerson, J.A. and Hannan, P. (2001). Fast food restaurant use among adolescents: associations with nutrient intake, food choices and behavioral and psychosocial variables. *International Journal of Obesity and Related Metabolic Disorders*, 25(12): 1823–33.

Frewer, L., Fischer, A., Scholderer, J. and Verbeke, W. (2005). Food safety and consumer behavior. In Jongen, W.M.F. and Meulenberg, M.T.G. (eds), *Innovation in agri-food systems, product quality and consumer acceptance*. Wageningen, The Netherlands: Wageningen Academic Publishers.

Frewer, L., Lassen, J., Kettlitz, B., Scholderer, J., Beekman, V. and Berdal, K.G. (2004). Societal aspects of genetically modified foods. *Food and Chemical Toxicology*, 42: 1181–93.

Frewer, L.J., Raats, M.M. and Shepherd, R. (1993). Modelling the media: the transmission of risk information in the British quality press. *IMA Journal of Mathematics Applied in Business and Industry*, 5: 235–47.

Frewer, L.J., Shepherd, R. and Sparks, P. (1994). The inter-relationship between perceived knowledge, control and risk associated with a range of food-related hazards targeted at the individual, other people and society. *Journal of Food Safety*, 14: 19–40.

Friedman, C.R., Neimann, J., Wegener, H.C. and Tauxe, R.V. (2000). Epidemiology of *Campylobacter jejuni* infections in the United States and other industrialized nations. In Nachamkin, I. and Blaser, M.J. (eds), *Campylobacter* (Second ed.) Washington, DC: American Society for Microbiology Press: 121–38.

Friedman, M. (2003). Chemistry, biochemistry and safety of acrylamide. A review. *Journal of Agricultural and Food Chemistry*, 51: 4504–26.

Friel, S. (2009). *Health equity in Australia: a policy framework based on action on the social determinants of obesity, alcohol and tobacco*. Canberra, Australia: The Australian National Preventative Health Taskforce. Accessed on 7 May 2015 at: www.health.gov.au/internet/preventativehealth/publishing.nsf/Content/0FBE20 3C1C547A82CA257529000231BF/$File/commpaper-hlth-equity-friel.pdf.

Furedi, F. (2005). *Politics of fear: beyond left and right*. London, United Kingdom: Continuum Press.

Furlong, V. (2011). Your guide to alcohol. *Australian Healthy Food Guide*. Accessed on 24 February 2015 at: www.healthyfoodguide.com.au/articles/2011/december/ your-guide-to-alcohol.

Furtado, A., Lupoi, J.S., Hoang, N.V., Healey, A., Singh, S., Simmons, B.A. and Henry, R.J. (2014). Modifying plants for biofuel and biomaterial production. *Plant Biotechnology Journal*, 12(9): 1246–58.

Gaby, A.R. (2005). Adverse effects of dietary fructose. *Alternative Medicine Review*, 10(4): 294–306.

Gahche, J., Bailey, R., Burt, V., Hughes, J., Yetley, E., Dwyer, J., Picciano, M.F., McDowell M. and Sempos, C. (2011). Dietary supplement use among U.S. adults has increased since NHANES III (1988–1994). *National Center for Health Statistics Data Brief*, 61: 1–8.

Gamboa da Costa, G., Churchwell, M.I., Hamilton, L.P., Von Tungeln, L.S., Beland, F.A., Marques, M.M. and Doerge, D.R. (2003). DNA adduct formation from acrylamide via conversion to glycidamide in adult and neonatal mice. *Chemical Research in Toxicology*, 16(10): 1328–37.

Garcia-Bailo, B., Toguri, C., Eny, K.M. and El-Sohemy, A. (2009). Genetic variation in taste and its influence on food selection. *OMICS*, 13: 69–80.

Gard, M. and Wright, J. (2005). *The Obesity Epidemic: science, morality and ideology*. London, United Kingdom: Routledge.

Gasparro, A. and Jargon, J. (2014). The problem with portions. *The Wall Street Journal*, 24 June. Accessed on 7 May 2015 at: www.wsj.com/articles/the-problem-w ith-portions-1403656205.

Gassmann, A.J., Petzold-Maxwell, J.L., Keweshan, R.S. and Dunbar, M.W. (2011). Field-evolved resistance to Bt maize by western corn rootworm. *PLoS One*, 6(7): e22629: 1–7.

Gately, I. (2008). *Drink: a cultural history of alcohol*. New York, NY: Gotham Books.

Gelatti, U., Covolo, L., Franceschini, M., Pirali, F., Tagger, A., Ribero, M.L., Trevisi, P., Martelli, C., Nardi, G. and Donato, F. (2005). Coffee consumption reduces the risk of hepatocellular carcinoma independently of its aetiology: a case-control study. *Journal of Hepatology*, 42: 528–34.

Gerhardt, K.E., Huang, X.-D., Glick, B.R. and Greenberg, B.M. (2009). Phytoremediation and rhizoremediation of organic soil contaminants: potential and challenges. *Plant Science*, 176(1): 20–30.

Gerlach, G., Herpertz, S. and Loeber, S. (2015). Personality traits and obesity: a systematic review. *Obesity Reviews,* 16(1): 32–63.

Germov, J. and Williams, L. (1996). The epidemic of dieting women: the need for a sociological approach to food and nutrition. *Appetite*, 27(2): 97–108.

Germov, J. and Williams, L. (1999). *A sociology of food and nutrition: the social appetite.* Oxford, United Kingdom: Oxford University Press.

Ghaliouqui, P. (1979). Fermented beverages in antiquity. In Gastineau, C.F., Darby, W.J. and Turner, T.B. (eds), *Fermented food beverages in nutrition.* New York, NY: Academic Press.

Giacosa, A., Barale, R., Bavaresco, L., Faliva, M.A., Gerbi, V., La Vecchia, C., Negri, E., Opizzi, A., Perna, S., Pezzotti, M. and Rondanelli, M. (2014). Mediterranean way of drinking and longevity. *Critical Reviews in Food Science and Nutrition* (Epub 10 September 2014).

Gibson, E.L. (2006). Emotional influences on food choice: sensory, physiological and psychological pathways. *Physiology & Behavior*, 89: 53–61.

Giddens, A. (1984). *The constitution of society.* Berkeley and Los Angeles, CA: University of California Press.

Giddens, A. (1990). *The consequences of modernity.* Cambridge, United Kingdom: Polity Press.

Giddens, A. ([1991]2002). *Modernity and self-identity: self and society in the late modern age.* Cambridge, United Kingdom: Polity Press in association with Basil Blackwell.

Giddens, A. (1994a) Living in a post-traditional society. In Beck, U., Giddens, A. and Lash, S. (eds), *Reflexive modernization: politics, tradition and aesthetics in the modern social order.* Cambridge, United Kingdom: Polity Press: 56–109.

Giddens, A. (1994b). *Beyond left and right.* Cambridge, United Kingdom: Polity Press.

Giddens, A. (1998). Risk society: the context of British politics. In Franklin, J. (ed.), *The politics of risk society.* Cambridge, United Kingdom: Polity Press.

Giddens, A. (1999). Risk and responsibility. *The Modern Law Review*, 62(1): 1–10.

Gifford, K. and Bernard, J.C. (2005). Influencing consumer purchase likelihood of organic food. *International Journal of Consumer Studies*, 30(2): 155–63.

Gilbert, K. and Bruszik, A. (2005). *Biodiversity and the food sector – an initial review of the extent to which biodiversity is protected through food standards in Europe.* Tilburg, The Netherlands: European Centre for Nature Conservation.

Gilbert, R.M., Marshman, J.A., Schwieder, M. and Berg, R. (1976). Caffeine content of beverages as consumed. *Canadian Medical Association Journal*, 114(3): 205–8.

Giles, E.L. and Brennan, M. (2014). Trading between healthy food, alcohol and physical activity behaviours. *BMC Public Health*, 14: 1231–42.

Gilman, S.L. (2008). *Diets and dieting: a cultural encyclopedia.* New York, NY/London, United Kingdom: Routledge.

Giskes, K., Turrell, G., Patterson, C. and Newman, B. (2002). Socio-economic differences in fruit and vegetable consumption among Australian adolescents and adults. *Public Health Nutrition*, 5: 663–9.

Giskes, K., van Lenthe, F., Avendano-Pabon, M. and Brug, J. (2011). A systematic review of environmental factors and obesogenic dietary intakes among adults: are we getting closer to understanding obesogenic environments? *Obesity Review*, 12(5): e95–e106.

Glass, R.I., Parashar, U.D. and Estes, M.K. (2009). Norovirus gastroenteritis. *New England Journal of Medicine*, 361: 1776–85.

Goldberg, D.M., Hoffman, B., Yang, J. and Soleas, G.J. (1999). Phenolic constituents, furans, and total antioxidant status of distilled spirits. *Journal of Agricultural and Food Chemistry*, 47(10): 3978–85.

Goñi, I., Díaz-Rubio, M.E. and Saura-Calixto, F. (2009). Dietary fiber in beer: content, composition, colonic fermentability, and contribution to the diet. In Preedy, V.R. (ed.), *Beer in health and disease prevention*. Burlington, MA: Elsevier: 299–307.

Goto, K., Asai, T., Hara, S., Namatame, I., Tomoda, H., Ikemoto, M. and Oku, N. (2005). Enhanced antitumour activity of xanthohumol, a diacylglycerol acyltransferas inhibitor under hypoxia. *Cancer Letters*, 219: 215–22.

Gough, B. (2007). 'Real men don't diet': an analysis of contemporary newspaper representations of men, food and health. *Social Science & Medicine*, 64(2): 326–37.

Gough, B. and Conner, M.T. (2006). Barriers to healthy eating amongst men: a qualitative analysis. *Social Science & Medicine*, 62(2): 387–95

Gould, D. (2014). Organic guarantee systems – an EC evolving landscape. In Willer, H. and Lernoud, J. (eds), *The world of organic agriculture. Statistics and emerging trends 2014*. Frick, Switzerland and Bonn, Germany: Research Institute of Organic Agriculture (FiBL), and International Federation of Organic Agriculture Movements (IFOAM).

Graham, H. (1984). Tea: the plant and its manufacture: chemistry and conception of the beverage. In Spiler, G.A. (ed.), *The methylxanthine beverages and foods: chemistry, consumption and health effects*. New York, NY: Alan R. Liss: 29–74.

Graham, H.N. (1992). Green tea composition, consumption, and polyphenol chemistry. *Preventive Medicine*, 21(3): 334–50.

Grass, J.E., Gould, L.H. and Mahon, B.E. (2013). Epidemiology of foodborne disease outbreaks caused by *Clostridium perfringens*, United States, 1998–2010. *Foodborne Pathogens and Disease*, 10(2): 131–6.

Gravani, R.B. (2009). The role of good agricultural practices in produce safety. In Fan, X., Niemira, B.A., Doona, C.J., Feeherry, F.E. and Gravani, R.B. (eds), *Microbial safety of fresh produce*. Oxford, United Kingdom: Wiley-Blackwell.

Greene, C., Dimitri, C., Lin, B.-H., McBride, W., Oberholtzer, L. and Smith, T.A. (2009). *Emerging issues in the U.S. organic industry* (Economic Information Bulletin No. EIB-55). Washington, DC: U.S. Department of Agriculture, Economic Research Service. Accessed on 7 December 2014 at: www.ers.usda.gov/publications/ eib-economic-information-bulletin/eib55.aspx.

Greenfield, L.A. (1998). *Alcohol and crime: an analysis of national data on the prevalence of alcohol involvement in crime* (Report prepared for the Assistant Attorney General's National Symposium on Alcohol Abuse and Crime). Washington, DC: US Department of Justice.

Greening, G.E. and Wolf, S. (2010). Calicivirus environmental contamination. In Hansman, G.S., Jiang, X.J. and Green, K.Y. (eds), *Caliciviruses: molecular and cellular virology*. Poole, United Kingdom: Caister Academic Press: 25–44.

Greenstone, G. (2009). The roots of evidence-based medicine. *British Columbia Medical Journal*, 51(8): 342–4.

Griffith, C.J., Worsfold, D. and Mitchell, R. (1998). Food preparation, risk communication and the consumer. *Food Control*, 9(4): 225–32.

Grigg, M., Bowman, J. and Redman, S. (1996). Disordered eating and unhealthy weight reduction practices among adolescent females. *Preventive Medicine*, 25(6): 748–56.

Grodstein, F., O'Brien, J., Kang, J.H., Dushkes, R., Cook, N.R., Okereke, O., Manson, J.E., Glynn, R.J., Buring, J.E., Gaziano, J.M. and Sesso, H.D. (2013). Long-term multivitamin supplementation and cognitive function in men. A randomized trial. *Annals of Internal Medicine*, 159: 806–14.

Groves, B. (2003). *William Banting father of the low-carbohydrate diet.* Washington, DC:TheWestonA.PriceFoundation.Accessedon5March2015at:www.westonaprice. org/know-your-fats/william-banting-father-of-the-low-carbohydrate-diet.

Gruère, G.P. and Rao, S.R. (2007). A review of international labeling policies of genetically modified food to evaluate India's proposed rule. *AgBioForum*, 10(1): 51–64.

Gu, X., Creasy, L., Kester, A. and Zeece, M. (1999). Capillary electrophoretic determination of resveratrol in wines. *Journal of Agricultural and Food Chemistry,* 47(8): 3223–27.

Guallar, E., Stranges, S., Mulrow, C., Appel, L.J. and Miller, E.R. (2013). Enough is enough: stop wasting money on vitamin and mineral supplements. *Annals of Internal Medicine*, 159(12): 850–51.

Gudorf, C.E. (2013). *Comparative religious ethics: everyday decisions for our everyday lives.* Minneapolis, MN: Fortress Press.

Guenther, H., Hoenicke, K., Biesterveld, S., Gerhard-Rieben, E. and Lantz, I. (2010). Furan in coffee: pilot studies on formation during roasting and losses during production steps and consumer handling. *Food Additives and Contaminants. Part A, Chemistry, Analysis, Control, Exposure and Risk Assessment*, 27(3): 283–90.

Guerin, K. (2014). *Where's the beef? (With vegans): a qualitative study of vegan-omnivore conflict.* Undergraduate Honors Thesis. Boulder, CO: University of Colorado.

Guerrero, R.F., García-Parrilla, M.C., Puertas, B. and Cantos-Villar, E. (2009). Wine, resveratrol and health: a review. *Natural Products Communication*, 4(5): 635–58.

Guillen, M.D., Sopelana, P. and Partearroyo, M.A. (1997). Food as a source of polycyclic aromatic carcinogens. *Reviews on Environmental Health*, 12: 133–46.

Gusfield, J.R. (1987). Passage to play: rituals of drinking time in American society. In Douglas, M. (ed.), *Constructive drinking: perspectives on drink from anthropology.* Cambridge, United Kingdom: Cambridge University Press.

Guyton, A.C. and Hall, J.E. (eds) (2001). *Textbook in medical physiology* (Tenth ed.). Philadelphia, PA: W.B. Saunders.

Hale, S. (2000). *The great American barbecue and grilling manual.* London, United Kingdom: Abacus Publishing.

Hall, C. (2007). GM technology in forestry: lessons from the GM food 'debate'. *International Journal of Biotechnology*, 9(5): 436–47.

Hall, G., Kirk, M.D., Becker, N., Gregory, J.E., Unicomb, L., Millard, G., Stafford, R. and Lalor, K. (2005). Estimating foodborne gastroenteritis, Australia. *Emerging Infectious Diseases*, 11(8): 1257–64.

Hall, H. (2014). Food myths: what science knows (and does not know) about diet and nutrition. *Skeptic*, 19(4): 10–19.

Hallman, W.K., Hebden, W.C., Aquino, H.L., Cutie, C.L. and Lang, J.T. (2003). *Public perceptions of genetically modified foods: a national study of American knowledge and opinion* (Food Policy Institute Publication RR-1003–004). New Brunswick, NJ: Rutgers University.

Hamilton, C., Adolphs, S. and Nerlich, B. (2007). The meanings of 'risk': a view from corpus linguistics. *Discourse & Society*, 18: 163–81.

Hammerstone, J.F., Lazarus, S.A. and Schmitz, H.H. (2000). Procyanidin content and variation in some commonly consumed foods. *Journal of Nutrition*, 130(8): 2086S–2092S.

Hamstra, M.R.W., Bolderdijk, J.W. and Veldstra, J.L. (2011). Everyday risk taking as a function of regulatory focus. *Journal of Research in Personality*, 45: 134–7.

Hanson, D.J. (1995). *Preventing alcohol abuse: alcohol, culture, and control*. Westport, CT: Praeger.

Harnack, L., Stang, J. and Story, M. (1999). Soft drink consumption among US children and adolescents: nutritional consequences. *Journal of American Dietetic Association*, 99: 436–41.

Haroldsen, V.M., Paulino, G., Chi-ham, C. and Bennett, A.B. (2012). Research and adoption of biotechnology strategies could improve California fruit and nut crops. *California Agriculture*, 66(2): 62–9.

Harper, G.C. and Makatouni, A. (2002). Consumer perception of organic food production and farm animal welfare. *British Food Journal*, 104: 287–99.

Harrabin, R., Coote, A. and Allen, J. (2003). *Health in the news*. London, United Kingdom: Kings Fund.

Harris, E.D. (1997). Copper. In O'Dell, B.L. and Sunde, R.A. (eds), *Handbook of nutritionally essential mineral elements*. New York, NY: Marcel Dekker: 231–73.

Harris, J.L. and Graff, S.K. (2011). Protecting children from harmful food marketing: options for local government to make a difference. *Preventing Chronic Disease*, 8(5): A92–A100.

Harris, J.L., Sarda, V., Schwartz, M.B. and Brownell, K.D. (2013). Redefining "child-directed advertising" to reduce unhealthy television food advertising. *American Journal of Preventive Medicine*, 44(4): 358–64.

Harrison, K. (2013). *The 5:2 diet book*. London, United Kingdom: Orion Publishing Group.

Harvey, P. (1994). Gender, community and confrontation: power relations in drunkenness in Ocongate (Southern Peru). In McDonald, M. (ed.), *Gender, drink and drugs*. Oxford, United Kingdom: Berg.

Haslam, D. (2007). Obesity: a medical history. *Obesity Reviews*, 8(s1): 31–6.

Haslam, D.W. and James, W.P. (2005). Obesity. *Lancet*, 366(9492): 1197–209.

Hatton, T.J. (2014). How have Europeans grown so tall? *Oxford Economic Papers*, 66 (2): 349–72.

Hawkes, C. (2013). *Promoting healthy diets through nutrition education and changes in the food environment: an international review of actions and their effectiveness*. Rome, Italy: Food and Agriculture Organization of the United Nation.

Hayashi, P.H., Barnhart, H., Fontana, R.J., Chalasani, N., Davern, T.J., Talwalkar, J.A., Reddy, K.R., Stolz, A.A., Hoofnagle, J.H. and Rockey, D.C. (2015). Reliability of causality assessment for drug, herbal and dietary supplement hepatotoxicity in the Drug-Induced Liver Injury Network (DILIN). *Liver International*, 35(5): 1623–32.

Headey, D. (2011). Turning economic growth into nutrition-sensitive growth (Conference Paper No. 6). New Delhi, India: 2020 Conference on Leveraging Agriculture for Improving Nutrition and Health, 10–12 February 2011.

Hearty, A.P., McCarthy, S.N., Kearney, J.M. and Gibney, M.J. (2007). Relationship between attitudes toward healthy eating and dietary behaviour, lifestyle and demographic factors in a representative sample of Irish adults. *Appetite*, 48: 1–11.

Heath, D.B. (1958). Drinking patterns of the Bolivian Camba. *Quarterly Journal of Studies on Alcohol*, 19(3): 491–508.

Heath, D.B. (1995). Some generalizations about alcohol and culture. In Heath, D.B. (ed.), *International handbook on alcohol and culture*. Westport, CT: Greenwood Press: 348–61.

Heckman, M.A., Weil, J. and Gonzalez de Mejia, E. (2010). Caffeine (1, 3, 7-trimethylxanthine) in foods: a comprehensive review on consumption, functionality, safety, and regulatory matters. *Journal of Food Science*, 75(3): R77–R87.

Heimer, K.A., Hart, A.M., Martin, L.G. and Rubio-Wallace, S. (2009). Examining the evidence for the use of vitamin C in the prophylaxis and treatment of the common cold. *Journal of the American Academy of Nurse Practitioners*, 21(5): 295–300.

Hensrud, D.D., Weinsier, R.L., Darnell, B.E. and Hunter, G.R. (1994). A prospective study of weight maintenance in obese participants reduced to normal body weight without weight-loss training. *American Journal for Clinical Nutrition*, 60: 688–94.

Hering-Hanit, R. and Gadoth, N. (2003). Caffeine-induced headache in children and adolescents. *Cephalalgia*, 23(5): 332–5.

Herman, C.P., Roth, D.A. and Polivy, J. (2003). Effects of the presence of others on food intake: a normative interpretation. *Psychological Bulletin*, 129: 873–86.

Herman, E.M., Helm, R.M., Jung, R. and Kinney, A.J. (2003). Genetic modification removes an immunodominant allergen from soybean. *Plant Physiology*, 132(1): 36–43.

Heron, M.P. (2007). *Deaths: leading causes for 2004* (National vital statistics reports, 56[5]). Hyattsville, MD: National Center for Health Statistics.

Hess, A. (1986). The origins of McDonald's golden arches. *Journal of the Society of Architectural Historians*, 45(1): 60–67.

Hicks, M.B., Hsieh, Y-H.P. and Bell, L.N. (1996). Tea preparation and its influence on methylxanthine concentration. *Food Research International*, 29(3–4): 325–30.

Hilgartner, S. (1990). The dominant view of popularisation: conceptual problems, political issues. *Social Studies of Science*, 20: 519–39.

Hjelmar, U. (2011). Consumers' purchase of organic food products. A matter of convenience and reflexive practices. *Appetite*, 56: 336–44.

Hogan, M.J. and Strasburger, V.C. (2008). Body image, eating disorders, and the media. *Adolescent Medicine*, 19: 521–46.

Hogervorst, J.G.F., Baars, B.J., Schouten, L.J., Konings, E.J.M., Goldbohm, R.A. and van den Brandt, P.A. (2010). The carcinogenicity of dietary acrylamide intake: a comparative discussion of epidemiological and experimental animal research. *Critical Reviews in Toxicology*, 40: 485–512.

Holick, M.F. (2004). Sunlight and vitamin D for bone health and prevention of autoimmune diseases, cancers, and cardiovascular disease. *American Journal of Clinical Nutrition*, 80(6 Suppl): 1678S–1688S.

Holm, L. and Kildevang, H. (1996). Consumers' views on food quality. A qualitative interview study. *Appetite*, 27: 1–14.

Hong, F. (2004). History of medicine in China. *McGill Journal of Medicine*, 8(1): 74–84.

Honkanen, P., Verplanken, B. and Olsen, S.O. (2006). Ethical values and motives driving organic food choice. *Journal of Consumer Behavior*, 5: 420–30.

Horsch, R.B., Fraley, R.T., Rogers, S.G., Sanders, P.R., Lloyd, A. and Hoffmann, N. (1984). Inheritance of functional foreign genes in plants. *Science*, 223: 496–8.

Howard, S., Adams, J. and White, M. (2012). Nutritional content of supermarket ready meals and recipes by television chefs in the United Kingdom: cross sectional study. *BMJ*, 345: e7607–e7617.

Howarth, A. (2012). *Discursive intersections of newspapers and policy elites: a case study of genetically modified food in Britain, 1996–2000*. London, United Kingdom: London School of Economics and Political Science.

Huang, H.Y., Caballero, B., Chang, S., Alberg, A.J., Semba, R.D., Schneyer, C.R., Wilson, R.F., Cheng, T.Y., Vassy, J., Prokopowicz, G., Barnes, G.J. II and Bass, E.B. (2006). The efficacy and safety of multivitamin and mineral supplement use to prevent cancer and chronic disease in adults: a systematic review for a National Institutes of Health state-of-the-science conference. *Annals of Internal Medicine*, 145: 372–85.

Huang, R., Moudon, A.V., Cook, A.J. and Drewnowski, A. (2014). The spatial clustering of obesity: does the built environment matter? *Journal of Human Nutrition and Dietetics* (Epublish): 1–9.

Huber, B. and Schmid, O. (2014). Standards and regulations. In Willer, H. and Lernoud, J. (eds), *The world of organic agriculture. statistics and emerging trends 2014*. Frick, Switzerland and Bonn, Germany: Research Institute of Organic Agriculture (FiBL), and International Federation of Organic Agriculture Movements (IFOAM).

Huber, M., de Vijver, L.P.L.V., Parmentier, H., Savelkoul, H., Coulier, L., Wopereis, S., Verheij, E., van der Greef, J., Nierop, D. and Hoogenboom, R.A.P. (2010). Effects of organically and conventionally produced feed on biomarkers of health in a chicken model. *British Journal of Nutrition*, 103(5): 663–76.

Hughner, R.S., McDonagh, P., Prothero, A., Schultz, C.J. and Stanton, J. (2007). Who are organic food consumers? A compilation and review of why people purchase organic food. *Journal of Consumer Behavior*, 6: 94–110.

Humphrey, T., O'Brien, S. and Madsen, M. (2007). Campylobacters as zoonotic pathogens: a food production perspective. *International Journal of Food Microbiology*, 117(3): 237–57.

Hunt, L. (2004). Factors determining the public understanding of GM technologies. *AgBiotechNet*, 6(128): 1–8.

Hunter, J.E., Zhang, J., Kris-Etherton, P.M. (2010). Cardiovascular disease risk of dietary stearic acid compared with trans, other saturated, and unsaturated fatty acids: a systematic review. *American Journal of Clinical Nutrition*, 91(1): 46–63.

Hussain, K. and El-Serag, H.B. (2009). Epidemiology, screening, diagnosis and treatment of hepatocellular carcinoma. *Minerva Gastroenterologica e Dietologica*, 55(2): 123–38.

Imamura, F., Micha, R., Khatibzadeh, S., Fahimi, S., Shi, P., Powles, J. and Mozaffarian, D. (2015). Dietary quality among men and women in 187 countries in 1990 and 2010: a systematic assessment. *Lancet Glob Health*, 3: e132–42.

Inoue, M., Yoshimi, I., Sobue, T. and Tsugane, S. (2005). Influence of coffee drinking on subsequent risk of hepatocellular carcinoma: a prospective study in Japan. *Journal of the National Cancer Institute*, 97: 293–300.

Institute of Medicine (1997). *Dietary Reference Intakes: Calcium, Phosphorus, Magnesium, Vitamin D and Fluoride*. Washington, DC: National Academy Press.

Institute of Medicine (1998). *Dietary reference intakes for thiamine, riboflavin, niacin, vitamin B6, folate, vitamin B12, pantothenic acid, biotin, and choline*. Washington, DC: National Academy Press.

Institute of Medicine (2000). *Dietary Reference Intakes: vitamin C, vitamin E, selenium, and carotenoids*. Washington, DC: National Academy Press.

Institute of Medicine (2001). *Dietary Reference Intakes for vitamin A, vitamin K, arsenic, boron, chromium, copper, iodine, iron, manganese, molybdenum, nickel, silicon, vanadium, and zinc*. Washington, DC: National Academy Press.

International Agency for Research on Cancer [IARC] (1973). *Certain polycyclic aromatic hydrocarbons and heterocyclic compounds. IARC Monographs on the evaluation of the carcinogenic risk of chemicals to humans*, 3.

International Agency for Research on Cancer [IARC] (1978). *Some N-nitroso compounds. IARC Monographs on the evaluation of the carcinogenic risk of chemicals to humans*, 17.

International Agency for Research on Cancer [IARC] (1987). *Overall evaluation of carcinogenicity: An updating of IARC Monographs volumes 1 to 42. IARC Monographs on the evaluation of carcinogenic risks to humans*, Supplement 7.

International Agency for Research on Cancer [IARC] (1993). Heterocyclic aromatic amines. In *Some Naturally Occurring Substances: Food Items and Constituents, Heterocyclic Aromatic Amines and Mycotoxins. IARC Monographs on the evaluation of carcinogenic risks to humans*, 56: 163–242.

International Agency for Research on Cancer [IARC] (1994). Acrylamide. In *Some industrial chemicals. Summary of data reported and evaluation. IARC Monographs on the evaluation of carcinogenic risks to humans*, 60: 389–91.

International Agency for Research on Cancer [IARC] (1995). Furan. In *Dry cleaning, some chlorinated solvents and other industrial chemicals. IARC Monographs on the evaluation of carcinogenic risks to humans*, 63: 394–407.

International Agency for Research on Cancer [IARC] (2003). *Fruit and Vegetables. IARC handbooks of cancer prevention*, 8: 1–368. Lyon, France: International Agency for Research on Cancer.

International Agency for Research on Cancer [IARC] (2010). *Alcohol consumption and ethyl carbamate. IARC Monographs on the Evaluation of Carcinogenic Risks to Humans*, 96.

International Assessment of Agricultural Knowledge, Science and Technology for Development [IAASTD] (2009). *Agriculture at a crossroads. Synthesis report.* Washington, DC: Island Press.

International Federation of Organic Agriculture Movements [IFOAM] (2005). Principles of organic agriculture. Accessed on 12 January 2013 at: www.ifoam.org/sites/default/files/ifoam_poa.pdf.

International Programme on Chemical Safety [IPCS]. (1998). *Selected non-heterocyclic polycyclic aromatic hydrocarbons* (Environmental Health Criteria No. 202). Geneva, Switzerland: International Programme on Chemical Safety, World Health Organization.

International Programme on Chemical Safety [IPCS] (2002). *Global assessment of the state-of-the-science of endocrine disruptors*. Geneva, Switzerland: World Health Organization.

International Programme on Chemical Safety [IPCS] (2004). *IPCS risk assessment terminology*. Geneva, Switzerland: World Health Organization.

Isenhour, C. (2014). Trading fat for forests: on palm oil, tropical forest conservation, and rational consumption. *Conservation and Society*, 12(3): 257–67.

Jabed, A., Wagner, S., McCracken, J., Wells, D.N. and Laible, G. (2012). Targeted microRNA expression in dairy cattle directs production of β-lactoglobulin-free, high-casein milk. *PNAS*, 109(42): 16811–16.

Jabs, J. and Devine, C.M. (2006). Time scarcity and food choices: an overview. *Appetite*, 47(2): 196–204.

Jabs, J., Devine, C.M., Bisogni, C.A., Farrell, T.J., Jastran, M. and Wethington, E. (2007). Trying to find the quickest way: employed mothers' constructions of time for food. *Journal of Nutrition Education and Behavior*, 39(1): 18–25.

Jackson, P. (2010). Food stories: consumption in an age of anxiety. *Cultural Geographies*, 17: 147–65.

Jackson, P., Watson, M. and Piper, N. (2013). Locating anxiety in the social: the cultural mediation of food fears. *European Journal of Cultural Studies*, 16: 24–42.

Jacob, R.A. and Sotoudeh, G. (2002). Vitamin C function and status in chronic disease. *Nutrition in Clinical Care*, 5(2): 66–74.

James, C. (2010). *Global status of commercialized biotech/GM crops: 2010* (ISAAA Brief 42). Ithaca, NY: ISAAA.

James, C. (2012). *Global status of commercialized biotech/GM crops: 2012* (ISAAA Brief 44). Ithaca, NY: ISAAA.

James, J., Thomas, P., Cavan, D. and Kerr, D. (2004). Preventing childhood obesity by reducing consumption of carbonated drinks: cluster randomised controlled trial. *BMJ*, 328: 1237–43.

James, J.E. (1997). *Understanding caffeine: a biobehavioral analysis*. Thousand Oaks, CA: Sage Publications.

Janssen, M. and Hamm, U. (2012). The mandatory EU logo for organic food: consumer perceptions. *British Food Journal*, 114(3): 335–52.

Jeffery, R.W. and French, S.A. (1998). Epidemic obesity in the United States: are fast foods and television viewing contributing? *American Journal of Public Health*, 88(2): 277–80.

Jenkins, S. (2013). Genetic engineering and seed banks: impacts on global crop diversity. *Macquarie Journal of International and Comparative Environmental Law*, 9(1): 67–77.

Jennings, A.A. (2012). Worldwide regulatory guidance values for surface soil exposure to carcinogenic or mutagenic polycyclic aromatic hydrocarbons. *Journal of Environmental Management*, (Epub) 28 June 2012.

Jevšnik, M., Hlebec, V. and Raspor, P. (2008). Consumers' awareness of food safety from shopping to eating. *Food Control*, 19: 737–45.

Joghataie, M.T., Roghani, M., Negahdar, F. and Hashemi, L. (2004). Protective effect of caffeine against neurodegeneration in a model of Parkinson's disease in rat: behavioral and histochemical evidence. *Parkinsonism & Related Disorders*, 10: 465–8.

Johansson, E., Hussain, A., Kuktaite, R., Andersson, S.C. and Olsson, M.E. (2014). Contribution of organically grown crops to human health. *International Journal of Environmental Research and Public Health*, 11: 3870–93.

Johansson, L., Thelle, D.S., Solvoll, K., Bjorneboe, G.E. and Drevon, C.A. (1999). Healthy dietary habits in relation to social determinants and lifestyle factors. *British Journal of Nutrition*, 81: 211–20.

Johnson, S.R., Strom, S. and Grillo, K. (2008). *Quantification of the impacts on US agriculture of biotechnology-derived crops planted in 2006*. Washington, DC: National Center for Food and Agricultural Policy. Accessed on 1 July 2015 at: www.ncfap. org./documents/2007biotech_report/Quantification_of_the_Impacts_on_US_ Agriculture_of_Biotechnology_Executive_Summary.pdf.

Johnston, K.L. and White, K.M. (2004). Beliefs underlying binge-drinking in young female undergraduate students: a theory of planned behaviour perspective. *Youth Studies Australia*, 23(2): 22–30.

Jonas, D.A., Elmadfa, I., Engel, K-H., Heller, K.J., Kozianowski, G., König, A., Müller, D., Narbonne, J.F., Wackernagel, W. and Kleiner, J, (2001). Safety considerations of DNA in food. *Annals of Nutrition & Metabolism*, 45: 235–54.

Jones, M., Freeth, E.C., Hennessy-Priest, K. and Costa, R.J.S. (2013). A systematic cross-sectional analysis of British based celebrity chefs' recipes: is there cause for public health concern? *Food and Public Health*, 3(2): 100–10.

Joosten, M.M., Chiuve, S.E., Mukamal, K.J., Hu, F.B., Hendriks, H.F.J. and Rimm, E.B. (2011). Changes in alcohol consumption and subsequent risk of type 2 diabetes in men. *Diabetes*, 60(1): 74–9.

Kamphuis, C.B.M., van Lenthe, F.J., Giskes, K., Brug, J. and Mackenbach, J.P. (2007). Perceived environmental determinants of physical activity and fruit and vegetable consumption among low and high socioeconomic groups in the Netherlands. *Health Place*, 13(2): 493–503.

Kang, J.X. (2005). From fat to fat-1: a tale of omega-3 fatty acids. *The Journal of Membrane Biology*, 206(2): 165–72.

Kant, A.K. (2000). Consumption of energy-dense, nutrient-poor foods by adult Americans: nutritional and health implications. The third National Health and Nutrition Examination Survey, 1988–1994. *American Journal of Clinical Nutrition*, 72(4): 929–36.

Kantiani, L., Llorca, M., Sanchís, J., Farré, M. and Barceló, D. (2010). Emerging food contaminants: a review. *Analytical and Bioanalytical Chemistry*, 398 (6): 2413–27.

Kaptan, G., Fischer, A.R.H. and Frewer, L.J. (2014). *Extrapolating understanding of food risk perceptions to emerging food safety cases*. Cambridge, MA: Harvard University Workshop. Accessed on 26 January 2016 at: https://cdn1.sph.harvard. edu/wp-content/uploads/sites/1273/2014/02/Risk-Perception-Kaptan-et-al.pdf.

Kasperson, R.E. (1992). The social amplification of risk: progress in developing an integrative framework in social theories of risk. In Krimsky, S. and Golding, D. (eds), *Social theories of risk*. Santa Barbara, CA: Praeger: 53–178.

Katz, S.H. and Voigt, M.M. (1987). Bread and beer: the early use of cereals in the human diet. *Expedition*, 28: 23–34.

Keast, R.S.J., Swinburn, B.A., Sayompark, D., Whitelock, S. and Riddell, L.J. (2015). Caffeine increases sugar-sweetened beverage consumption in a free-living population: a randomised controlled trial. *British Journal of Nutrition*, 113: 366–71.

Kechidi, M. (2005). La théorie de la structuration. *Relations Industrielles/Industrial Relations*, 60(2): 348–69.

Kelly, J.P., Kaufman, D.W., Koff, R.S., Laszlo, A., Wilholm, B.E. and Shapiro, S. (1995). Alcohol consumption and the risk of major upper gastrointestinal bleeding. *American Journal of Gastroenterology*, 90(7): 1058–64.

Kennedy, J.A., Matthews, M.A. and Waterhouse, A.L. (2002). Effect of maturity and vine water status on grape skin and wine flavonoids. *American Journal of Enology and Viticulture*, 53(4): 268–74.

Kessler, A. and Baldwin, I.T. (2002). Plant responses to insect herbivory: the emerging molecular analysis. *Annual Review of Plant Physiology and Plant Molecular Biology*, 53: 299–328.

Ketchum, C. (2005). The essence of cooking shows. How the food network constructs consumer fantasies. *Journal of Communication Inquiry*, 29(3): 217–34.

Key, S., Ma, J.K. and Drake, P.M. (2008). Genetically modified plants and human health. *Journal of the Royal Society of Medicine*, 101(6): 290–98.

Khan, E.U. and Liu, J-H. (2009). Plant biotechnological approaches for the production and commercialization of transgenic crops. *Biotechnology & Biotechnological Equipment*, 23(3): 1281–8.

Kher, S.V., de Jonge, J., Wentholt, M.T.A., Deliza, R., Cunha de Andrade, J., Cnossen, H.J., Luijckx, N.B.L. and Frewer, L.J. (2013). Consumer perceptions of risks of chemical and microbiological contaminants associated with food chains: a cross-national study. *International Journal of Consumer Studies*, 37(1): 73–83.

Kiefer, I., Rathmanner, T. and Kunze, M. (2005). Eating and dieting differences in men and women. *Journal of Men's Health and Gender*, 2(2): 194–201.

Kimmel, C.A., Kimmel, G.L., White, C.G., Grafton, T.F., Young, J.F. and Nelson C.J. (1984). Blood flow changes and conceptual development in pregnant rats in response to caffeine. *Fundamental and Applied Toxicology*, 4: 240–47.

Kirchmann, H., Thorvaldsson, G., Bergström, L., Gerzabek, M., Andrén, O., Eriksson, L.-O. and Winninge, M. (2008). Fundamentals of organic agriculture – past and present. In Kirchmann, H. and Bergström, L. (eds), *Organic crop production – ambitions and limitations*. Dordrecht, The Netherlands: Springer: 13–38.

Kitzinger, J. (1999). Researching risk and the media. *Health, Risk and Society*, 1(1): 55–69.

Kizil, M., Oz, F. and Besler, H.T. (2011). A review on the formation of carcinogenic/ mutagenic heterocyclic aromatic amines. *Journal of Food Processing and Technology*, 2: 120–24.

Kjærnes, U., Harvey, M. and Warde, A. (2007). *Trust in food: a comparative and institutional analysis*. Hampshire, United Kingdom: Palgrave Macmillan.

Kjeldgaard, D. and Ostberg, J. (2007). Coffee grounds and the global cup: glocal consumer culture in Scandinavia. *Consumption, Markets and Culture*, 10(2): 175–87.

Kleiman, S., Ng, S.W. and Popkin, B. (2011). Drinking to our health: can beverage companies cut calories while maintaining profits? *Obesity Review*, 13: 258–74.

Klein, E.A., Thompson, I.M. Jr, Tangen, C.M., Crowley, J.J., Lucia, M.S., Goodman, P.J., Minasian, L.M., Ford, L.G., Parnes, H.L., Gaziano, J.M., Karp, D.D., Lieber, M.M., Walther, P.J., Klotz, L., Parsons, J.K., Chin, J.L., Darke, A.K., Lippman, S.M., Goodman, G.E., Meyskens, F.L. Jr, and Baker, L.H. (2011). Vitamin E and the risk of prostate cancer: the selenium and vitamin E cancer prevention trial (SELECT). *JAMA*, 306(14): 1549–56.

Klein, G.B. (2001). *The world's first insurance company*. Dallas, TX: International Risk Management Institute (IRMI). Accessed on 15 February 2011 at: www.irmi.com/ expert/articles/2001/klein07.aspx.

Klein, H. (1991). Cultural determinants of alcohol use in the United States. In Pittman, D.J. and White, H.R. (eds), *Society, culture and drinking patterns reexamined*. New Brunswick, Canada: Rutgers Center of Alcohol Studies.

Klein, S. (2013). Does grilling cause cancer? How to make grilling healthier and safer. *Huffington Post*, 24 May. Accessed on 9 July 2015 at: www.huffingtonpost. com/2013/05/24/does-grilling-cause-cance_n_3326194.html.

Knight, C.A., Knight, I. and Mitchell, D.C. (2006). Beverage caffeine intakes in young children in Canada and the US. *Canadian Journal of Dietetic Practice and Research*, 67(2): 96–9.

Knize, M.G. and Felton, J.S. (2005). Formation and human risk of carcinogenic heterocyclic amines formed from natural precursors in meat. *Nutrition Reviews*, 63: 158–65.

Knize, M.G., Salmon, C.P., Pais, P. and Felton, J.S. (1999). Food heating and the formation of heterocyclic aromatic amine and polycyclic aromatic hydrocarbon mutagens/carcinogens. *Advances in Experimental Medicine and Biology*, 459: 179–93.

Kolbert, E. (2014). Stone soup. How the Paleolithic life style got trendy. Annals of Alimentation. *The New Yorker*, 28 July. Accessed on 15 May 2015 at: www. newyorker.com/magazine/2014/07/28/stone-soup.

Komirenko, Z., Veeman, M.M. and Unterschultz, J.R. (2010). Do Canadian consumers have concerns about genetically modified animal feeds? *AgBioForum*, 13(3): 242–50.

Kondo, K. (2004). Beer and health: preventive effects of beer components on lifestyle-related diseases. *Biofactors*, 22: 303–10.

Kopicki, A. (2013). Strong support for labeling modified foods. *International New York Times*, 27 July. Accessed on 6 November 2014 at: www.nytimes.com/2013/07/28/science/strong-support-for-labeling-modified-foods.html.

Kratky, R. and Buiatti, S. (2008). Beer in health and disease prevention. In Preedy, V.R. (ed.), *The chemical nature of flavor in beer*. London, United Kingdom: Elsevier Science & Technology: 73–84.

Krause, M., Josefsen, M.H., Lund, M., Jacobsen, N.R., Brorsen, L., Moos, M., Stockmarr, A. and Hoorfar, J. (2006). Comparative, collaborative, and on-site validation of a Taqman PCR method as a tool for certified production of fresh, *Campylobacter*-free chickens. *Applied and Environmental Microbiology*, 72(8): 5463–8.

Kuiper, H.A., Kleter, G.A., Noteburn, H.P.J.M. and Kok, E.J. (2001). Assessment of the food safety issues related to genetically modified foods. *The Plant Journal*, 27: 503–28.

Kulnik, D. and Elmadfa, I. (2008). Assessment of the nutritional situation of elderly nursing home residents in Vienna. *Annals of Nutrition and Metabolism*, 52 (Suppl 1): 51–3.

Kumar, G.B.S., Ganapathi, T.R., Revathi, C.J., Srinivas, L. and Bapat, V.A. (2005). Expression of hepatitis B surface antigen in transgenic banana plants. *Planta*, 222(3): 484–93.

Kundakovic, M. and Champagne, F.A. (2011). Epigenetic perspective on the developmental effects of bisphenol A. *Brain, Behavior and Immunity*, 25(6): 1084–93.

Kurtz, E. (2013). *Not God: a history of alcoholics anonymous*. Center City, MI: Hazelden Publishing.

Kushi, L.H., Doyle, C., McCullough, M., Rock, C.L., Demark-Wahnefried, W., Bandera, E.V., Gapstur, S., Patel, A.V., Andrews, K. and Gansler, T. (2012). American Cancer Society guidelines on nutrition and physical activity for cancer prevention. *A Cancer Journal for Clinicians*, 62(1): 30–67.

Kyle, U.G., Bosaeus, I., De Lorenzo, A.D., Deurenberg, P., Elia, M., Gómez, J.M., Heitmann, B.L., Kent-Smith, L., Melchior, J-C., Pirlich, M., Scharfetter, H., Schols, A.M.W.J. and Pichard, C. (2004). Bioelectrical impedance analysis – part I: review of principles and methods. *Clinical Nutrition*, 23(5): 1226–43.

Laaksonen, M., Prattala, R., Helasoja, V., Uutela, A. and Lahelma, E. (2003). Income and health behaviours. Evidence from monitoring surveys among Finnish adults. *Journal of Epidemiology and Community Health*, 57: 711–17.

Lachenmeier, D.W., Ganss, S., Rychlak, B., Rehm, J., Sulkowska, U., Skiba, M. and Zatonski, W. (2009a). Association between quality of cheap and unrecorded alcohol products and public health consequences in Poland. *Alcoholism, Clinical and Experimental Research*, 33(10): 1757–69.

Lachenmeier, D.W., Leitz, J., Schoeberl, K., Kuballa, T., Straub, I. and Rehm, J. (2011). Quality of illegally and informally produced alcohol in Europe: results from the AMPHORA project. *Adicciones*, 23(2): 133–40.

Lachenmeier, D.W., Lima, M.C., Nóbrega, I.C., Pereira, J.A., Kerr-Corrêa, F., Kanteres, F. and Rhem, J. (2010). Cancer risk assessment of ethyl carbamate in alcoholic beverages from Brazil with special consideration to the spirits cachaça and tiquira. *BMC Cancer*, 10: 266–81.

Lachenmeier, D.W., Rehm, J. and Gmel, G. (2007). Surrogate alcohol: what do we know and where do we go? *Alcohol*, 31(10): 1613–24.

Lachenmeier, D.W., Sarsh, B. and Rehm, J. (2009b). The composition of alcohol products from markets in Lithuania and Hungary, and potential health consequences: a pilot study. *Alcoholism, Clinical and Experimental Research*, 44(1): 93–102.

Lachenmeier, D.W., Schehl, B., Kuballa T., Frank, W. and Senn, T. (2005). Retrospective trends and current status of ethyl carbamate in German stone-fruit sprits. *Food Additives and Contaminants*, 22: 397–405.

Lairon, D. (2009). Nutritional quality and safety of organic food. A review. *Agronomy for Sustainable Development*, 30: 33–4.

Lamers, Y. (2011). Folate recommendations for pregnancy, lactation, and infancy. *Annals of Nutrition and Metabolism*, 59(1): 32–7.

Lampel, K.A., Al-Khaldi, S. and Cahill, S.M. (eds) (2012). *Bad bug book, foodborne pathogenic microorganisms and natural toxins* (Second ed.). Silver Springs, MD: Food and Drug Administration. Accessed on 24 November 2004 at: www.fda.gov/downloads/Food/FoodborneIllnessContaminants/UCM297627.pdf.

Lane, S. and Bruhn, C.G. (1991). *Food safety: consumer concerns and consumer behaviour* (Working Paper No. 593). Berkeley, CA: California Agricultural Experiment Station, University of California.

Lappalainen, R., Saba, A., Holm, L., Mykkanen, H., Gibney, M.J. and Moles, A. (1997). Difficulties in trying to eat healthier: descriptive analysis of perceived barriers for healthy eating. *European Journal of Clinical Nutrition*, 51(S2): S36–S40.

Lara, D.R. (2010). Caffeine, mental health, and psychiatric disorders. *Journal of Alzheimer's Disease*, 20(Suppl) 1: S239–S248.

Lash, S. (1994). Reflexivity and its doubles: structure, aesthetics, community. In Beck, U., Giddens, A. and Lash, S. (eds), *Reflexive modernization, politics, tradition and aesthetics in the modern social order*. Cambridge, United Kingdom: Polity Press: 110–73.

Lash, S. ([2000] 2007). Risk culture. In Adam, B., Beck, U. and van Loon, J. (eds), *The risk society and beyond*. London, United Kingdom: Thousand Oaks: 47–62.

Latour, B. (1995). *Wir sind nie modern gewesen: versuch einer symmetrischen Anthropologie*. Berlin, Germany: Akademie Verlag.

Latour, B. (1999). *Pandora's hope: essays on the reality of science studies*. Cambridge, MA: Harvard University Press.

Latruffe, N. and Rifler, J.P. (2013). Bioactive polyphenols from grapes and wine emphasized with resveratrol. *Current Pharmaceutical Design*, 19(34): 6053–63.

Lauridsen, C., Young, C., Halekoh, U., Bügel, S.H., Brandt, K., Christensen, L.P. and Jorgensen, H. (2008). Rats show differences in some biomarkers of health when eating diets based on ingredients produced with three different cultivation strategies. *Journal of the Science of Food and Agriculture*, 88(4): 720–32.

Lawrence, R.G., Lyons, K. and Wallington, T. (eds) (2009). *Food security, nutrition and sustainability*. Stirling, VA: Penguin.

Lawrence, L. (2004). *How big media uses technology and the law to lock down culture and control creativity*. New York, NY: Penguin Group.

Lechner, L., Brug, J., De Vries, H. (1997). Misconceptions of fruit and vegetable consumption: differences between objective and subjective estimation of intake. *Journal of Nutrition Education*, 29: 313–20.

Lee, H. (2013). *The making of the obesity epidemic – how food activism led public health astray.* Oakland, CA: The Breakthrough Institute. Accessed on 7 May 2015 at: thebreakthrough.org/index.php/journal/past-issues/issue-3/the-making-of-the-obesity-epidemic.

Lee, J. (2015). Labels to show country of origin on food following frozen berry hepatitis A outbreak. *Sydney Morning Herald* 22 July, p. 9. Accessed on 22 July 2015 at: www.smh.com.au/federal-politics/political-news/labels-to-show-country-of-origin-on-food-following-frozen-berry-hepatitis-a-outbreak-20150721-gih1g9.html.

Lee, K.W., Lee, H.J., Surh, Y-J. and Lee, C.Y. (2003). Vitamin C and cancer chemoprevention: reappraisal. *American Journal of Clinical Nutrition*, 78(6): 1074–8.

Lemaux, P.G. (2008). Genetically engineered plants and foods: a scientist's analysis of the issues (Part I). *Annual Review of Plant Biology*, 59: 771–812.

Lentzos, F. and Rose, N. (2009). Governing insecurity: contingency planning, protection, resilience. *Economy and Society*, 38(2): 230–54.

Leonard, K. (2001). Domestic violence and alcohol: what is known and what do we need to know to encourage environmental interventions? *Journal of Substance Use*, 6(4): 235–47.

Lesher, S.D.H. and Lee, Y.T.M. (1989). Acute pancreatitis in a military hospital. *Military Medicine*, 154(11): 559–64.

Levidow, L., Murphy, J. and Carr, S. (2007). Recasting "substantial equivalence": transatlantic governance of GM food. *Science, Technology and Human Values*, 32(1): 26–64.

Levine, A.S., Kotz, C.M. and Gosnell, B.A. (2003). Sugars and fats: the neurobiology of preference. *Journal of Nutrition*, 133(3): 831S–834S.

Li, F., Gong, Q., Dong, H. and Shi, J. (2012). Resveratrol, a neuroprotective supplement for Alzheimer's disease. *Current Pharmaceutical Design*, 18(1): 27–33.

Lianou, A. and Sofos, J.N. (2007). A review of the incidence and transmission of *Listeria monocytogenes* in ready-to-eat products in retail and food service environments. *Journal of Food Protection*, 70(9): 2172–98.

Lichtenstein, A. and Ludwig, D. (2010). Bring back home economics education. *Journal of the American Medical Association*, 303(18): 1857–8.

Lichtenstein, A.H., Appel, L.J., Brands, M., Carnethon, M., Daniels, S., Franch, H.A., Franklin, B., Kris-Etherton, P., Harris, W.S., Howard, B., Karanja, N., Lefevre, M., Rudel, L., Sacks, F., Van Horn, L., Winston, M. and Wylie-Rosett, J. (2006). Diet and lifestyle recommendations revision 2006. A scientific statement from the American Heart Association Nutrition Committee. *Circulation*, 114: 82–96.

Lichtenstein, A.H. and Russell, R.M. (2005). Essential nutrients: food or supplements? Where should the emphasis be? *JAMA*, 294(3): 351–8.

Lieber, C.S. (1998). Hepatic and other medical disorders of alcoholism: from pathogenesis to treatment. *Journal of Studies on Alcohol*, 59: 9–25.

Lijinsky, W. (1991). The formation and occurrence of polynuclear aromatic hydrocarbons associated with food. *Mutation Research*, 259: 251–61.

Lijinsky, W. and Ross, A.E. (1967). Production of carcinogenic polynuclear hydrocarbons in the cooking of food. *Food and Cosmetics Toxicology*, 5: 343–7.

Lim, S.S., Vos, T., Flaxman, A.D., Danaei, G., Shibuya, K., Adair-Rohani, H., AlMazroa, M.A. *et al.* (2012). A comparative risk assessment of burden of disease and injury attributable to 67 risk factors and risk factor clusters in 21 regions, 1990–2010: a systematic analysis for the Global Burden of Disease Study 2010. *Lancet*, 380: 2224–60.

Lima, G.P.P. and Vianello, F. (2011). Review on the main differences between organic and conventional plant-based foods. *International Journal of Food Science & Technology*, 46 (1): 1–13.

Lin, J.S., O'Connor, E., Rossom, R.C., Perdue, L.A. and Eckstrom, E. (2013). Screening for cognitive impairment in older adults: a systematic review for the U.S. Preventive Services Task Force. *Annals of Internal Medicine*, 159: 601–12.

Lindsay, J.O. (2010). Healthy living guidelines and the disconnect with everyday life. *Critical Public Health*, 20(4): 475–87.

Lindtner, O., Ehlscheid, N., Berg, K., Blume, K., Dusemund, B., Ehlers, A., Niemann, B., Rüdiger, T., Heinemeyer, G. and Greiner, M. (2013). *Anlassbezogene Befragung von Hochverzehrern von Energy-Drinks.* Berlin, Germany: Bundesinstitut für Risikobewertung.

Lineback, D.R., Coughlin, J.R. and Stadler, R.H. (2012). Acrylamide in foods: a review of the science and future considerations. *Annual Review of Food Science and Technology*, 3: 15–35.

Lineback, D.R. and Stadler, R.H. (2008). Introduction to food process toxicants. In Stadler, R.H. and Lineback, D.R. (eds), *Process-induced food toxicants: occurrence, formation, mitigation, and health risks.* Hoboken, NJ: John Wiley & Sons.

Lipworth, L., Sonderman, J.S., Tarone, R.E. and McLaughlin, J.K. (2012). Review of epidemiologic studies of dietary acrylamide intake and the risk of cancer. *European Journal of Cancer Prevention*, 21: 375–86.

Liu, B.L., Zhang, X., Zhang, W. and Zhen, H.N. (2007). New enlightenment of French Paradox: resveratrol's potential for cancer chemoprevention and anti-cancer therapy. *Cancer biology & Therapy*, 6(12): 1833–6.

Liu, C., Zhao, M., Sun, W. and Ren, J. (2013). Effects of high hydrostatic pressure treatments on haemagglutination activity and structural conformations of phytohemagglutinin from red kidney bean (*Phaseolus vulgaris*). *Food Chemistry*, 136(3–4): 1358–63.

Liu, M., Hansen, P.E., Wang, G., Qiu, L., Dong, J., Yin, H., Qian, Z., Yang, M. and Miao, J. (2015). Pharmacological profile of xanthohumol, a prenylated flavonoid from hops (*Humulus lupulus*). *Molecules*, 20: 754–79.

Lofstedt, R.E. and Frewer, L. (eds) (1998). *The Earthscan Reader in risk and modern society.* London, United Kingdom: Earthscan Publications.

Lopez-Garcia, E., van Dam, R.M., Li, T.Y., Rodriguez-Artalejo, F. and Hu, F.B. (2008). The relationship of coffee consumption with mortality. *Annals of Internal Medicine*, 148: 904–14.

Lopman, B.A., Reacher, M.H., Vipond, I.B., Sarangi, J. and Brown, D.W. (2004). Clinical manifestation of norovirus gastroenteritis in health care settings. *Clinical Infectious Diseases*, 39: 318–24.

Loureiro, L.L., McCluskey, J.J. and Mittelhammer, R.C. (2001). Assessing consumer preferences for organic, eco-labeled, and regular apples. *Journal of Agricultural and Resource Economics*, 26(2): 404–16.

Lucia, S.P. (1963). The antiquity of alcohol in diet and medicine. In Lucia, S.P. (ed.), *Alcohol and civilization.* New York, NY: McGraw-Hill.

Ludwig, D.S., Peterson, K.E. and Gortmaker, S.L. (2001). Relation between consumption of sugar-sweetened drinks and childhood obesity: a prospective, observational analysis. *Lancet*, 357(9255): 505–8.

Luhmann, N. (1990). Risiko und Gefahr. *Soziologische Aufklärung*, 5:137–169.

Luhmann, N. (1993). *Risk: a sociological theory.* New York, NY: Aldine de Gruyter.

Luning, P.A., Marcelis, W.J. and Jongen, W.M. (2005). *Zarządzanie jakością żywności. Ujęcie technologiczno-menadżerskie.* Warsaw, Poland: Wydawnictwo Naukowo-Techniczne.

Lupton, D. (1999). *Risk.* London, United Kingdom: Routledge and Kegan Paul.

Lupton, D. (2006). Sociology and risk. In Mythen, G. and Walklate, S. (eds), *Beyond the risk society critical reflections on risk and human security.* Berkshire, United Kingdom: Open University, McGraw-Hill: 11–24

Lusser, M., Parisi, C., Plan, D. and Rodriguez-Cerezo, E. (2012). Deployment of new biotechnologies in plant breeding. *Nature Biotechnology*, 30: 231–9.

Ma, J., Betts, N.M., Horacek, T., Georgiou, C., White, A. and Nitzke, S. (2002). The importance of decisional balance and self-efficacy in relation to stages of change for fruit and vegetable intakes by young adults. *American Journal of Health Promotion*, 163: 157–66.

Ma, J.K.-C., Christou, P., Chikwamba, R., Haydon, H., Paul, M., Ferrer, M.P., Ramalingam, S., Rech, E., Rybicki, E., Wigdorowitz, A., Yang, D.-C. and Thangaraj, H. (2013). Realising the value of plant molecular pharming to benefit the poor in developing countries and emerging economies. *Plant Biotechnology Journal*, 11: 1029–33.

Macdonald, S. (1994). Whisky, women and the Scottish drinking problem. A view from the Highlands. In McDonald, M. (ed.), *Gender, drink and drugs.* Oxford, United Kingdom: Berg.

Macfarlane, A. and Macfarlane, I. (2009). *The empire of tea.* New York, NY: Overlook Press.

Macfarlane, R. (2002). Integrating the consumer interest in food safety: the role of science and other factors. *Food Policy*, 27: 65–80.

Maga, J.A. and Katz, I. (1979). Furan in foods. *CRC Critical Reviews in Food Science and Nutrition*, 11(4): 355–400.

Magkos, F., Arvaniti, F. and Zampelas, A. (2006). Organic food: buying more safety or just peace of mind? A critical review of the literature. *Critical Reviews in Food Science and Nutrition*, 46(1): 23–56.

Magnusson, M.K., Arvola, A., Hursti, U.K., Åberg, L. and Sjödén, P.O. (2003). Choice of organic foods is related to perceived consequences for human health and to environmentally friendly behaviour. *Appetite*, 40(2): 109–17.

Malik, V.S., Schulze, M.B. and Hu, F.B. (2006). Intake of sugar-sweetened beverages and weight gain: a systematic review. *American Journal of Clinicla Nutrition*, 84: 274–88.

Malinauskas, B.M., Aeby, V.G., Overton, R.F., Carpenter-Aeby, T. and Barber-Heidal, K. (2007). A survey of energy drink consumption patterns among college students. *Nutrition Journal*, 6: 35–43.

Mandal, S. and Stoner, G.D. (1990). Inhibition of N-nitrosobenzylmethylamine-induced esophageal tumorigenesis in rats by ellagic acid. *Carcinogenesis*, 11(1): 55–61.

Mandelbaum, D.G. (1965). Alcohol and culture. *Current Anthropology*, 6(3): 281–93.

Marks, L., Kalaitzandonakes, N. and Zakharova, L. (2003). Media coverage of agrobiotechnology: did the butterfly have an effect? *Journal of Agribusiness*, 21: 1–20.

Marks, P.J., Vipond, I.B., Carlisle, D., Deakin, D., Fey, R.E. and Caul, E.O. (2000). Evidence for airborne transmission of norwalk-like virus (NLV) in a hotel restaurant. *Epidemiology of Infections*, 124(3): 481–7.

Mars, G. and Altman, Y. (1987). Alternative mechanism of distribution in a Soviet economy. In Douglas, M. (ed.), *Constructive drinking: perspectives on drink from anthropology*. Cambridge, United Kingdom: Cambridge University Press.

Marsden, E. (2003). Risk and regulation: US regulatory policy on genetically modified food and agriculture. *Boston College Law Review*, 44(3): 733–87.

Martin-Gronert, M.S. and Ozanne, S.E. (2013). Early life programming of obesity. *Medycyna Wieku Rozwojowego*, 17(1): 7–12.

Martinez-Poveda, A., Molla-Bauza, M.B., Gomis, F.J.C. and Martinez, L.M.C. (2009). Consumer-perceived risk model for the introduction of genetically modified food in Spain. *Food Policy*, 34: 519–28.

Marwick, C. (2002). Adverse reactions to dietary supplements under investigation by FDA. *BMJ*, 325(7539): 298.

Mask, L., Blanchard, C.M. and Baker, A. (2014). Do portrayals of women in action convey another ideal that women with little self-determination feel obligated to live up to? Viewing effects on body image evaluations and eating behaviors. *Appetite*, 83: 277–86.

Matt, D., Rembiałkowska, E., Peetsmann, E. and Pehme, S. (2011). *Quality of organic vs. conventional food and effects on health*. Tartu, Estonia: Estonian University of Life Sciences.

Maughan, R.J. and Griffin, J. (2003). Caffeine ingestion and fluid balance: a review. *Journal of Human Nutrition and Dietetics*, 16(6): 411–20.

May, P.A., Baete, A., Russo, J., Elliott, A.J., Blankenship, J., Kalberg, W.O., Buckley, D., Brooks, M., Hasken, J., Abdul-Rahman, O., Adam, M.P., Robinson, L.K., Manning, M. and Hoyme, H.E. (2014). Prevalence and characteristics of fetal alcohol spectrum disorders. *Pediatrics*, 134(5): 855–66.

Mayer, O., Simon, J. and Rosolova, H. (2001). A population study of the influence of beer consumption on folate and homocysteine concentrations. *European Journal of Clinical Nutrition*, 55(7): 605–9.

McCluskey, J.J. and Swinnen, J.F.M. (2004). Political economy of the media and consumer perceptions of biotechnology. *American Journal of Agricultural Economics*, 86: 1230–37.

McCluskey, J. and Swinnen, J. (2011). The media and food-risk perceptions. *EMBO Report*, 12(7): 624–9.

McCrory, M.A., Fuss, P.J., Hays, N.P., Vinken, A.G., Greenberg, A.S. and Roberts, S.B. (1999). Overeating in America: association between restaurant food consumption and body fatness in healthy adult men and women aged 19 to 80. *Obesity Research & Clinical Practice*, 7: 564–71.

McDonald's Corporation (2014). *Getting to know us*. Oak Brook, IL: McDonald's Corporation. Accessed on 7 May 2015 at: www.aboutmcdonalds.com/mcd/our_company.html.

McGovern, P.E., Zhang, J., Tang, J., Zhang, Z., Hall, G.R., Moreau, R.A., Nuñez, A., Butrym, E.D., Richards, M.P., Wang, C., Cheng, G., Zhao, Z. and Wang C. (2004). Fermented beverages of pre- and proto-historic China. *Proceedings of the National Academy of Sciences*, 101(51): 17593–8.

McKenna, K.E. and Dawson, J.F. (1993). Scurvy occurring in a teenager. *Journal of Clinical and Experimental Dermatology*, 18(1): 75–7.

McKim, W.A. and Hancock, S.D. (2012). *Drugs and behavior: an introduction to behavioral pharmacology*. London, United Kingdom: Prentice Hall.

McLaren, L. (2007). Socioeconomic status and obesity. *Epidemiologic Reviews*, 29(1): 29–48.

McLellan, T.M. and Lieberman, H.R. (2012). Do energy drinks contain active components other than caffeine? *Nutrition Reviews*, 70(12): 730–44.

Meagher, R.B. (2000). Phytoremediation of toxic elemental and organic pollutants. *Current Opinion in Plant Biology*, 3(2): 153–62.

Meier, B. (2012). Caffeinated drink cited in reports of 13 deaths. *New York Times*. Accessed on 20 June 2015 at: www.nytimes.com/2012/11/15/business/5-hour-energy-is-cited-in-13-death-reports.html?_r=0.

Meister, M. (2001). Cultural feeding, good life science, and the TV Food Network. *Mass Communication & Society*, 4(2): 165–82.

Mela, D.J. (1999). Food choice and intake: the human factor. *Proceedings of the Nutrition Society*, 58: 513–21.

Mensink, G.B., Fletcher, R., Gurinovic, M., Huybrechts, I., Lafay, L., Serra-Majem, L., Szponar, L., Tetens, I., Verkaik-Kloosterman, J., Baka, A. and Stephen, A.M. (2013). Mapping low intake of micronutrients across Europe. *British Journal of Nutrition*, 110(4): 755–73.

Merritt, C., Bazinet, M.L., Sullivan, J.H. and Robertson, D.H. (1963). Mass spectrometric determination of the volatile components from ground coffee. *Journal of Agricultural and Food Chemistry*, 11(2): 152–5.

Meyer-Rochow, V.B. (2009). Food taboos: their origins and purposes. *Journal of Ethnobiology and Ethnomedicine*, 5: 18–28.

Migicovsky, Z. and Kovalchuk, I. (2011). Epigenetic memory in mammals. *Frontiers in Genetics*, 2: 28–40.

Mikkila, V., Rasanen, L., Raitakari, O.T., Pietinen, P. and Viikari, J. (2004). Longitudinal changes in diet from childhood into adulthood with respect to risk of cardiovascular diseases: the Cardiovascular Risk in Young Finns Study. *European Journal of Clinical Nutrition*, 58: 1038–45.

Miles, S., Braxton, D. and Frewer, L. (1999). Public perceptions about microbiological hazards in food. *British Food Journal*, 101: 744–62.

Miles, S. and Frewer, L.J. (2001). Investigating specific concerns about different food hazards. *Food Quality and Preference*, 12: 47–61.

Miller, E.R. III, Juraschek, S., Pastor-Barriuso, R., Bazzano, L.A., Appel, L.J. and Guallar, E. (2010). Meta-analysis of folic acid supplementation trials on risk of cardiovascular disease and risk interaction with baseline homocysteine levels. *The American Journal of Cardiology*, 106(4): 517–27.

Miller, E.R. III, Pastor-Barriuso, R., Dalal, D., Riemersma, R.A., Appel, L.J. and Guallar, E. (2005). Meta-analysis: high-dosage vitamin E supplementation may increase all-cause mortality. *Annals of Internal Medicine*, 142: 37–46.

Miller, K.E. (2008). Energy drinks, race, and problem behaviors among college students. *The Journal of Adolescent Health*, 43(5): 490–97.

Mizen, J. (2014). Coffee cup size leads to caffeine confusion. *Scientific American*, 23 July. Accessed on 24 July 2015 at: www.scientificamerican.com/article/coffee-cup-size-leads-to-caffeine-confusion/.

Monsivais, P., Aggarwal, A. and Drewnowski, A. (2014). Time spent on home food preparation and indicators of healthy eating. *American Journal of Preventive Medicine*, 47(6): 796–802.

Montella, M., Polesel, J., La Vecchia, C., Dal Maso, L., Crispo, A., Crovatto, M., Casarin, P., Izzo, F., Tommasi, L.G., Talamini, R. and Franceschi, S. (2007). Coffee and tea consumption and risk of hepatocellular carcinoma in Italy. *International Journal of Cancer*, 120: 1555–9.

Montewka, J., Goerlandt, F. and Kujala, P. (2014). On a systematic perspective on risk for formal safety assessment (FSA). *Reliability Engineering & System Safety*, 127: 77–85.

Montizaan, G.K., Kramers, P.G.N., Janus, J.A. and Posthumus, R. (1989). *Integrated criteria document polynuclear aromatic hydrocarbons (PAH): effects of 10 selected compounds* (Appendix to RIVM Report no. 758474007). Bilthoven, The Netherlands: Rijksinstituut voor de Volksgezondheid en Milieuhygiene.

Moon, W. and Balasubramanian, S.K. (2004). Public attitudes toward agrobiotechnology: the mediating role of risk perceptions on the impact of trust, awareness, and outrage. *Applied Economic Perspective and Policy*, 26(2): 186–208.

Mooney, C. (1990). Cost and availability of healthy food choices in a London health district. *Journal of Human Nutrition and Dietetics*, 3: 111–20.

Moore, A. (2003). Food fights. *EMBO Report*, 4(7): 647–9.

Moore, R. and Pearson, T. (1986). Moderate alcohol consumption and coronary artery disease. *Medicine*, 65(4): 242–67.

Moro, S., Chipman, J.K., Wegener, J-W., Hamberger, C., Dekant, W. and Mally, A. (2012). Furan in heat-treated foods: formation, exposure, toxicity, and aspects of risk assessment. *Molecular Nutrition and Food Research*, 56: 1197–211.

Morris, J.G. Jr. (2011). How safe is our food? *Emerging Infectious Diseases*, 17(1): 126–8.

Mortensen, D.A., Egan, J.F., Maxwell, B.D., Ryan, M.R. and Smith R.G. (2012). Navigating a critical juncture for sustainable weed management. *BioScience*, 62(1): 75–84.

Mostofsky, E., Rice, M.S., Levitan, E.B. and Mittleman, M.A. (2012). Habitual coffee consumption and risk of heart failure: a dose-response meta-analysis. *Circulation. Heart Failure*, 5: 401–5.

Mou, Y. and Lin, C.A. (2014). Communicating food safety via the social media. The role of knowledge and emotions on risk perception and prevention. *Science Communication* 36(5): 593–616.

Ministry for Primary Industries [MPI] (2012). Importing genetically modified organisms. Accessed on 3 November 2014 at: www.biosecurity.govt.nz/regs/imports/plants/gmo.

Mukamal, K.J. (2003). Alcohol use and prognosis in patients with coronary heart disease. *Preventive Cardiology*, 6(2): 93–8.

Muñoz, P., Rojas, L., Bunsow, E., Saez, E., Sánchez-Cambronero, L., Alcalá, L., Rodríguez-Creixems, M. and Bouza, E. (2012). Listeriosis: an emerging public health problem especially among the elderly. *Journal of Infection*, 64(1): 19–33.

Murcott, A. (1983). *The sociology of food and eating.* Aldershot, United Kingdom: Gower.

Murcott, A. (1988). Sociological and social anthropological approaches to food and eating. *World Review of Nutrition and Dietetics*, 55: 1–40.

Murcott, A. (1995). Social influences on food choice and dietary change: a sociological attitude. *Proceedings of the Nutrition Society*, 54: 729–35.

Murcott, A. (1998). *The nation's diet: the social science of food choice.* New York, NY: Addison Wesley Longman.

Mursu, J., Robien, K., Harnack, L.J., Park, K. and Jacobs, D.R Jr. (2011). Dietary supplements and mortality rate in older women: the Iowa Women's Health Study. *Archives of Internal Medicine*, 171(18): 1625–33.

Mustad, V.A., Etherton, T.D., Cooper, A.D., Mastro, A.M., Pearson, T.A., Jonnalagadda, S.S. and Kris-Etherton P.M. (1997). Reducing saturated fat intake is associated with increased levels of LDL receptors on mononuclear cells in healthy men and women. *Journal of Lipid Research*, 38(3): 459–68.

Mythen, G. (2005). Employment, individualization and insecurity: rethinking the risk society perspective. *The Sociological Review*, 53(1): 129–49.

Nagao, M., Honda, M., Seino, Y., Yahagi, T. and Sugimura, T. (1977). Mutagenicities of smoke condensates and the charred surface of fish and meat. *Cancer Letters*, 2(4–5): 221–6.

Nahoum-Grappe, V. (1995). France. In Heath, D.B. (ed.), *International handbook on alcohol and culture*. Westport, CT: Greenwood.

Nanu, C., Tăut D. and Băban, A. (2014). Why adolescents are not happy with their body image? *Analize – Journal of Gender and Feminist Studies*, 2(16): 37–56.

National Cancer Institute (2010). Chemicals in meat cooked at high temperatures and cancer risk. Accessed on 23 April 2015 at: www.cancer.gov/cancertopics/causes-prevention/risk/diet/cooked-meats-fact-sheet.

National Cancer Institute (2014). *Mean intake of energy and mean contribution (kcal) of various foods among US population, by age, NHANES 2005–06*. Bethesda, MD: National Cancer Institute. Accessed on 7 May 2015 at: appliedresearch.cancer.gov/diet/foodsources/energy/table1a.html.

National Health Service (2011). *Supplements who needs them?* London, United Kingdom: National Health Service. Accessed on 25 July 2015 at: www.nhs.uk/news/2011/05may/documents/BtH_supplements.pdf.

Nauta, M.J., Fischer, A.R.H., van Asselt, E.D., de Jonge, A.E.I., Frewer, L.J. and de Jonge, R. (2008). Food safety in the domestic environment: the effect of consumer risk information on human disease risks. *Risk Analysis*, 28(1): 179–92.

Navarro, V.J., Barnhart, H., Bonkovsky, H.L., Davern, T., Fontana, R.J., Grant, L., Reddy, K.R., Seeff, L.B., Serrano, J., Sherker, A.H., Stolz, A., Talwalkar, J., Vega, M. and Vuppalanchi, R. (2014). Liver injury from herbals and dietary supplements in the US Drug-Induced Liver Injury Network. *Hepatology*, 60(4): 1399–408.

Nawrot, P., Jordan, S., Eastwood, J., Rotstein, J., Hugenholtz, A. and Feeley, M. (2003). Effects of caffeine on human health. *Food Additives & Contaminants*, 20(1): 1–30.

Nehlig, A. (2010). Is caffeine a cognitive enhancer? *Journal of Alzheimer's Disease*, 20 (Suppl 1): S85–94.

Nehlig, A., Daval, J.L. and Debry, G. (1992). Caffeine and the central nervous system: mechanisms of action, biochemical, metabolic and psychostimulant effects. *Brain Research Review*, 17(2): 139–70.

Neumark-Sztainer, D., Wall, M., Story, M. and Standish, A.R. (2012). Dieting and unhealthy weight control behaviors during adolescence: associations with 10-year changes in body mass index. *Journal of Adolescent Health*, 50(1): 80–86.

Newell, D.G., Koopmans, M., Verhoef, L., Duizer, E., Aidara-Kane, A., Sprong, H., Opsteegh, M., Langelaar, M., Threfall, J., Scheutz, F., van der Giessen, J. and Kruse, H. (2010). Food-borne diseases – the challenges of 20 years ago still persist while new ones continue to emerge. *International Journal of Food Microbiology*, 139: S3–S15.

Newmaster, S.G., Grguric, M., Shanmughanandhan, D., Ramalingam, S. and Ragupathy, S. (2013). DNA barcoding detects contamination and substitution in North American herbal products. *BMC Medicine*, 11: 222–35.

Ng, M., Fleming, T., Robinson, M., Thomson, B., Graetz, N., Margono, C., Mullany, E. *et al.* (2014). Global, regional, and national prevalence of overweight and obesity in children and adults during 1980–2013: a systematic analysis for the Global Burden of Disease Study 2013. *Lancet*, 384(9945): 766–81.

Ngokwey, N. (1987). Varieties of palm wine among the Lele of the Kasai. In Douglas, M. (ed.) *Constructive drinking: perspectives on drink from anthropology*. Cambridge, United Kingdom: Cambridge University Press.

Nichter, M. (2003). Harm reduction: a core concern for medical anthropology. In Harthorn, B.H. and Oaks, L. (eds), *Risk, culture, and health inequality: shifting perceptions of danger and blame*. Westport, CT: Praeger: 13–33.

Nichter, M. and Thompson, J.J. (2006). For my wellness, not just my illness: North Americans' use of dietary supplements. *Culture, Medicine and Psychiatry*, 30: 175–222.

Nicolia, A., Manzo, A., Veronesi. F. and Rosellini, D. (2014). An overview of the last 10 years of genetically engineered crop safety research. *Critical Reviews in Biotechnology*, 34(1): 77–88.

Nieburg, O. (2013). Interactive map: top 20 chocolate consuming nations of 2012. Accessed on 20 June 2015 at: www.confectionerynews.com/Markets/Interactive-Map-Top-20-chocolate-consuming-nations-of-2012.

Nielsen, S.J. and Popkin, B.M. (2003). Patterns and trends in food portion sizes, 1977–1998. *Journal of the American Medical Association*, 289: 450–53.

Nielsen, S.J. and Popkin, B.M. (2004). Changes in beverage intake between 1977 and 2001. *American Journal of Preventive Medicine*, 27: 205–10.

Nielsen, T., Jørgensen, H.E., Larsen, J.C. and Poulsen, M. (1996). City air pollution of polycyclic aromatic hydrocarbons and other mutagens: occurrence, sources and health effects. *Science of the Total Environment*, 189/190: 41–9.

Northbourne, L. (1940). *Look to the land*. London, United Kingdom: JM Dent.

Nowotny, H. (2000). Transgressive competence: the narrative of expertise. *European Journal of Social Theory*, 3(1): 5–21.

Nowotny, H., Scott, P. and Gibbons, M. (2001). *Re-thinking science: knowledge and the public in an age of uncertainty*. Cambridge, United Kingdom: Polity Press.

NSW Food Authority (2006). *Dioxins in seafood in Port Jackson and its tributaries*. Report of the Expert Panel, 24 February 2006. NSW Food Authority, Sydney, NSW, Australia.

National Toxicology Program [NTP] (1993). *Toxicology and carcinogenesis studies of furan in F344 rats and B6C3F1 mice (gavage studies)* (NTP Technical Report No. 402). Research Triangle Park, NC: National Institute of Environmental Health Sciences.

O'Beirne, K. (2003). Poor and fat. A special problem in America. *National Review*, 10 February. Accessed on 7 May 2015 at: www.nationalreview.com/article/206054/poor-and-fat-kate-obeirne?target=author&tid=900157.

O'Brien, M.C., McCoy, T.P., Rhodes, S.D., Wagoner, A. and Wolfson, M. (2008). Caffeinated cocktails: energy drink consumption, high-risk drinking, and alcohol-related consequences among college students. *Academic Emergency Medicine*, 15(5): 453–60.

O'Dea, K. (1991). Traditional diet and food preferences of Australian Aboriginal hunter- gatherers. *Philosophical Transactions of the Royal Society of London – Series B: Biological Sciences*, 334: 233–41.

O'Hara, L. and Gregg. J. (2010). Don't diet: adverse effects of the weight-centered health paradigm. In De Meester, F., Zibadi, S. and Watson, R.R. (eds), *Modern dietary fat intakes in disease promotion, nutrition and health*. New York, NY: Springer: 431–41.

O'Malley, P. (2010). Resilient subjects: uncertainty, warfare and liberalism, *Economy and Society*, 39(4): 488–509.

Organisation for Economic Co-operation and Development [OECD] (1992). *Safety considerations for biotechnology*. Paris, France: OECD Publishing.

Organisation for Economic Co-operation and Development [OECD] (1993). *Safety evaluation of foods derived by modern biotechnology: concepts and principles*. Paris, France: OECD Publishing.

Organisation for Economic Co-operation and Development [OECD] (2012). *Health at a glance: Europe 2012*. Paris, France: OECD Publishing. Accessed on 25 January 2016 at: http://ec.europa.eu/health/reports/docs/health_glance_2012_en.pdf.

Ogden, C.L., Carroll, M.D., Kit, B.K. and Flegal, K.M. (2012). *Prevalence of obesity in the United States, 2009–2010* (NCHS data brief, no 82). Hyattsville, MD: National Center for Health Statistics.

Okholm, D. (2014). *Dangerous passions, deadly sins learning from the psychology of ancient monks*. Ada, MI: Brazos Press.

Olesen, P., Olsen, A., Frandsen, H., Frederiksen, K., Overvad, K. and Tjønneland, A. (2008). Acrylamide exposure and incidence of breast cancer among postmenopausal women in the Danish Diet Cancer and Health Study. *International Journal of Cancer*, 122: 2094–100.

Oral, T. (1997). *A contemporary Turkish coffeehouse design based on historic traditions*. Thesis. Blacksburg, VA: Faculty of the Virginia Polytechnic Institute and State University.

Orrú, M., Guitart, X., Karcz-Kubicha, M., Solinas, M., Justinova, Z., Barodia, S.K., Zanoveli, J., Cortes, A., Lluis, C., Casado, V., Moeller, F.G. and Ferré, S. (2013). Psychostimulant pharmacological profile of paraxanthine, the main metabolite of caffeine in humans. *Neuropharmacology*, 67: 476–84.

Osaili, T.M., Obeidat, B.A., Jamous, D.O.A. and Bawadi, H.A. (2011). Food safety knowledge and practices among college female students in north of Jordan. *Food Control*, 22(2): 269–76.

Osler, M., Rasmussen, N.K. and Brønnum-Hansen, H. (1990). Voksne danskeres kostbevisthed [Dietary consciousness among Danish adults]. *Ugeskrift for Læger*, 152: 1577–80.

Ostapenko, Y.N. and Elkis, I.S. (2010). Alcohol and substitute poisoning: diagnosis and emergency medical care in the pre-hospital stage. *Therapeutic Archives*, 1: 18–24.

Oxford Dictionaries Online (2013). *Language matters*. Oxford, United Kingdom: Oxford University Press. Accessed on 25 November 2013 at: www.oxforddictionaries.com.

Oyebode, O., Gordon-Dseagu, V., Walker, A. and Mindell, J.S. (2014). Fruit and vegetable consumption and all-cause, cancer and CVD mortality: analysis of Health Survey for England data. *Journal of Epidemiology and Community Health*, 68(9): 856–62.

Paci, G., Lisi, E., Bagliacca, M. and Maritan, A. (2003). Reproductive performance in a local rabbit population reared under organic and conventional system. *Annali della Facoltà di Medicina Veterinaria*, LVI(20): 115–26.

Padel, S. and Foster, C. (2005). Exploring the gap between attitudes and behaviour. *British Food Journal*, 107: 606–25.

Palmieri, D., Pane, B., Barisione, C., Spinella, G., Garibaldi, S., Ghigliotti, G., Brunelli, C., Fulcheri, E. and Palombo, D. (2011). Resveratrol counteracts systemic and local inflammation involved in early abdominal aortic aneurysm development. *The Journal of Surgical Research*, 171: e237–e246.

Papagaroufali, E. (1992). Uses of alcohol among women: games of resistance, power and pleasure. In Gefou-Madianou, D. (ed.), *Alcohol, gender and culture*. London, United Kingdom: Routledge.

Parashar, U., Quiroz, E.S., Mounts, A.W., Monroe, S.S., Fankhauser, R.L., Ando, T., Noel, J.S., Bulens, S.N., Beard, S.R., Li, J.F., Bresee, J.S. and Glass, R.I. (2001). Norwalk-like viruses. Public health consequences and outbreak management. *Morbidity and Mortality Weekly Report, Recommendations and Reports*, 50(RR-9): 1–17.

Patel, M.M., Widdowson, M.-A., Glass, R.I., Akazawa K., Vinjé, J. and Parashar, U.D. (2008). Systematic literature review of role of noroviruses in sporadic gastroenteritis. *Emerging Infectious Diseases*, 14(8): 1224–31.

Patil, S.R., Morales, R., Cates, S., Anderson, D. and Kendal, D. (2004). An application of meta-analysis in food safety consumer research to evaluate consumer behaviours and practices. *Journal of Food Protection*, 67(11): 2587–95.

Patrick, C.H. (1952). *Alcohol, culture, and society*. Durham, North Carolina: Duke University Press: 12–13. Reprint edition by AMS Press, New York, 1970.

Patton, G.C., Johnson-Sabine, E., Wood, K., Mann, A.H. and Wakeling, A. (1990). Abnormal eating attitudes in London schoolgirls – a prospective epidemiological study: outcome at twelve month follow-up. *Psychological Medicine*, 20(2): 383–94.

Pauling, L. (1970). *Vitamin C and the common cold*. San Francisco, CA: W.H. Freeman and Company.

Paull, J. (2011a). Biodynamic agriculture: the journey from Koberwitz to the world, 1924–1938. *Journal of Organic Systems*, 6(1): 27–41.

Paull, J. (2011b). The uptake of organic agriculture: a decade of worldwide development. *Journal of Social and Development Sciences*, 2(3): 111–20.

Paull, J. and Lyons, K. (2008). Nanotechnology: the next challenge for organics. *Journal of Organic Systems*, 3(1): 3–22.

Payette, H. and Shatenstein, B. (2005). Determinants of healthy eating in the community-dwelling elderly people. *Canadian Journal of Public Health*, 96: S27–S31.

Payne, S. (2014). Constructing the gendered body? A critical discourse analysis of gender equality schemes in the health sector in England. *Current Sociology*, 62(7): 956–74.

Peacock, M. (2009). *Killer company: James Hardie exposed*. Sydney, Australia: Harper Collins.

Peck, J.D., Leviton, A. and Cowan, L.D. (2010). A review of the epidemiologic evidence concerning the reproductive health effects of caffeine consumption: a 2000–2009 update. *Food and Chemical Toxicology*, 48(10): 2549–76.

Pellizzoni, L. (2003). Uncertainty and participatory democracy. *Environmental Values*, 12(2): 195–224.

Perri, M.G. and Fuller, P.R. (1995). Success and failure in the treatment of obesity: where do we go from here? *Medicine, Exercise, Nutrition, and Health*, 4: 255–72.

Persson, T. and von Sydow, E. (1973). Aroma of canned beef: gas chromatographic and mass spectrometric analysis of the volatiles. *Journal of Food Science*, 38(3): 377–85.

Petty, R.E. and Cacioppo, J.T. (1996). *Communication and persuasion: central and peripheral routes to attitude change*. New York, NY: Springer.

Phillips, D.H. (1999). Polycyclic aromatic hydrocarbons in the diet. *Mutation Research*, 443(1–2): 139–47.

Phipps, R.G. (1977). *The Swanson story: when the chicken flew the coop*. Omaha, NE: Carl and Caroline Swanson Foundation.

Pidgeon, N., Kasperson, R.E. and Slovic, P. (eds) (2003). *The Social amplification of risk*. Cambridge, United Kingdom: Cambridge University Press.

Pietrykowski, B. (2004). You are what you eat: the social economy of slow food movement. *Review of Social Economy*, LXII(3): 307–21.

Pipitone, L. (2012). Situation and prospects for cocoa supply and demand. World Cocoa Conference 2012. Accessed on 9 January 2014 at: www.icco.org/about-us/international-cocoa-agreements/doc_download/364-laurent-pipitone-market-outlook.html.

Pitkin, R.M. (2007). Folate and neural tube defects. *American Journal of Clinical Nutrition*, 85(1): 285S–288S.

Pluhar, E.B. (2010). Meat and morality: alternatives to factory farming. *Journal of Agricultural and Environmental Ethics*, 23: 455–68.

Polivy, J. and Herman, C.P. (2007). Is the body the self? Women and body image. *Collegium Antropologicum*, 31(1): 63–7.

Pollard, J., Kirk, S.F.L. and Cade, J.E. (2002). Factors affecting food choice in relation to fruit and vegetable intake: a review. *Nutrition Research Reviews*, 15: 373–87.

Polley, S. (2006). The obesity problem in US hospitals. *The Hospitalist*, 1 August. Accessed on 7 May 2015 at: www.the-hospitalist.org/details/article/239101/The_Obesity_Problem_in_U_S_Hospitals.html.

Pope, L., Latimer, L. and Wansink, B. (2015). Viewers vs. doers. The relationship between watching food television and BMI. *Appetite*, 90: 131–5.

Popkin, B.M., Bray, G.A. and Hu, F. (2014). The role of high sugar foods and sugar-sweetened beverages in weight gain and obesity. In Gill, T. (ed.), *Managing and preventing obesity: behavioural factors and dietary interventions*. Cambridge, United Kingdom: Woodhead Publishing: 45–57.

Prakash, D., Verma, S., Bhatia, R. and Tiwary, B.N. (2011). Risks and precautions of genetically modified organisms. *ISRN Ecology*, 2011: 1–13.

Prättälä, R., Berg, M. and Puska, P. (1992). Diminishing or increasing contrasts? Social class variations in Finnish food consumption patterns, 1979–1990. *European Journal of Clinical Nutrition*, 46: 279–87.

Prättälä, R., Paalanen, L., Grinberga, D., Helasoja, V., Kasmel, A. and Petkeviciene, J. (2007). Gender differences in the consumption of meat, fruit and vegetables are similar in Finland and the Baltic countries. *The European Journal of Public Health*, 17(5): 520–25.

Puhl, R.M. and Heuer, C.A. (2010). Obesity stigma: important considerations for public health. *American Journal of Public Health*, 100(6): 1019–28.

Putnam, J., Allshouse, J., Kantor, L.S. (2002). US per capita food supply trends: more calories, refined carbohydrates, and fats. *FoodReview*, 25: 2–15.

Qazi, H.I.A. and Keval, H. (2013). At war with their bodies or at war with their minds? A glimpse into the lives and minds of female yo-yo dieters – the curtain has lifted in UK? *Journal of International Women's Studies*, 14(1): 311–32.

Raab, C. and Grobe, D. (2005). Consumer knowledge and perceptions about organic food. *Journal of Extension*, 43(4): 4RIB3. Accessed on 8 December 2014 at: www.joe.org/joe/2005august/rb3.php.

Ramachandran, A. and Snehalatha, C. (2010). Rising burden of obesity in Asia. *Journal of Obesity*, E-pub 2010: 868573: 1–8.

Ramaswamy, V., Cresence, V.M., Rejitha, J.S., Lekshmi, M.U., Dharsana, K.S., Prasad, S.P. and Vijila, H.M. (2007). *Listeria* – review of epidemiology and pathogenesis. *Journal of Microbiology, Immunology and Infection*, 40(1): 4–13.

Ramos, S. (2008). Cancer chemoprevention and chemotherapy: Dietary polyphenols and signalling pathways. *Molecular Nutrition & Food Research*, 52: 507–26.

Rasmussen, M., Krolner, R., Klepp, K.I., Lytle, L., Brug, J., Bere, E. and Due, P. (2006). Determinants of fruit and vegetable consumption among children and adolescents: a review of the literature. Part I: quantitative studies. *The International Journal of Behavioral Nutrition and Physical Activity*, 11(3): 22–41.

Rath, M. (2012). Energy drinks: what is all the hype? The dangers of energy drink consumption. *Journal of the American Academy of Nurse Practitioners*, 24(2): 70–76.

Raven, P.H. (2014). GM crops, the environment and sustainable food production. *Transgenic Research*, 23(6): 915–21.

Redmond, E.C., Griffith, C.J., Slader, J. and Humphrey, T.J. (2004). Microbiological and observational analysis of cross contamination risks during domestic food preparation. *British Food Journal*, 106(8): 581–97.

Rehm, J., Gmel, G., Sepos, C.T. and Trevisan, M. (2003). Alcohol-related morbidity and mortality. *Alcohol Research and Health*, 27(1): 39–51.

Rehm, J., Mathers, C., Popova, S., Thavorncharoensap, M., Teerawattananon, Y. and Patra, J. (2009). Global burden of disease and injury and economic cost attributable to alcohol use and alcohol use disorders. *Lancet*, 373: 2223–33.

Reissig, C.J., Strain, E.C. and Griffiths, R.R. (2009). Caffeinated energy drinks – a growing problem. *Drug and Alcohol Dependency*, 99(1–3): 1–10.

Rembiałkowska, E. (2007). Quality of plant products from organic agriculture. *Journal of the Science of Food and Agriculture*, 87: 2757–62.

Renaud, S. and de Lorgeril, M. (1992). Wine, alcohol, platelets, and the French paradox for coronary heart disease. *Lancet*, 339: 1523–6.

Renn, O. (2005). *Rational choice and risk research*. Learning about risk, SCARR Launch Conference, Canterbury, United Kingdom, 27 January 2015.

Resnicow, K., Smith, M., Baranowski, T., Baranowski, J., Vaughan, R. and Davis, M. (1998). 2-year tracking of children's fruit and vegetable intake. *Journal of the American Dietetic Association*, 98: 785–9.

Reuters (2013). Unapproved Monsanto GMO wheat found in Oregon. *CNBC*, 29 May. Accessed on 2 July 2015 at: www.cnbc.com/id/100774325.

Rice, S. (2014). Retrofitting hospitals for obese patients. *Modern Healthcare*, 8 February. Accessed on 7 May 2015 at: www.modernhealthcare.com/article/20140208/MAGAZINE/302089980.

Rietjens, I.M. and Alink, G.M. (2003). Nutrition and health – toxic substances in food. *Nederlands Tijdschrift voor Geneeskunde*, 147(48): 2365–70.

Ritson, C. and Oughton, L. (2007). Food consumers and organic agriculture. In: Cooper. J., Niggli, U. and Leifert, C. (eds) *Handbook of organic food safety and quality*. Cambridge, United Kingdom: CRC Press: 74–94.

Roberts, D., Crews, C., Grundy, H., Mills, C. and Matthews, W. (2008). Effect of consumer cooking on furan in convenience foods. *Food Additives and Contaminants: Part A Chemistry, Analysis, Control, Exposure and Risk Assessment*, 25(1): 25–31.

Rock, C.L. (2007). Multivitamin-multimineral supplements: who uses them? *American Journal of Clinical Nutrition*, 85(1): 277S–279S.

Roden, C. (1981). *Coffee*. London, United Kingdom: Penguin Books.

Roerecke, M. and Rehm, J. (2014). Alcohol consumption, drinking patterns, and ischemic heart disease: a narrative review of meta-analyses and a systematic review and meta-analysis of the impact of heavy drinking occasions on risk for moderate drinkers. *BMC Medicine*, 12(1): 182–93.

Rohrmann, B. (1999). *Risk perception research. Review and documentation*. Revised edtion, *Arbeiten zur Risiko-Kommunication*, Heft 69, Programmgruppe Mensch, Umwelt, Technik (MUT). Forschungszentrum Jülich, Jülich, pp.1-164. Accessed on 23 January 2016 at citeseerx.ist.psu.edu/viewdoc/download;jsessionid=E1E3865D9 6D202EA72DC3F22F04911AF?doi=10.1.1.194.8636&rep=rep1&type=pdf.

Roininen, K., Tuorila, H., Zandstra, E.H., de Graaf, C., Vehkalahti, K., Stubenitsky, K. and Mela, D.J. (2001). Differences in health and taste attitudes and reported behavior among Finnish, Dutch and British consumers: A cross-national validation of the Health and Taste Attitude Scales (HTAS). *Appetite*, 37: 33–45.

Rolls, B.J., Roe, L.S., Kral, T.V.E., Meengs, J.S. and Wall, D.E. (2004). Increasing the portion size of a packaged snack increases energy intake in men and women. *Appetite*, 42(1): 63–9.

Römer, L. and Scheibel, T. (2008). The elaborate structure of spider silk. Structure and function of a natural high performance fiber. *Prion*, 2(4): 154–61.

Roncone, D.P. (2006). Xerophthalmia secondary to alcohol-induced malnutrition. *Optometry*, 77(3): 124–33.

Rooney, J.F. (1991). Patterns of alcohol use in Spanish society. In Pittman, D.J. and White, H.R. (eds), *Society, culture and drinking patterns reexamined*. New Brunswick, Canada: Rutgers Center for Alcohol Studies.

Ropeik, D. (2007). Risk communication, an overlooked tool for improving public health. In Last, J. and Wallace, R. (eds), *Maxcy-Rosenau-Last public health and preventive medicine*. New Jersey, NJ: Prentice Hall International.

Rose, G. (1992). *The strategy of preventive medicine*. New York, NY: Oxford University Press.

Rose, N. (1990). *Governing the soul: the shaping of the private self*. Florence, KY: Taylor & Frances/Routledge.

Rose, N. (1996). Refiguring the territory of government. *Economy and Society*, 25(3): 327–56.

Rose, N. (1999). *Powers of freedom*. Cambridge, United Kingdom: Cambridge University Press.

Rose, N. and Miller, P. (1992). Political power beyond the state. *British Journal of Sociology*, 43(2): 173–205.

Roselli, M., Finamore, A., Brasili, E., Capuani, G., Kristensen, H.L., Micheloni, C. and Mengheri, E. (2012). Impact of organic and conventional carrots on intestinal and peripheral immunity. *Journal of the Science of Food and Agriculture*, 92(14): 2913–22.

Rosen, S.D. (2004). Physiological insights into Shechita. *Veterinary Record*, 154: 759–65.

Rosengren, A. and Lissner, L. (2008). The sociology of obesity. *Frontiers of Hormone Research*, 36: 260–70.

Rosenquist, H., Nielsen, N.L., Sommer, H.M., Nørrung, B. and Christensen, B.B. (2003). Quantitative risk assessment of human campylobacteriosis associated with thermophilic *Campylobacter* species in chickens. *International Journal of Food Microbiology*, 83: 87–103.

Rosin, O. (2008). The economic causes of obesity: a survey. *Journal of Economic Surveys*, 22(4): 617–47.

Rowe, S., Alexander, N., Almeida, N., Black, R., Burns, R., Bush, L., Crawford, P., Keim, N., Kris-Etherton, P. and Weaver, C. (2011). Food science challenge: translating the dietary guidelines for Americans to bring about real behavior change. *Journal of Food Science*, 76(1): R29–R37.

Rozin, P. (2006). The integration of biological, social, cultural and psychological influences on food choice. In Shepherd, R. and Raats, M. (eds), *The psychology of food choice*. Wallingford, United Kingdom: Cabi.

Rozin, P., Fischler, C. and Shields-Argelès, C. (2012). European and American perspectives on the meaning of natural. *Appetite*, 59(2): 448–55.

Rozin, P., Pelchat, M.L. and Fallon, A.E. (1986). Psychological factors influencing food choice. In Ritson, C., Gofton, L. and McKenzie, J. (eds), *The food consumer*. Chichester and New York, NY: John Wiley & Sons Ltd: 85–106.

Rude, R.K. (2010). Magnesium. In Coates, P.M., Betz, J.M., Blackman, M.R., Cragg, G.M., Levine, M., Moss, J. and White, J.D. (eds), *Encyclopedia of dietary supplements* (Second ed.) New York, NY: Informa Healthcare: 527–37.

Rudgley, R. (1994). *Essential substances: a cultural history of intoxicants in society*. New York, NY: Kodansha America, Inc.

Ruiz-Lopez, N., Haslam, R.P., Napier, J.A. and Sayanova O. (2014). Successful high-level accumulation of fish oil omega-3 long chain polyunsaturated fatty acids in a transgenic oilseed crop. *The Plant Journal*, 77: 198–208.

Rumble, J.N. and Leal, A. (2013). Public opinion of food in Florida (PIE2012/13–15). Gainesville, FL: University of Florida/IFAS Center for Public Issues Education.

Ryan, L., Hatfield, C. and Hofstetter, M. (2002). Caffeine reduces time-of-day effects on memory performance in older adults. *Psychological Science*, 13(1): 68–71.

Sabaté, J. (2004). Religion, diet and research. *British Journal of Nutrition*, 92: 199–201.

Sacert (2013). *Standards*. Bristol, United Kingdom: Soil Association Certification. Accessed on 3 December 2014 at: www.sacert.org/farming/standards.

Sacks, J.J., Roeber, J., Bouchery, E.E., Gonzales, K., Chaloupka, F.J. and Brewer, R. (2013). State costs of excessive alcohol consumption, 2006. *American Journal of Preventive Medicine*, 45: 474–85.

Salmon, A.G., Painter, P., Dunn, A.J., Wu-Williams, A., Monserrat, L. and Zeise, L. (1991). Carcinogenic effects. In Salmon, A.G. and Zeise, L. (eds), *Risks of carcinogenesis from urethane exposure*. Boca Raton, FL: CRC Press: 48–77.

Sanahuja, G., Banakar, R., Twyman, R.M., Capell, T. and Christou, P. (2011). *Bacillus thuringiensis*: a century of research, development and commercial applications. *Plant Biotechnology Journal*, 9: 283–300.

Sanap, M. and Chapman, M.J. (2003). Severe ethanol poisoning: a case report and brief review. *Critical Care and Resuscitation*, 5(2): 106–8.

Sandman, P.M., Sachsman, D.B. and Greenberg, M.R. (1992). *The environmental news source: providing environmental risk information to the media*. New Brunswick, NJ: Environmental Communication Research Program, Cook College, Rutgers University.

Sanz Alaejos, M., Ayala, J.H., González, V. and Afonso, A.M. (2008). Analytical methods applied to the determination of heterocyclic aromatic amines in foods.

Journal of Chromatography B Analytical Technologies in the Biomedical and Life Sciences, 862(1–2): 15–42.

Saremi, A. and Arora, R. (2008). The cardiovascular implications of alcohol and red wine. *American Journal of Therapeutics*, 15(3): 265–77.

Sassi, F. (2010). *Obesity and the economics of prevention: fit not fat*. Paris, France: OECD Publishing.

Savage, J.S., Fisher, J.O. and Birch, L.L. (2007). Parental influence on eating behaviour. Conception to adolescence. *The Journal of Law, Medicine & Ethics*, 35(1): 22–34.

Sayre, R., Beeching, J.R., Cahoon, E.B., Egesi, C., Fauquet, C., Fellman, J., Fregene, M., Gruissem, W., Mallowa, S., Manary, M., Maziya-Dixon, B., Mbanaso, A., Schachtman, D.P., Siritunga, D., Taylor, N., Vanderschuren, H. and Zhang, P. (2011). The biocassava plus program: biofortification of cassava for sub-Saharan Africa. *Annual Review of Plant Biology*, 62: 251–72.

Scallan, E., Hoekstra, R.M., Angulo, F.J., Tauxe, R.V., Widdowson, M.A., Roy, S.L., Jones, J.L. and Griffin, P.M. (2011). Foodborne illness acquired in the United States – major pathogens. *Emerging Infectious Diseases*, 17(1): 7–15.

Scharff, R.L. (2012). Economic burden from health losses due to foodborne illness in the United States. *Journal of Food Protection*, 75(1): 123–31.

Schehl, B., Senn, T., Lachenmeier, D.W., Rodicio, R. and Heinisch, J.J. (2007). Contribution of the fermenting yeast strain to ethyl carbamate generation in stone fruit sprits. *Applied Microbiology and Biotechnology*, 74: 843–50.

Schleenbecker, R. and Hamm, U. (2013). Consumers' perception of organic product characteristics. A review. *Appetite*, 71: 420–29.

Schlosser, E. (2001). *Fast food nation: the dark side of the all American meal*. New York, NY: Houghton Mifflin Company.

Schmidt, B.M., Ribnicky, D.M., Lipsky, P.E. and Raskin, I. (2007). Revisiting the ancient concept of botanical therapeutics. *Nature Chemical Biology*, 3: 360–66.

Schoenborn, C.A., Adams, P.F. and Barnes, P.M. (2002). Body weight status of adults: United States, 1997–98. *Advance Data* 330: 1–15.

Scientific Committee on Food [SCF] (2002). Opinion of the Scientific Committee on Food on the risks to human health of polycyclic aromatic hydrocarbons in food. Accessed on 10 July 2015 at: ec.europa.eu/food/fs/sc/scf/out153_en.pdf.

Scrinis, G. (2008). On the ideology of nutritionism. *Gastronomica: The Journal of Critical Food Studies*, 8(1): 39–48.

Searles, E. (2002). Food and the making of modern Inuit identities. *Food & Foodways: History & Culture of Human Nourishment*, 10: 55–78.

Sears, A., Baker, M.G., Wilson, N., Marshall, J., Muellner, P., Campbell, D.M., Lake, R.J. and French, N.P. (2011). Marked campylobacteriosis decline after interventions aimed at poultry, New Zealand. *Emerging Infectious Diseases*, 17(6): 1007–15.

Seifert, S.M., Schaechter, J.L., Hershorin, E.R. and Lipshultz, S.E. (2011). Health effects of energy drinks on children, adolescents, and young adults. *Pediatrics*, 127(3): 511–28.

Sekirov, I., Russell, S.L., Antunes, L.C.M. and Finlay, B.B. (2010). Gut microbiota in health and disease. *Physiological Reviews*, 90(3): 859–904.

Senellart, M. (ed.) (1978). *Michel Foucault. Security, territory, population* (Lectures at the Collège de France, 1977–78). Melbourne, Australia: Palgrave Macmillan.

Senghore, I. (2013). How to be a healthy vegetarian. *The Point*, 29 October. Accessed on 14 October 2014 at: thepoint.gm/africa/gambia/article/how-to-be-a-healthy-vegetarian.

Shankar, U. and Abrol, D.P. (2012). Integrated pest management in stored grains. In Abrol, D.P. and Shankar, U. (eds), *Integrated pest management: principles and practice.* Wallingford, United Kingdom: CABI Publishing. Chapter 14: 38–407.

Shayne, V. (2000). *Whole food nutrition: the missing link in vitamin therapy.* Lincoln, NE: iUniverse.

Shepherd, R., Sparks, P. and Guthrie, C.A. (1995). The application of the theory of planned behaviour to consumer food choice. *European Advances in Consumer Research*, 2: 360–65.

Shepherd, R., Magnusson, M. and Sjödén, P.O. (2005). Determinants of consumer behavior related to organic foods. *Ambio*, 34(4–5): 352–9.

Shield, K.D, Parry, C. and Rehm, J. (2013). Chronic diseases and conditions related to alcohol use. *Alcohol Research: Current Reviews*, 35(2): 155–73.

Shimazu, T., Tsubono, Y., Kuriyama, S., Ohmori, K., Koizumi, Y., Nishino, Y., Shibuya, D. and Tsuji, I. (2005). Coffee consumption and the risk of primary liver cancer: pooled analysis of two prospective studies in Japan. *International Journal of Cancer*, 116: 150–54.

Shirlow, M.J. and Mathers, C.D. (1985). A study of caffeine consumption and symptoms; indigestion, palpitations, tremor, headache and insomnia. *International Journal of Epidemiology*, 14(2): 239–48.

Shiva, V. (2000). *Stolen harvest: the hijacking of the global food supply.* Cambridge, MA: South End Press.

Shively, C.A. and Tarka, S.M. (1984). Methylxanthine composition and consumption patterns of cocoa and chocolate products. *Progress in Clinical and Biological Research*, 158: 149–78.

Siegrist, M. and Cvetkovich, G. (2001). Better negative than positive? Evidence of a bias for negative information about possible health dangers. *Risk Analysis*, 21: 199–206.

Simini, B. (2000). Serge Renaud: from French paradox to Cretan miracle. *Lancet*, 355(9197): 48.

Singh, R.P. and Wang C.Y. (1977). Quality of frozen foods – a review. *Journal of Food Process Engineering*, 1(2): 97–127.

Sinha, R. (2002). An epidemiologic approach to studying heterocyclic amines. *Mutation Research*, 506–507: 197–204.

Sinha, R., Rothman, N., Salmon, C.P., Knize, M.G., Brown, E.D., Swanson, C.A., Rhodes, D., Rossi, S., Felton, J.S. and Levander, O.A. (1998). Heterocyclic amine content in beef cooked by different methods to varying degrees of doneness and gravy made from meat drippings. *Food and Chemical Toxicology*, 36: 279–87.

Skakkebaek, N.E., Toppari, J., Söder, O., Gordon, C.M., Divall, S. and Draznin, M. (2011). The exposure of fetuses and children to endocrine disrupting chemicals: a European Society for Paediatric Endocrinology (ESPE) and Pediatric Endocrine Society (PES) call to action statement. *Journal of Clinical Endocrinology Metabolism*, 96(10): 3056–8.

Skaznik-Wikiel, M.E. and Polotsky, A.J. (2014). The health pros and cons of continuous versus intermittent calorie restriction: more questions than answers. *Maturitas*, 79(3): 275–8.

Slater, D. (2014). Who made that charcoal briquette? *New York Times*, 28 September, p. MM19. Accessed on 10 December 2014 at: www.nytimes.com/2014/09/28/magazine/who-made-that-charcoal-briquette.html?_r=0.

Slovic, P. (1986). Informing and educating the public about risk. *Risk Analysis*, 6(4): 403–15.

Slovic, P. (1987). Perception of risk. *Science*, 236: 280–86.

Slovic, P. (1993). Perceived risk, trust and democracy. *Risk Analysis*, 13(6): 675–82.

Slovic, P. (2000). *Perception of risk*. London, United Kingdom: Earthscan Publications.

Slovic, P., Fischhoff, B. and Lichtenstein, S. (1980). Facts and fears: understanding perceived risk. In Schwing, R.C. and Albers, W.A. Jr. (eds), *Societal risk assessment: how safe is safe enough?* New York, NY: Plenum Press.

Smed, S. (2012). Information and consumer perception of the "organic" attribute in fresh fruits and vegetables. *Agricultural Economics*, 43(Supplement s1): 33–48.

Smith, A. (2009). Effects of caffeine in chewing gum on mood and attention. *Human Psychopharmacology*, 24(3): 239–47.

Smith, E., Hay, P., Campbell, L. and Trollor, J.N. (2011). A review of the association between obesity and cognitive function across the lifespan: implications for novel approaches to prevention and treatment. *Obesity Reviews*, 12: 740–55.

Smith, G.S., Branas, C.C. and Miller, T.R. (1999). Fatal nontraffic injuries involving alcohol: a metaanalysis. *Annals of Emergency Medicine*, 33(6): 659–68.

Smith, L. and Foxcroft, D. (2009). *Drinking in the UK. An exploration of trends*. York, United Kingdom: Joseph Rowntree Foundation. Accessed on 26 February 2015 at: www.jrf.org.uk/sites/files/jrf/UK-alcohol-trends-FULL.pdf.

Smith, M.D., Asche, F., Guttormsen, A.G. and Wiener, J.B. (2010). Genetically modified salmon and full impact assessment. *Science*, 330: 1052–3.

Smith-Spangler, C., Brandeau, M.L., Hunter, G.E., Bavinger, J.C., Pearson, M., Eschbach, P.J., Sundaram, V., Liu, H., Schirmer, P., Stave, C., Olkin, I. and Bravata, D.M. (2012). Are organic foods safer or healthier than conventional alternatives? A systematic review. *Annals of Internal Medicine*, 157(5): 348–66.

Sobal, J. and Stunkard, A.J. (1989). Socioeconomic status and obesity: a review of the literature. *Psychological Bulletin*, 105(2): 260–75.

Soleri, D. and Cleveland, D.A. (2006). Transgenic maize and Mexican maize diversity: Risky synergy? *Agriculture and Human Values*, 23: 27–31.

Sooman, A., Macintyre, S. and Anderson, A. (1993). Scotland's health – a more difficult challenge for some? The price and availability of healthy foods in socially contrasting localities in the west of Scotland. *Health Bulletin (Edinburgh)*, 51: 276–84.

Sørensen, L.B., Møller, P., Flint, A., Martens, M. and Raben, A. (2003). Effect of sensory perception of foods on appetite and food intake: a review of studies on humans. *International Journal of Obesity*, 27: 1152–66.

Sørensen, M.P. and Christiansen, A. (2013). *Ulrich Beck. An introduction to the theory of second modernity and the risk society*. London, United Kingdom: Routledge, Taylor & Frances Group.

Sorenson, S.B., Manz, J.G.P. and Berk, R.A. (1998). News media coverage and the epidemiology of homicide. *American Journal of Public Health*, 88: 1510–14.

Sörqvist, P., Hedblom, D., Holmgren, M., Haga, A., Langeborg, L., Nöstl, A. and Kågström, J. (2013). Who needs cream and sugar when there is eco-labeling? Taste and willingness to pay for "eco-friendly" coffee. *PLoS One*, 8(12): e80719 (1–9).

Sparks, P., Conner, M., James, R., Shepherd, R. and Povey, R. (2001). Ambivalence about health-related behaviors: an exploration in the domain of food choice. *British Journal of Health Psychology*, 6: 53–68.

Speer, K., Steeg, E., Horstmann, P., Kühn, Th. and Montag, A. (1990). Determination and distribution of polycyclic aromatic hydrocarbons in native vegetable oils, smoked fish products, mussels and oysters, and bream from the river Elbe. *Journal of High Resolution Chromatography*, 13: 104–11.

Spellman, F.R. and Bieber, R.M. (2012). *Environmental health and science desk reference*. Lanham, MD: Government Institutes.

Stampfer, M.J., Kang, J.H., Chen, J., Cherry, R. and Grodstein, F. (2005). Effects of moderate alcohol consumption on cognitive function in women. *New England Journal of Medicine*, 352: 245–53.

Standing Committee on Foodstuffs [SCFS] (2001). Outcome of the expert group meeting on 3 October on ways to prevent contamination of olive residue oil and other oils with polycyclic aromatic hydrocarbons (PAH). Summary record of the 85th meeting of the Standing Committee on Foodstuffs, 25th October.

Stanfield, P.S. and Hui, Y.H. (2010). *Nutrition and diet therapy: self-instructional approaches*. Sudbury, MA: Jones & Bartlett Publishers.

Stavric, B., Klassen, R., Watkinson, B., Karpinski, K., Stapley, R. and Fried, P. (1988). Variability in caffeine consumption from coffee and tea: possible significance for epidemiological studies. *Food and Chemical Toxicology*, 26(2): 111–18.

Steiner, R. (1929). *Agriculture course* (printed for private circulation only; first English language edition; George Kaufmann translation). Dornach, Switzerland: Goetheanum.

Steptoe, A., Wardle, J., Cui, W., Bellisle, F., Zotti, A.M., Baranyai, R. and Sanderman, R. (2002). Trends in smoking, diet, physical exercise, and attitudes toward health in European university students from 13 countries, 1990–2000. *Preventive Medicine*, 35(2): 97–104.

Stevens, J.F., Taylor, A.W. and Deinzer, M.L. (1999). Quantitative analysis of xanthohumol and related prenylflavonoids in hops and beer by liquid chromatography-tandem mass spectrometry. *Journal of Chromatography*, A832: 97–107.

Stewart, M. (1992). I can't drink beer, I've just drunk water: alcohol, bodily substance and commensality among Hungarian Roma. In Gefou-Madianou, D. (ed.), *Alcohol, gender and culture*. London, United Kingdom: Routledge.

Stidworthy, M.F., Bleakley, J.S., Cheeseman, M.T. and Kelly, D.F. (1997). Chocolate poisoning in dogs. *Veterinary Record*, 141(1): 28.

Stinner, D.H. (2007). The science of organic farming. In Lockeretz, W. (ed.), *Organic farming: an international history*. Oxfordshire, United Kingdom & Cambridge, MA: CAB International (CABI).

Stoffelsma, J., Sipma, G, Kettenes, D.K. and Pypker, J. (1968). New volatile compounds of roasted coffee. *Journal of Agricultural and Food Chemistry*, 16: 1000–04.

Stroebele, N. and De Castro, J.M. (2004). Effect of ambience on food intake and food choice. *Nutrition*, 20: 821–38.

Sturm, R. (2008). Disparities in the food environment surrounding US middle and high schools. *Public Health*, 122(7): 681–90.

Sullivan, A. and Brown, M. (2013). *Overweight and obesity in mid-life: evidence from the 1970 British Cohort Study at age 42*. London, United Kingdom: Centre for Longitudinal Studies. Accessed on 5 March 2015 at: www.cls.ioe.ac.uk/shared/get-file.ashx?itemtype=document&id=1748.

Surgeoner, B.V., Chapman, B. and Powell, D.A. (2009). University students' hand hygiene practice during a gastrointestinal outbreak in residence: what they say they do, and what they actually do. *Journal of Environmental Health*, 72(2): 24–8.

SUTLA (2014). Slimming soap. Accessed on 9 October 2014 at: www.sutlaflawlesscebu. com/index.php?route=product/product&product_id=73.

Svirbely, J.L. and Szent-Györgyi, A. (1932). The chemical nature of vitamin C. *The Biochemical Journal*, 26(3): 865–70.

Swedish National Food Administration (2002). *Acrylamide in food*. Uppsala, Sweden: Swedish National Food Administration.

Sweeting, H., Anderson, A. and West, P. (1994). Socio-demographic correlates of dietary habits in mid to late adolescence. *European Journal of Clinical Nutrition*, 48: 736–48.

Swinburn, B. and Egger, G. (2004). The runaway weight gain train: too many accelerators, not enough brakes. *BMJ*, 329(7468): 736–9.

Swinburn, B., Gill, T. and Kumanyika, S. (2005). Obesity prevention: a proposed framework for translating evidence into action. *Obesity Reviews*, 6(1): 23–33.

Swinburn, B.A., Sacks, G., Hall, K.D., McPherson, K., Finegood, D.T., Moodie, M.L. and Gortmaker, S.L. (2011). The global obesity pandemic: shaped by global drivers and local environments. *Lancet*, 378(9793): 804–14.

Tabashnik, B.E., Brévault, T. and Carrière, Y. (2013). Insect resistance to Bt crops: lessons from the first billion acres. *Nature Biotechnology*, 31(6): 510–21.

Takahashi, O., Ichikawa, H. and Sasaki, M. (1990). Hemorrhagic toxicity of d-alpha-tocopherol in the rat. *Toxicology*, 63: 157–65.

Talavera-Bianchi, M., Chambers, E., Carey, E.E. and Chambers, D.H. (2010). Effect of organic production and fertilizer variables on the sensory properties of pac choi (*Brassica rapa* var. Mei Qing Choi) and tomato (*Solanum lycopersicum* var. Bush Celebrity). *Journal of the Science of Food and Agriculture*, 90(6): 981–8.

Tanaka, H., Nakazawa, K., Arima, M. and Iwasaki, S. (1984). Caffeine and its dimethyl-xanthines and fetal cerebral development in rat. *Brain Development*, 6: 355–61.

Tanaka, K., Hara, M., Sakamoto, T., Higaki, Y., Mizuta, T., Eguchi, Y., Yasutake, T., Ozaki, I., Yamamoto, K., Onohara, S., Kawazoe, S., Shigematsu, H. and Koizumi, S. (2007). Inverse association between coffee drinking and the risk of hepatocellular carcinoma: a case-control study in Japan. *Cancer Science*, 98: 214–18.

Tareke, E., Rydberg, P., Karlsson, P., Eriksson, S. and Törnqvist, M. (2002). Analysis of acrylamide, a carcinogen formed in heated foodstuffs. *Journal of Agricultural and Food Chemistry*, 50: 4998–5006.

Tate, D.F., Turner-McGrievy, G., Lyons, E., Stevens, J., Erickson, K., Polzien, K., Diamond, M., Wang, X. and Popkin, B. (2012). Replacing caloric beverages with water or diet beverages for weight loss in adults: main results of the Choose Healthy Options Consciously Everyday (CHOICE) randomized clinical trial. *American Journal of Clinical Nutrition*, 95: 555–63.

Taubes, G. (2014). Why nutrition is so confusing. *New York Times*, 8 February. Accessed on 5 March 2015 at: www.nytimes.com/2014/02/09/opinion/sunday/why-nutrition-is-so-confusing.html?_r=0.

Taylor, C. (2010). Foucault and the ethics of eating. *Foucault Studies*, 9: 71–88.

Taylor-Gooby, P. and Zinn, J. (2006). *Risk in social science*. Oxford, United Kingdom: Oxford University Press.

Temple, J.L. (2009). Caffeine use in children: what we know, what we have left to learn, and why we should worry. *Neuroscience & Biobehavioral Reviews*, 33(6): 793–806.

The Guardian (2008). Chinese figures show five fold rise in babies sick from contaminated milk. *The Guardian*, 2 December. Accessed on 27 November 2013 at: www.theguardian.com/world/2008/dec/02/china/print.

The Social Issues Research Centre (1998). *Social and cultural aspects of drinking. A report to the European Commission.* Oxford, United Kingdom: The Social Issues Research Centre.

Thoma, M.K., Murray, R., Flockhart, L., Pintar, K., Pollari, F., Fazil, A., Nesbitt, A. and Marshall, B. (2013). Estimates of the burden of foodborne illness in Canada for 30 specified pathogens and unspecified agents, circa 2006. *Foodborne Pathogens and Disease,* 10(7): 639–48.

Thompson, G.D. and Kidwell, J. (1998). Explaining the choice of organic produce: cosmetic defects, prices, and consumer preferences. *American Journal of Agricultural Economics,* 80(2): 277–87.

Thompson, R.L., Margetts, B.M., Speller, V.M. and McVey, D. (1999). The Health Education Authority's health and lifestyle survey 1993: who are the low fruit and vegetable consumers? *Journal of Epidemiology and Community Health,* 53: 294–9.

Thorn, C.F., Aklillu, E., McDonagh, E.M., Klein, T.E. and Altman, R.B. (2012). PharmGKB summary: caffeine pathway. *Pharmacogenetics and Genomics,* 22(5): 389–95.

Tomé-Carneiro, J., Larrosa, M., González-Sarrías, A., Tomás-Barberán, F.A., García-Conesa, M.T. and Espín, J.C. (2013). Resveratrol and clinical trials: the crossroad from in vitro studies to human evidence. *Current Pharmaceutical Design,* 19(34): 6064–93.

Tonsor, G.T., Schroeder, T.C. and Pennings, J.M.E. (2009). Factors impacting food safety risk perceptions. *Journal of Agricultural Economics,* 60(3): 625–44.

Topper, M.D. (1985). Navajo "alcoholism". In Bennett, L.A. and Ames, G.M. (eds), *The American experience with alcohol: contrasting cultural perspectives.* New York, NY: Plenum Publishing Corporation: 227–51.

Townsend, B. (1991). Consumers don't always do what they say. *American Demographics,* 13(4): 12–13.

Trenberth, K.E., Fasullo, J.T. and Balmaseda, M.A. (2014). Earth's energy imbalance. *Journal of Climate,* 27: 3129–44.

Trevitt, J., Vallance, C., Harris, A. and Goode, T. (2009). Adenosine antagonists reverse the cataleptic effects of haloperidol: implications for the treatment of Parkinson's disease. *Pharmacology Biochemistry and Behavior,* 92: 521–7.

Tsochatzis, E.A., Bosch, J. and Burroughs, A.K. (2014). Liver cirrhosis. *Lancet,* 383(9930): 1749–61.

Tuck, S.P. and Datta, H.K. (2007). Osteoporosis in the aging male: treatment options. *Clinical Intervention Aging,* 2(4): 521–36.

Tulloch, J. and Lupton, D. (2003). *Risk and everyday life.* London, United Kingdom: Sage.

Tuso, P.J., Ismail, M.H., Ha, B.P. and Bartolotto, C. (2013). Nutritional update for physicians: plant-based diets. *The Permanente Journal,* 17(2): 61–6.

Twigg, J. (1984). Vegetarianism and the meanings of meat. In: Murcott, A. (ed.), *The sociology of food and eating: essays on the sociological significance of food.* Aldershot, United Kingdom: Gower: 18–30.

Ukers, W.H. (1922). All about coffee. New York, NY: Tea and Coffee Trade Journal Company. Accessed on 24 June 2015 at: www.gutenberg.org/files/28500/28500-h/28500-h.htm.

United Kingdom Food Standards Agency [UK FSA] (2010). *The joint government and industry target to reduce Campylobacter in UK produced chickens by 2015.* London, United Kingdom: UK Food Standards Agency. Accessed on 2 July, 2015 at: www.food.gov.uk/sites/default/files/multimedia/pdfs/campytarget.pdf.

United Kingdom Food Standards Agency [UK FSA] (2014). *A microbiological survey of Campylobacter contamination in fresh whole UK produced chilled chickens at retail sale – an interim report to cover Quarters 1 & 2.* London, United Kingdom: UK Food Standards Agency. Accessed on 12 March 2015 at: www.food.gov.uk/sites/default/files/campylobacter-survey-q2-report.pdf.

United Nations (2008). *Organic agriculture and food security in Africa.* UNEP-UNCTAD Capacity-building Task Force on Trade, Environment and Development. New York and Geneva: United Nations.

United Nations Department of Economic and Social Affairs, Population Division (2015). *World population prospects: the 2015 revision, key findings and advance tables* (Working Paper No. ESA/P/WP.241). New York, NY: United Nations.

United States Department of Agriculture [USDA] (2013). *National nutrient database for standard reference* (Release 26). Beltsville, MD: Agricultural Research Service, United States Department of Agriculture. Accessed on 15 March 2004 at: www.ars.usda.gov/Services/docs.htm?docid=24936.

United States Department of Agriculture [USDA] (2014). *Pesticide data program: annual summary, calendar year 2012.* Washington, DC: Department of Agriculture. Accessed on 4 August 2015 at: www.ams.usda.gov/AMSv1.0/getfile?dDocName=stelprdc5106521.

United States Environmental Protection Agency [US EPA] (1984). *Carcinogen assessment of coke oven emissions* (EPA-600/6-82-003F). Washington, DC: U.S. Environmental Protection Agency, Office of Health and Environmental Assessment.

United States Food and Drug Administration [FDA] (2004). *Exploratory data on furan in food.* Washington, DC: US Food and Drug Administration. Accessed on 9 July 2015 at: www.fda.gov/ohrms/dockets/ac/04/briefing/4045b2_09_furan data.pdf.

United States Food and Drug Administration [FDA/NIH] (2002). *Healthy people 2010 – volume II. Objectives for improving health, nutrition and overweight.* Bethesda, MD: National Institutes of Health: 15. Accessed on 7 May 2015 at: www.healthypeople.gov/2010/document/pdf/Volume2/19Nutrition.pdf.

Unnikrishnan, A.G., Kalra, S. and Garg, M.K. (2012). Preventing obesity in India: weighing the options. *Indian Journal of Endocrinology and Metabolism*, 16(1): 4–6.

Unusan, N. (2007). Consumer food safety knowledge and practices in the home in Turkey. *Food Control*, 18(1): 45–51.

Urban, M., Kavvadias, D., Riedel, K., Scherer, G. and Tricker, A.R. (2006). Urinary mercapturic acids and a hemoglobin adduct for the dosimetry of acrylamide exposure in smokers and nonsmokers. *Inhalation Toxicology*, 18: 831–9.

Urry, J. (2014a). *Offshoring.* Cambridge, United Kingdom: Polity.

Urry, J. (2014b). Preface in Beck, U. (ed.). Ulrich Beck pioneer in cosmopolitan sociology and risk society. *Springer Briefs on Pioneers in Science and Practice*, 18: v–xi.

Uzogara, S.G. (2000). The impact of genetic modification of human foods in the 21st century: a review. *Biotechnology Advances*, 18: 179–206.

van Beilen, J.B. and Poirier, Y. (2008). Production of renewable polymers from crop plants. *The Plant Journal*, 54: 684–701.

van den Eede, G., Aarts, H., Buhk, H.J., Corthier, G., Flint, H.J., Hammes, W., Jacobsen, B., Midtvedt, T., van der Vossen, J., von Wright, A., Wackernagel, W. and Wilcks, A. (2004). The relevance of gene transfer to the safety of food and feed derived from genetically modified (GM) plants. *Food and Chemical Toxicology*, 42(7): 1127–56.

Vattem, D.A. and Shetty, K. (2005). Biological functionality of ellagic acid: a review. *Journal of Food Biochemistry*, 29(3): 234–66.

Vaughan, E.J. (1997). *Risk management*. New York, NY: Wiley.

Verbeke, W. (2005). Agriculture and the food industry in the information age. *European Review of Agricultural Economics*, 32: 347–68.

Verbeke, W., Frewer, L.J., Scholderer, J. and de Brabander, H.F. (2007). Why consumers behave as they do with respect to food safety and risk information. *Analytica Chimica Acta*, 586(1–2): 2–7.

Verhagen, H., Buijsse, B., Jansen, E. and Bueno-de-Mesquita, B. (2006). The State of antioxidant affairs. *Nutrition Today*, 41: 244–50.

Vikström, A.C., Abramsson-Zetterberg, L., Naruszewicz, M., Athanassiadis, I., Granath, F.N. and Törnqvist, M.A. (2011). In vivo doses of acrylamide and glycidamide in humans after intake of acrylamide-rich food. *Toxicological Sciences*, 119(1): 41–9.

Vinson, J.A., Mandarano, M., Hirst, M., Trevithick, J.R. and Bose, P. (2003). Phenol antioxidant quantity and quality in foods: beers and the effect of two types of beer on an animal model of atherosclerosis. *Journal of Agricultural and Food Chemistry*, 51: 5528–33.

Vogel, E. and Mol, A. (2014). Enjoy your food: on losing weight and taking pleasure. *Sociology of Health & Illness*, 36(2): 305–17.

Vogt Yuan, A.S. (2010). Body perceptions, weight control behavior, and changes in adolescents' psychological well-being over time: a longitudinal examination of gender. *Journal of Youth and Adolescence*, 39(8): 927–39.

Voytas, D.F. and Gao, C. (2014). Precision genome engineering and agriculture: opportunities and regulatory challenges. *PLoS Biology*, 12(6): e1001877 (1–6).

Wadolowska, L., Babicz-Zielinska, E. and Czarnocinska, J. (2008). Food choice models and their relation with food preferences and eating frequency in the Polish population: POFPRES study. *Food Policy*, 33(2): 122–34.

Waltz, E. (2009). GM crops: battlefield. *Nature*, 461: 27–32.

Wan, P., Huang, Y., Wu, H., Huang, M., Cong, S., Tabashnik, B.E. and Wu, K. (2012). Increased frequency of pink bollworm resistance to Bt toxin Cry1Ac in China. *PLoS One*, 7(1): e29975 (1–9).

Wandel, M. (1994). Understanding consumer concern about food-related health risks. *British Food Journal*, 96(7): 35–40.

Wang, Y., Beydoun, M.A., Liang, L., Caballero, B. and Kumanyika, S.K. (2008). Will all Americans become overweight or obese? Estimating the progression and cost of the US obesity epidemic. *Obesity*, 16(10): 2323–30.

Wang, Y., Chen, H-J., Shaikh, S. and Mathur, P. (2009). Is obesity becoming a public health problem in India? Examine the shift from under- to overnutrition problems over time. *Obesity Review*, 10(4): 456–74.

Wang, Y.C., McPherson, K., Marsh, T., Gortmaker, S.L. and Brown, M. (2011). Health and economic burden of the projected obesity trends in the USA and the UK. *Lancet*, 378: 815–25.

Wardle, J., Haase, A.M., Steptoe, A., Nillapun, M., Jonwutiwes, K. and Bellisie, F. (2004). Gender differences in food choice: the contribution of health beliefs and dieting. *Annals of Behavioral Medicine*, 27(2): 107–16.

Warin, M., Turner, K., Moore, V. and Davies, M. (2007). Bodies, mothers and identities: rethinking obesity and the BMI. *Sociology of Health and Illness*, 30(1): 97–111.

Watanabe, F., Yabuta, Y., Bito, T. and Teng, F. (2014). Vitamin B_{12}-containing plant food sources for vegetarians. *Nutrients*, 6(5): 1861–73.

Webb, P. and Block, S. (2004). Nutrition information and formal schooling as inputs to child nutrition. *Economic Development and Cultural Change*, 52(4): 801–20.

Weinberg, B.A. and Bealer, B.K. (2001). *The world of caffeine: the science and culture of the world's most popular drug*. New York, NY: Routledge.

Weiss, E.C., Galuska, D.A., Khan, L.K. and Serdula, M.K. (2006). Weight-control practices among US adults, 2001–2002. *American Journal of Preventive Medicine*, 31(1): 18–24.

Weng, H.H., Bastian, L.A., Taylor, D.H., Moser, B.K. and Ostbye, T. (2004). Number of children associated with obesity in middle-aged women and men: results from the health and retirement study. *Journal of Women's Health*, 13(1): 85–91.

Westerterp-Plantenga, M.S. and Verwegen, C.R.T. (1999). The appetizing effect of an aperitif in overweight and normal-weight humans. *American Journal of Clinical Nutrition*, 69: 205–12.

Wikswo, M.E., Cortes, J., Hall, A.J., Vaughan, G., Howard, C., Gregoricus, N. and Cramer, E.H. (2011). Disease transmission and passenger behaviors during a high morbidity norovirus outbreak on a cruise ship, January 2009. *Clinical Infectious Diseases*, 52: 1116–22.

Wildavsky, A. and Dake, K. (1990). Theories of risk perception: who fears what and why? *Daedalus*, 119(4): 41–60.

Wilkinson, I. (2001). Social theories of risk perception: at once indispensable and insufficient. *Current Sociology*, 49(1): 1–22.

Wilkinson, R.G. and Pickett, K.E. (2009). Income inequality and social dysfunction. *Annual Review of Sociology*, 35: 493–511.

Willer, H. and Lernoud, J. (eds) (2014). *The world of organic agriculture. Statistics and emerging trends 2014*. Frick, Switzerland and Bonn, Germany: Research Institute of Organic Agriculture (FiBL), and International Federation of Organic Agriculture Movements (IFOAM).

Willer, H., Lernoud, J. and Schlatter, B. (2014). Current statistics on organic agriculture worldwide: organic area, producers and market. In Willer, H. and Lernoud, J. (eds), *The world of organic agriculture. Statistics and emerging trends 2014*. Frick, Switzerland and Bonn, Germany: Research Institute of Organic Agriculture (FiBL), and International Federation of Organic Agriculture Movements (IFOAM).

Willett, W. (1998). *Nutritional epidemiology*. New York, NY: Oxford University Press.

Willett, W.C. and Leibel, R.L. (2002). Dietary fat is not a major determinant of body fat. *American Journal of Medicine*, 113(Suppl 9B): 47S–59S.

Willis, W.T., Dallman, P.R. and Brooks, G.A. (1988). Physiological and biochemical correlates of increased work in trained iron-deficient rats. *Journal of Applied Physiology*, 65: 256–63.

Wills, W.J., Backett-Milburn, K., Gregory, S. and Lawton, J. (2005). The influence of the secondary school setting on the food practices of young teenagers from disadvantaged backgrounds in Scotland. *Health Education Research*, 20(4): 458–65.

Wilson, D.J., Gabriel, E., Leatherbarrow, A.J.H., Cheesbrough, J., Gee, S., Bolton, E., Fox, A., Fearnhead, P., Hart, C.A. and Diggle, P.J. (2008). Tracing the source of campylobacteriosis. *PLoS Genetics*, 4(9): e1000203: 1–9.

Winkler, E. and Turrell, G. (2010). Confidence to cook vegetables and the buying habits of Australian households. *Journal of the American Dietetic Association*, 110(5S): S52–S61.

Winter, C.K. and Davis, S.H. (2006). Organic foods. *Journal of Food Science*, 71(9): 117–24.

Wolk, B.J., Ganetsky, M. and Babu, K.M. (2012). Toxicity of energy drinks. *Current Opinion in Pediatrics*, 24(2): 243–51.

Wolsko, P.M., Solondz, D.K., Phillips, R.S., Schachter, S.C. and Eisenberg, D.M. (2005). Lack of herbal supplement characterization in published randomized controlled trials. *American Journal of Medicine*, 118(10): 1087–93.

Woolf, A., Watson, W., Smolinske, S. and Litovitz, T. (2005). The severity of toxic reactions to ephedra: comparisons to other botanical products and national trends from 1993–2002. *Clinical Toxicology (Philadelphia, PA)*, 43 (5): 347–55.

Woese, K., Lange, D., Boess, C. and Bögl, K.W. (1997). A comparison of organically and conventionally grown foods. Results of a review of the relevant literature. *Journal of Science of Food and Agriculture*, 74(3): 281–293.

World Bank (2007). *From agriculture to nutrition: pathways, synergies and outcomes* (Report No. 40196-GLB). Washington, DC: World Bank.

World Cancer Research Fund/American Institute for Cancer Research [WCRF/AICR] (2007). *Food, nutrition, physical activity, and the prevention of cancer: a global perspective*. Washington, DC: American Institute for Cancer Research.

World Health Organization [WHO] (1990). *Diet, nutrition, and the prevention of chronic diseases*. (Report of a WHO Study Group – Technical Report Series 797). Geneva, Switzerland: World Health Organization.

World Health Organization [WHO] (2000). *Obesity: preventing and managing the global epidemic*. (Technical Report Series 894). Geneva, Switzerland: World Health Organization.

World Health Organization [WHO] (2002). *WHO traditional medicine strategy 2002–2005*. Geneva, Switzerland: World Health Organization.

World Health Organization [WHO] (2003). *Diet, nutrition and the prevention of chronic diseases*. (Report of the Joint WHO/FAO Expert Consultation – Technical Report Series 916). Geneva, Switzerland: World Health Organization.

World Health Organization [WHO] (2004a). *Vitamin and mineral requirements in human nutrition*. Report of a joint FAO/WHO expert consultation. Bangkok, Thailand, 21–30 September. Geneva, Switzerland: World Health Organization.

World Health Organization [WHO] (2004b). *Global strategy on diet, physical activity and health*. Geneva, Switzerland: World Health Organization.

World Health Organization [WHO] (2005). *Dietary intake of fruit and vegetables and management of body weight*. Geneva, Switzerland: World Health Organization.

World Health Organization [WHO] (2007). *WHO initiative to estimate the global burden of foodborne diseases*. Geneva, Switzerland: World Health Organization.

World Health Organization [WHO] (2009). *Global health risks: mortality and burden of disease attributable to selected major risks*. Geneva, Switzerland: World Health Organization.

World Health Organization [WHO] (2011a). *Global status report on alcohol and health*. Geneva, Switzerland: World Health Organization.

World Health Organization [WHO] (2011b). *Safety evaluation of certain contaminants in food* (WHO Food Additives Series: 63/FAO JECFA Monographs 8) Geneva, Switzerland: World Health Organization.

World Health Organization [WHO] (2012). *Variant Creutzfeldt-Jakob disease* (Fact Sheet no 180). Geneva, Switzerland: World Health Organization.

World Health Organization [WHO] (2013a). *Diarrhoeal disease* (Fact Sheet no 330). Geneva, Switzerland: World Health Organization.

World Health Organization [WHO] (2013b). *Salmonella (non-typhoidal)* (Fact Sheet no 139). Geneva, Switzerland: World Health Organization.

World Health Organization [WHO] (2014a). *Obesity and overweight* (Fact Sheet No 311). Geneva, Switzerland: World Health Organization.

World Health Organization [WHO] (2014b). *Global database on body mass index.* Geneva, Switzerland: World Health Organization. Accessed on 18 August 2014 at: apps.who.int/bmi/index.jsp?introPage=intro_1.html.

World Health Organization [WHO] (2014c). *Global status report on alcohol and health 2014.* Geneva, Switzerland: World Health Organization.

World Health Organization [WHO] (2015). *Global health observatory data repository.* Geneva, Switzerland: World Health Organization. Accessed on 19 July 2015 at: apps.who.int/gho/data/node.main.A904?lang=en.

Worth, T. (2010). How to make grilling safer. *CNN*, 2 July. Accessed on 23 April 2015 at: edition.cnn.com/2010/HEALTH/07/02/how.make.grilling.safe/.

Worthington, V. (2001). Nutritional quality of organic versus conventional fruits, vegetables, and grains. *The Journal of Alternative and Complementary Medicine*, 7(2): 161–73.

Wrangham, R. and Conklin-Brittain, N. (2003). Cooking as a biological trait. *Comparative Biochemistry and Physiology Part A*, 136: 35–46.

Wunderlich, S., Zürcher, A. and Back, W. (2005). Enrichment of xanthohumol in the brewing process. *Molecular Nutrition & Food Research*, 49(9): 874–81.

Wynne, B. (1992). Public understanding of science research. *Public Understanding of Science*, 1(1): 37–43.

Wynne, B. (1996). May the sheep safely graze? In Lash, S., Szerszinski, B. and Wynne, B. (eds). *Risk, environment and modernity*. London, United Kingdom: Sage: 44–83.

Xu, G.R. and Bao, T.F. (2000). *Grandiose survey of Chinese alcoholic drinks and beverages.* Wuxi, Jiangsu Province, China: School of Biotechnology, Wuxi University of Light Industry.

Yang, B., Wang, J., Tang, B., Liu, Y., Guo, C., Yang, P., Yu, T., Li, R., Zhao, J., Zhang, L., Dai, Y. and Li, N. (2011). Characterization of bioactive recombinant human lysozyme expressed in milk of cloned transgenic cattle. *PLoS One*, 6(3): e17593 (1–10).

Yang, L. and Colditz, G.A. (2015). Prevalence of overweight and obesity in the United States, 2007–2012. *JAMA Internal Medicine*, published online 22 June 2015.

Yanovski, S. (2003). Sugar and fat: cravings and aversions. *Journal of Nutrition*, 133: 835S–837S.

Yates, J. and Murphy, C. (2006). A cost benefit analysis of weight management strategies. *Asia Pacific Journal of Clinical Nutrition*, 15(Suppl): 74–9.

Yaylayan, V.A. (2006). Precursors, formation and determination of furan in food. *Zeitschrift für Verbraucherschutz und Lebensmittelsicherheit*, 1: 5–9.

Yeomans, M.R. and Gray R.W. (2002). Opioid peptides and the control of human ingestive behaviour. *Neuroscience & Biobehavioral Reviews*, 26(6): 713–28.

Yetley, E.A. (2007). Multivitamin and multimineral dietary supplements: definitions, characterization, bioavailability, and drug interactions. *American Journal of Clinical Nutrition*, 85(1): 269S–276S.

Yeung, R.M.W. and Morris, J. (2001a). Food safety risk – consumer perception and purchase behaviour. *British Food Journal*, 103(3): 170–86.

Yeung, R.M.W. and Morris, J. (2001b). Consumer perception of food risk in chicken meat. *Nutrition & Food Science*, 31(6): 270–79.

Young, L.R. and Nestle, M. (2002). The contribution of expanding portion sizes to the US obesity epidemic. *American Journal of Public Health*, 92(2): 246–9.

Zadoks, J.C. (1989). *Development of farming systems. Evaluation of the five-year period 1980–1988*. Wageningen, The Netherlands: Pudoc.

Zador, P.L., Krawchuk, S.A. and Voas, R.B. (2000). Alcohol-related relative risk of driver fatalities and driver involvement in fatal crashes in relation to driver age and gender: an update using 1996 data. *Journal of Studies on Alcohol*, 61(3): 387–95.

Zenith International (2012). Global energy drinks report. Accessed on 29 June 2015 at: www.zenithinternational.com/reports_data/146/Global+Energy+Drinks+Report+2012.

Zhang, Q. and Wang, Y. (2004). Trends in the association between obesity and socioeconomic status in US adults: 1971 to 2000. *Obesity Research*, 12: 1622–32.

Zhang, X., Lu, G., Long, W., Zou, X., Li, F. and Nishio, T. (2014). Recent progress in drought and salt tolerance studies in *Brassica* crops. *Breeding Science*, 64(1): 60–73.

Zhang, Y. and Zhang, Y. (2007). Formation and reduction of acrylamide in Maillard reaction: a review based on the current state of knowledge. *Critical Reviews in Food Science and Nutrition*, 47: 521–42.

Zhao, X., Chambers, E., Matta, Z., Loughin, T.M. and Carey, E.E. (2007). Consumer sensory analysis of organically and conventionally grown vegetables. *Journal of Food Science*, 72(2): S87–S91.

Zheng, W. and Lee, S.A. (2009). Well-done meat intake, heterocyclic amine exposure, and cancer risk. *Nutrition and Cancer*, 61: 437–46.

Zimmerli, B. and Schlatter, J. (1991). Ethyl carbamate: analytical methodology, occurrence, formation, biological activity and risk assessment. *Mutation Research*, 259: 325–50.

Zinn, J.O. (2010). Risk as discourse: interdisciplinary perspectives. *Critical Approaches to Discourse Analysis across Disciplines*, 4(2): 106–24.

Zivković, R. (2000). Coffee and health in the elderly. *Acta Medica Croatica: Casopis Hravatske Akademije Medicinskih Znanosti*, 54(1): 33–6.

Zurbriggen, M.D., Hajirezaei, M.-R. and Carrillo, N. (2010). Engineering the future. Development of transgenic plants with enhanced tolerance to adverse environments. *Biotechnology and Genetic Engineering Reviews*, 27(1): 33–56.

Index

For Product Safety Concerns and Information please contact our EU representative GPSR@taylorandfrancis.com Taylor & Francis Verlag GmbH, Kaufingerstraße 24, 80331 München, Germany

Printed and bound by CPI Group (UK) Ltd, Croydon, CR0 4YY

01/05/2025

01858509-0003